Pathways to Illness

Angele McGrady · Donald Moss

Pathways to Illness, Pathways to Health

Springer

Angele McGrady, Ph.D.
Department of Psychiatry
University of Toledo
Toledo, OH, USA

Donald Moss, Ph.D.
School of Mind-Body Medicine
Saybrook University
San Francisco, CA, USA

ISBN 978-1-4899-9760-9   ISBN 978-1-4419-1379-1 (eBook)
DOI 10.1007/978-1-4419-1379-1
Springer New York Heidelberg Dordrecht London

© Springer Science+Business Media New York 2013
Softcover re-print of the Hardcover 1st edition 2013
This work is subject to copyright. All rights are reserved by the Publisher, whether the whole or part of the material is concerned, specifically the rights of translation, reprinting, reuse of illustrations, recitation, broadcasting, reproduction on microfilms or in any other physical way, and transmission or information storage and retrieval, electronic adaptation, computer software, or by similar or dissimilar methodology now known or hereafter developed. Exempted from this legal reservation are brief excerpts in connection with reviews or scholarly analysis or material supplied specifically for the purpose of being entered and executed on a computer system, for exclusive use by the purchaser of the work. Duplication of this publication or parts thereof is permitted only under the provisions of the Copyright Law of the Publisher's location, in its current version, and permission for use must always be obtained from Springer. Permissions for use may be obtained through RightsLink at the Copyright Clearance Center. Violations are liable to prosecution under the respective Copyright Law.
The use of general descriptive names, registered names, trademarks, service marks, etc. in this publication does not imply, even in the absence of a specific statement, that such names are exempt from the relevant protective laws and regulations and therefore free for general use.
While the advice and information in this book are believed to be true and accurate at the date of publication, neither the authors nor the editors nor the publisher can accept any legal responsibility for any errors or omissions that may be made. The publisher makes no warranty, express or implied, with respect to the material contained herein.

Springer is part of Springer Science+Business Media (www.springer.com)

Foreword

It is becoming increasingly clear that optimal therapeutic approaches for people with chronic emotional and physical problems must be comprehensive, integrative, and carefully individualized. Sometimes with acute conditions, particularly ones that have obvious physical causes, a single clinician-administered intervention is sufficient: the appropriate antibiotic for a bacterial infection, adrenaline or a steroid to break the hold of a severe allergic reaction, a word of therapeutic wisdom and reassurance in a moment of confusion. But this is rarely the case in a society increasingly plagued by chronic illness and unhappiness, and with the long-term emotional distress and the chronic physical problems for which most people seek clinical and specifically psychotherapeutic and behavioral help. Here is where we need guidance in combining the self-care strategies which all of us should be using to prevent and treat chronic illnesses and conditions, with clinician-directed therapies individualized for each person and his or her specific problems. And here is where *Pathways to Illness, Pathways to Health* serves us well.

Angele McGrady and Donald Moss are a research physiologist/counselor and a clinical health psychologist, respectively, with long experience in developing these comprehensive care plans and in teaching others to do so. And they begin, like the good teachers they are, by orienting us to the problem and its solution with chapters on the genetic, psychosocial, and psychophysiological factors which predispose us to becoming ill. They also let us know from the beginning that each of these factors can also offer us, if we address them wisely, hope for healing.

The chapter on assessment which follows provides a way for us to evaluate the importance of each of these factors – and the spiritual as well – in each person's life. It also positions us to make good use of the three levels of intervention which the authors then describe, reestablishing normal rhythms, skill building, and multicomponent professional interventions. In the following chapters, Moss and McGrady share with us the levels one and two self-care and skill-building techniques they have long used – deep breathing, movement, mindful eating, and guided imagery among them – and show how they may be combined with approaches drawn from a variety of therapeutic orientations, including dynamic and cognitive behavioral therapy, dialectical behavior therapy, biofeedback, and clinical hypnosis.

And here, as McGrady and Moss offer us case histories, is where *Pathways* becomes especially valuable. They take us step by step from an initial clinical history, to the development of a therapeutic plan, through the implementation of that plan over time. They show us how people – even and perhaps especially those who had been regarded as "treatment resistant" – can be actively engaged in developing their own comprehensive therapeutic intervention and in their own care. As McGrady and Moss clearly show us, people who feel respected and who are treated as active partners rather than passive patients and clients often begin to respect and take care of themselves. McGrady and Moss also help us to evaluate when level three interventions are necessary and show us how the clinical interactions these approaches demand can easily be integrated with the guiding and coaching functions of self-regulation and skill building. And they demonstrate how this can work with condition after condition, including anxiety and depression, cardiovascular disease, chronic pain, and gastrointestinal disorders.

Pathways is clearly written, well referenced, and immensely practical. It offers clinicians the kind of reliable guidance they are looking for as they try to make what they offer useful and acceptable to ever larger numbers of people with complex chronic problems. *Pathways* will also, I believe, be an important text in helping all of us to create the holistic and integrative models of care which are necessary to effectively address our current worldwide crisis of chronic illness

James S. Gordon, MD
The Center for Mind-Body Medicine,
School of Mind-Body Medicine,
Saybrook University, San Francisco, CA, USA
Author, *Unstuck: Your Guide to the*
Seven Stage Journey Out of Depression

Acknowledgments

I deeply appreciate Patrick, Michele, Kevin and Brandy for their love and encouragement throughout the process of gathering ideas and completing the project. I am most grateful to my "girlfriends" for their support and good humor.

I give thanks to my colleagues in the UT Department of Psychiatry for their insights as the book took shape and to my secretary Bonnie for her tireless efforts in my behalf. I have also been blessed with mentors, beginning in high school, in college, graduate school, and throughout my career.

I thank my clients who shared their personal stories with me, trusted me, and prayed for me during our hours together. The cases used in this book are composites of many of those stories. I also thank the medical, nursing, graduate, and physician assistant students at University of Toledo who motivated me to stay up to date and challenged me with new ideas.

Finally, this book is dedicated to the memory of Fernand and Santina Vial, professors, authors, and parents.

Angele McGrady

I thank my wife Nancy, for her love, her tireless pursuit of health in spite of cancer, and her occasional nudges to write that next chapter.

I thank my research assistants, Erica Shane Hamilton and Jennifer Heintzman, for their invaluable assistance. I thank my colleagues at Saybrook University, especially Stanley Krippner, James Gordon, Lyn Freeman, Fred Shaffer, and Eric Willmarth, for their encouragement, example, and inspiration.

I thank my clients, who implemented so many of the pathways interventions described in this book, and shared their triumphs and setbacks with me. The case narratives are composites from their lives, modified for anonymity, but preserving, I hope, their sense of determination to move toward restored well-being.

Finally, this book is dedicated to the memory of Jeanne Achterberg, who continues to shine as a spiritual light for many of her students and friends.

Donald Moss

Contents

Foreword.. v

Part I Basic Concepts of Health and Illness

1 Introducing the Pathways Model... 3
   Introduction: The Pathway to Illness 3
      The New Face of Illness.. 4
      The Leading Causes of Death 5
      The Leading Causes of Disability.. 6
   Major Factors in Illness Onset 7
   The Continuum of Health and Illness 9
   Rethinking Health and Disease... 11
   The Geography of Illness: Exporting Western Health Risks 12
   Wellness Is an Option 13
   Conclusion: Pathways to Health 14
   References.. 15

2 Genetic Etiology of Illness 19
   Definitions.. 19
   Genetics and Personality 20
   Genetics and Risk 21
   Genetics and Environment 22
   Genetics and Psychiatric Illness.. 23
   Genetics and Physical Illness.. 24
   Genetic Factors in Coexisting Disorders 25
   Summary 26
   References.. 26

3	**Psychosocial Etiology of Illness**	29
	Introduction	29
	Life Events, Trauma, and Health	30
	The Psychosomatic History	30
	Stressful Life Events and Health	31
	The Role of Trauma in Later Illness	32
	Negative Coping, Health Risk Behaviors, and Risky Lifestyles	35
	Psychosocial Pathways to Health	36
	Social Supports	36
	Positive Coping, Health Supportive Behaviors, and Well Lifestyles	38
	Pathways Interventions: The Case of Esther	39
	Initial Visit and Assessment	40
	Initial Pathway Interventions	41
	Summary	43
	References	43
4	**Psychophysiological Etiology of Illness**	47
	Introduction	47
	Models of Mind–Body Interactions	49
	Association Between Psychological Stress and Illness	49
	Somatization and Medically Unexplained Symptoms	50
	Risk and Resilience Factors	56
	Personal Mastery and Optimism Promote Resilience	58
	Summary	59
	References	59
5	**Assessment in the Pathways Model**	63
	Goals of Assessment	63
	Self-Assessment	64
	Professional Assessment	66
	Preparation for Intervention	69
	Assessment of the Client's Readiness for Change	69
	Summary	71
	References	72
6	**Interventions in the Pathways Model**	75
	Introduction	75
	Level One Interventions	76
	Mindful Breathing	76
	Nutrition and Feeding Behavior	77
	Sleep and Rest	78
	Self-Soothing	79
	Movement	80
	Level Two Interventions	81
	Progressive Relaxation	82

Physical Exercise	82
Cognitive Renewal	82
Pause: Introducing a Moment of Awareness	83
Mindfulness	84
Communication	85
Level Three Interventions	86
Psychotherapy	86
Applied Psychophysiological Therapy	88
Biofeedback	88
Guided Imagery	89
Hypnosis	89
Conclusion	89
References	90

Part II Applications to Common Illnesses

7 Substance Abuse Disorders 95
Introduction	95
Substance Abuse Prevalence and Costs	96
Paradigms for Substance Abuse Problems	97
The Health Problem Model for Substance Abuse: An Acute Versus Chronic Disease Model?	98
The Pathways Model: The Case of Alice	102
References	106

8 Depression 109
Introduction	109
Clinical Depression: Incidence and Costs	110
Mechanisms and Models for Depression	111
Genetics	111
Neurochemical and Neuroscience Models of Depression	111
Environmental Factors	112
Comorbidity with Other Disorders	112
Interventions	114
Medication	114
Psychotherapy	115
Exercise	117
Nutrition	117
Mind-Body Therapies	119
Integrative Treatment Combining Multiple Interventions	121
Pathways Interventions: The Case of Abigail	122
Initial Visit and Assessment	122
Pathways Interventions	124
Abigail Today	127
References	128

9 Anxiety ... 133
Introduction ... 133
Brief Descriptions of the Anxiety Disorders ... 134
Psychological and Physiological Characteristics of Anxiety ... 135
The Case of Suzette ... 135
Intervention Plan ... 136
    Education and Level One Intervention ... 136
    Level Two Interventions ... 137
    Level Three Interventions ... 137
Case Summary ... 138
The Case of Bernie ... 138
    Interventions: Level One ... 140
    Interventions: Level Two ... 140
    Interventions: Level Three ... 141
Case Summary ... 142
References ... 142

10 Diabetes and Obesity ... 145
Definitions and Standard Management ... 145
Psychophysiological Etiology ... 146
The Case of Rosa ... 149
Case Summary ... 153
References ... 153

11 Hypertension and Neurocardiogenic Syncope ... 157
Introduction ... 157
Regulation of Blood Pressure ... 158
Essential Hypertension ... 158
    Psychosocial Factors Influencing Blood Pressure ... 159
Case of Marquise ... 160
    Case Summary ... 163
Dysautonomia: Autonomic Nervous System Disorders ... 163
    Etiology of ANS Disorders ... 163
    Case of Gabriella (Gaby) ... 164
Case Summary ... 166
References ... 167

12 Headache and Back Pain ... 171
Chronic Pain and Quality of Life ... 171
Migraine Headache ... 172
Tension-Type Headache ... 173
Assessment of the Patient with Chronic Pain ... 173
The Case of Melinda ... 173
    Case Summary ... 175
Research Support for Case Interventions ... 175
Psychophysiological Basis for Transition from Acute
to Chronic Pain ... 176

	The Case of Peter...	177
	Pathways Interventions in the Case of Peter...........................	178
	Case Summary...	180
	References..	181
13	**Fibromyalgia Syndrome**..	185
	Understanding the Fibromyalgia Syndrome.......................................	185
	Definition of the Fibromyalgia Syndrome..............................	185
	Prevalence of the Disorder...	186
	Mechanisms and Models for Fibromyalgia...	187
	The Case of Elizabeth..	189
	Case Summary...	194
	References..	196
14	**Gastrointestinal Disorders**..	199
	Overview of Gastrointestinal Function..	199
	Functional GI Disorders...	201
	Irritable Bowel Syndrome..	202
	Functional Dyspepsia...	204
	Functional Abdominal Pain Syndrome..	204
	The Case of Rod..	205
	Case Summary...	208
	References..	209
15	**Sleep Disorders**...	211
	Introduction: Normal Sleep...	211
	Sleep Deprivation and Its Effects..	212
	The Case of Brandon	213
	Case Summary	216
	The Case of Cerise	216
	Case Summary	218
	References..	219

Part III Personalizing the Path to Health and Wellness

16	**Simple Pathways to Health and Wellness**.....................................	223
	Introduction..	223
	Simple Pathways I: Autogenic Training..	224
	Simple Pathways II: Thermal Biofeedback...	227
	Simple Pathways III: Emotional Journaling..	229
	Simple Pathways IV: Heart Rate Variability Biofeedback...................	231
	Simple Pathways V: Audio-Visual Entrainment..................................	234
	Simple Pathways VI: Mindfulness...	236
	Simple Pathways VII: Expressive Dance...	237
	Simple Pathways VIII: Psychoeducation...	238
	Simple Pathways: Conclusion..	238
	References..	239

17	**Developing a Wellness Plan**	243
	Types of Wellness Programs	243
	The Case of Philip	244
	Case Summary	247
	References	248
18	**Seeking Professional Help**	249
	Finding a Provider for Pathways Interventions	249
	The Well-Informed, Critical Health-Care Consumer	251
About the Authors		255
Index		257

Part I
Basic Concepts of Health and Illness

Chapter 1
Introducing the Pathways Model

> *"Midway in this mortal life I found myself astray, in a dark wood. Ah, who can say how terrible it was!"*
>
> (Divine Comedy, Dante Alleghieri, 1265–1321)

Abstract The demographics and etiologies of illness have changed in the past century. The most common causes of mortality and morbidity today are diseases of lifestyle, behavior, and adaptation; stress-related conditions; chronic illnesses and impairments; and complex biopsychosocial conditions. No illness is purely physical or emotional, but rather illness emerges from heredity and personality, through choices in consumption and activity, forged by life stress and environment. The Pathways Model introduces a stepwise program for improving well behaviors, addressing body, mind, and spirit through Level One changes in everyday health behaviors, Level Two self-regulation skills, and Level Three professional complementary and integrated interventions. The aim of this model is to educate health-care professionals to recognize the signposts on the path to illness so that the consumer can be assisted in reestablishing normal rhythms and modifying maladaptive behaviors, to assist ill individuals to identify the factors that have contributed to the onset and escalation of the disease, and to discover new choices and well behaviors to enable the recovery of health.

Keywords Geography of mortality and morbidity • Illness onset • Pathways principles • Intervention model

Introduction: The Pathway to Illness

In his Divine Comedy, Dante introduced the idea that human beings go astray in life and can rediscover their way. Dante's text suggests the image of life as a journey and a process and also suggests the need for a guide to rediscover one's path.

The Pathways Model suggests that individuals can go astray in health as well, through lifestyle choices and turning points that induce illness. Homeostasis and health are lost at multiple levels, and the result is a dysregulation of body, emotion, and spirit. Health is also a journey, and illness is a caution light that one has gone astray in health and life. The Pathways Model suggests that with a guide, sick individuals can rediscover a new pathway to health, involving positive choices, new turning points, and restored balance in body, mind, and spirit.

The Pathways Model is not simply a metaphor. In the present chapter, and throughout the book, we will present evidence from the demographics of illness, from functional medicine, and from a variety of other sources that most illness is not a discrete event. Rather it is truly a pathway, a process involving a continuum from complete health to mild insufficiencies, to concerning deficiencies, and to diagnosed disease. Mainstream health care, which identifies a problem to address only when the individual's health is grossly impaired and diagnostic criteria are met, misses multiple opportunities to intervene in less expensive ways and to sustain optimal wellness.

The aim of the Pathways Model is twofold: (1) to educate health-care professionals and the general public to recognize earlier on the signs that one is on a pathway directed toward illness, allowing one to correct that path earlier in the process, and (2) to assist those already in a state of disease to identify those past and present lifestyle choices and turning points, which have contributed to the onset and escalation of the disease, and to discover new choices and well behaviors to enable the recovery of health.

The New Face of Illness

Fundamental changes in the face of human health have reinforced the importance of the Pathways Model. The face of illness has changed dramatically, in the course of only a century. In 1900, physicians faced the scourge of acute medical conditions, which often killed quickly: infectious diseases, bacterial parasites, and unhealed physical trauma. The powerful tools of public health, immunization, and antibiotic medication have marginalized the illnesses of the past in health care. Today's Western primary care physician rarely encounters typhoid, cholera, smallpox, or polio. Clean water, effective waste management, and childhood vaccinations have brought such diseases under control, except for occasional instances where travelers carry infections back from journeys abroad.

Today illness presents a new face. The primary care clinic today is busy with diseases of lifestyle and adaptation, stress-related conditions, chronic illnesses and impairments, and complex biopsychosocial conditions. The most common illnesses are those linked to specific behaviors, such as smoking, inactivity, and substance abuse.

Table 1.1 Top ten causes of death (Lynn, 2004)

Ranking	1900	2000
1	Pneumonia	Heart disease
2	Tuberculosis	Cancer
3	Diarrhea and enteritis	Stroke
4	Heart disease	Emphysema and chronic bronchitis
5	Liver disease	Unintentional injuries
6	Injuries	Diabetes
7	Stroke	Pneumonia and influenza
8	Cancer	Alzheimer's disease
9	Senility	Kidney failure
10	Diptheria	Septicemia

The Leading Causes of Death

Table 1.1 shows the contrast between the leading causes of death in 1900 and those of the year 2000 (Lynn, 2004, p. 6). The top three killers in 1900 were pneumonia, tuberculosis, and diarrhea/enteritis, and of these three only pneumonia remains in the top ten. Tuberculosis is preventable and treatable, and the more serious diarrheal conditions have been greatly reduced by public health measures and antibiotics. On the other hand, heart disease has moved from the fourth position to the very first. Further, heart disease has become more gender-neutral in distribution. As women's roles have changed occupationally and economically, women have come to suffer cardiovascular disease in ever greater numbers. The Centers for Disease Control *Chronic Disease Overview* reported that over half of the persons who die each year of heart disease are now women (CDC, 2005). Cancer has also increased greatly as a cause of death, moving from the eighth position to the second. Diabetes, which was not in the top ten leading causes of death in 1900, was in the sixth position in year 2000 and unfortunately continues to increase as a health problem worldwide. As lifestyles change, so does disease.

There is a substantial difference in death rates among ethnic and racial groups, reflecting the interaction of genetic and lifestyle differences, as well as socioeconomic factors affecting access to care. In 2004, the age-adjusted death rate for the White population was significantly less (about 30%) than that of the Black population. Death rates in the self-identified Hispanic population are lower than the non-Hispanic group, but it is believed that Hispanic origin may be underreported or that migrants are healthy when they reside in the USA and return home when elderly or seriously ill. There continue to be differences in life expectancy by gender and among the ethnic groups. Although life expectancy continues to rise in all groups, data for all Whites (78.3 years) continues to exceed that for Blacks (73.1 years). All females' life expectancy is 80.4 years, and for all males, it is 75.2 years (Minino, Heron, Murphy, & Kochanek, 2007).

Table 1.2 Ten projected leading causes of disability in developed regions in 2020, as measured by disability adjusted years (Murry & Lopez, 1996)

Ranking	Causes of disability
1.	Ischemic heart disease
2.	Unipolar major depression
3.	Road traffic accidents
4.	Cerebrovascular disease
5.	Chronic obstructive pulmonary disease
6.	Lower respiratory infections
7.	Tuberculosis
8.	War injuries
9.	Diarrheal disease
10.	HIV/AIDS

Death rates (age adjusted) due to heart disease, stroke, and cancer have decreased steadily during the past decade for both genders and all ethnic groups (Minino et al., 2007). However, the number of deaths from heart disease and stroke remained almost twice as high for African-Americans compared to Whites (OMH, 2009), perhaps due to access to care or socioeconomic factors, such as education, income, and occupation.

The Leading Causes of Disability

If we change our focus from causes of death to the burden of disability, the same shifts in prevailing health problems are evident. The Harvard School of Public Health carried out a massive 5-year study for the World Health Organization and the World Bank, on the "global burden of disease," and this data was used to establish projections for the year 2020 (Murry & Lopez, 1996; Fleishman, 2002, 2003). Table 1.2 shows the top ten conditions which are expected to cause individuals to lose years of their life and/or spend years of their life in disability. The composite index is called DALY—"disability-adjusted life years."

As Table 1.2 shows, the top three conditions causing disability are ischemic heart disease, cardiovascular diseases, and unipolar major depression! Each of these is a condition impacted by genetic vulnerability but also by lifestyle, diet, and accumulated life stress.

Pathways Principle: The Pathways Model conceives of illness as a pathway emanating from genetic predisposition through dietary choices and level of physical activity, through a series of lifestyle choices, and through the impact of life and work stress, culminating in medical conditions that are largely avoidable and that in many cases can be reversed.

Understanding the Pathways Model challenges the reader to move beyond one-cause conceptualizations to a multicausal paradigm. This model rejects such questions as:

Is it genetics or diet that causes diabetes?
Is hypertension dietary or stress related?
Is fibromyalgia medical or is it really psychiatric?

The linear and polarizing cognitive style has little place in understanding health and disease. Each medical condition has some greater or lesser genetic loading, yet a host of environmental conditions, dietary factors, lifestyle variables, and environmental stress also contribute to the onset of a full-fledged disease. For example, even families with the strongest genetic disposition toward depression do not exhibit depression in each family member. Similarly, the pathway to a restoration of health involves many steps, and multiple interventions are often more effective in moderating chronic illness than are single-treatment regimens. Understanding the overlap or comorbidity between physiological and psychological factors in onset of illness facilitates design of more effective, multimodal interventions. In contrast, relying only on medical management of type 2 diabetes or solely on psychotherapy in anxiety disorders ignores scientific evidence for shared etiological pathways in these disorders.

Major Factors in Illness Onset

In the following discussion, we will draw on demographic figures from the year 2000 and more recent figures as available. Many of these numbers are actually worsening by the year, as unhealthy lifestyles spread and increase their impact.

Obesity, Inactivity, and Smoking. Obesity in the USA doubled between 1987 and 2004 (Thorpe, Florence, Howard, & Joski, 2004). Thirty-four percent of adults in the USA are now overweight and 31% obese. This leaves only 35% of adults in the health-conducive weight range! The numbers of overweight adults and children are increasing, and the impact of obesity and overweight on health is fast approaching the impact of tobacco, according to a study supported by the Centers for Disease Control (Mokdad, Marks, Stroup, & Gerberding, 2004). Anyone with a body mass index (BMI) of 25 or above is considered overweight, and anyone with a BMI of 30 or above is regarded as obese. To translate this from a BMI measure into height and weight, a person of 5 feet 4 inches and weighing 145 pounds will typically qualify as overweight, and a person of 5 feet 6 inches and weighing 186 pounds will usually be considered obese. More recent data from Flegal, Carroll, Ogden, and Curtin (2010) confirm that this trend toward widespread obesity in the US population continued from 1999 to 2008, with 32% of men and 35.5% obese in 2007–2008. The figures are worse when we examine specific age and racial/ethnic groups. If we examine the non-Hispanic Black population, ages 40–59, 39.7% of the men are obese and 51.7% of the women. In the Hispanic population, ages 40–59, 37.4% of the men are obese and 35.7% of the women.

In 2000, poor diet and physical inactivity caused 400,000 US deaths, making the combination of overweight and sedentary lifestyle the number 2 killer in the USA. Tobacco contributed to 435,000 deaths in the same time period, or 18% of all deaths in the USA. Using a database drawn from the USA and international studies, increasing BMI and smoking had additive effects on risk; each increase of 5 kg/m^2 was associated with about 30% higher mortality (PSC, 2009).

Overweight and physical inactivity are major contributors to the top three causes of death—heart disease, cancer, and cerebrovascular diseases, including stroke. The World Health Organization estimates that 80% of deaths from heart disease could be eliminated through healthy diet, regular exercise, and the elimination of smoking (WHO, 2009). Obesity and inactivity are also major contributors to diabetes, the sixth leading cause of death.

As we adopt a point of view emphasizing lifestyle and a continuum of disease, some of the statistical emphasis on discrete illnesses and distinct lifestyle factors seems misplaced. For example, medical researchers have identified the metabolic syndrome as a major threat to health in the Western world. The metabolic syndrome involves a convergent cluster of conditions, including obesity, hypertension, hyperglycemia, and hyperlipidemia. These are actually not separate diseases, but overlapping conditions, rooted in the lifestyle factors of poor nutritional choices, sedentary ways of life, and a continuum of metabolic changes. The ultimate result is the development of diabetes, hypertension, heart disease, and a heightened risk for stroke. Later chapters will be devoted to diabetes/obesity and hypertension/heart disease.

Additional Lifestyle Factors. Alcohol abuse contributes to liver disease and to a lack of proper diet, causing an estimated 85,000 deaths in the USA in the year 2000, or 3.5% of all deaths (Mokdad et al., 2004). Car accidents caused 43,00 deaths, firearms 29,000 deaths, sexual diseases 20,000 deaths, and illegal drug use 17,000 deaths. None of these conditions approach the impact of the major triad of lifestyle factors: obesity, inactivity, and smoking. Together this triad of major factors contributed to approximately one third of the deaths in the USA in 2000.

Emotional Illness. The presence of psychological distress or frank psychiatric illness also increases risk for medical illness. Depression interferes with the diabetic patient's motivation to maintain exercise and decreases compliance to treatment (Fisher, Thorpe, DeVellis, & DeVellis, 2007). Anxious reactions to stressful situations worsen the risk for syncope in young adults (McGrady & McGinnis, 2005). Mortality and morbidity from cardiac causes are so strongly influenced by depression and anxiety that these negative psychological states are monitored during routine cardiac rehabilitation (Todaro, Biing-Jiun, Niaura, & Tilemeier, 2005; Davidson et al., 2006). Unfortunately, management of mood or anxiety disturbances in medical clinics is often not optimal. Our most compromised citizens, the severely mentally ill, demonstrate a significantly higher risk for serious physical illness. Common etiology for chronic psychiatric and certain medical illnesses, such as cardiovascular disease, has been suggested but not confirmed. Nonetheless, decision-making ability in this group is questionable, and faulty decisions lead to poor food choices, inappropriate use of substances, and difficulties managing medicines (Newcomer & Hennekens, 2007).

Running parallel to the worldwide increase in disorders of behavior, the prevalence of psychological illnesses continues to rise. During a lifetime, the risk of anxiety disorders is 28%, mood disorders is 20%, and substance abuse disorders stands at 14%; the prevalence for all psychiatric disorders now approaches 40% (Kessler, Berglund, Demler, Jin, & Walters, 2005). Although services are available for most people with depression, for example, the stigma of mental illness still forms a barricade to seeking help. People remain symptomatic for many months despite the availability of effective drugs and behavioral therapies (Wang et al., 2005).

The sufferer's reluctance to access mental health services not only affects productivity in the workplace and increases family stress but also burdens the primary care network. For example, people with anxiety disorders often have comorbid gastrointestinal and musculoskeletal symptoms. They worry about slight discomfort, imagining the barely discernable as potentially catastrophic and consequently contact their primary care medicine physician frequently (Levy, Maselko, Bauer, Richman, & Kubzansky, 2007).

Pathways Principle: The Pathways Model considers physical, emotional, social, behavioral, and spiritual variables to be interrelated throughout the lifespan. No illness is purely physical and none only emotional. Thus, the individual beginning on the pathway to health learns which of the variables facilitated illness onset and then assesses what is needed to return to health. Persons who can clearly see their role in illness creation, through past choices and lifestyle habits, can better dedicate themselves to regaining health and wellness through new pathways.

The Continuum of Health and Illness

Figure 1.1 shows the continuum of health and illness. The figure emphasizes that there are health risk behaviors that move the individual toward illness and well behaviors that move the individual toward health and wellness. Many individuals do not seek health care until they are suffering daily and chronically at the disease end of the spectrum. The ultimate goal of the Pathways Model is to provide education and intervention much earlier on that continuum, preventing chronic illness.

Figure 1.2, provided by Sheila Dean (2009), shows another view of the continuum of health and disease, emphasizing the movement from health to insufficiency to deficiency to disease. Dean is a specialist in functional medicine. Her continuum includes biological markers and symptomatic markers, showing that as the individual moves from health to insufficiency, he or she might begin to feel stiff and achy. At the insufficiency stage, such conditions as migraine, fatigue, pain, and weight gain will be observed, and one might see a mildly elevated fasting blood sugar. At the deficiency stage, several lab values may show abnormality, with an elevated TSH (thyroid-stimulating hormone) value, elevated homocysteine, and with

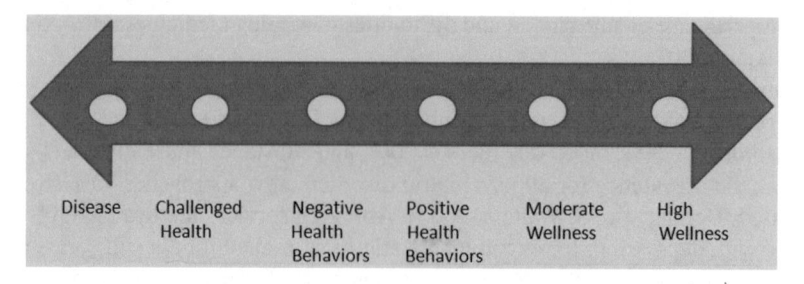

Fig. 1.1 The continuum of health and disease

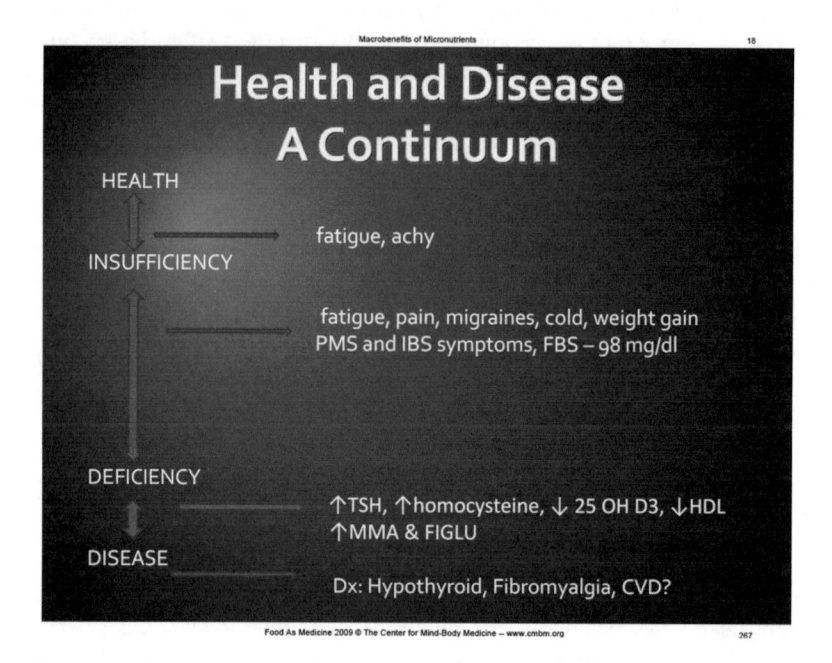

Fig. 1.2 Health and disease: a continuum (Dean, 2009)

lowered HDL (high-density lipoprotein or "good cholesterol") and other markers. At the disease level are found diagnosed illnesses and conditions, such as cardiovascular disease, fibromyalgia, or a hypothyroid condition.

In many cases individuals are already situated at the illness end of the continuum when they seek assistance. The Pathways Model emphasizes identifying and reducing health risk behaviors that are present in the individual's lifestyle and identifying positive well behaviors that appear both possible and relevant for improving this individual's overall health. The stepwise organization of Pathways interventions will be discussed in Chap. 5, but a brief glimpse of the intervention model is relevant here. The emphasis in the Pathways Model is to begin with self-guided Level

One interventions, such as increasing movement, practicing mindful breathing, and obtaining adequate sleep and rest. Each of these basic interventions is designed to facilitate restoration of normal body rhythms (McEwen & Lasley, 2003). Level Two interventions consist of learning self-regulation skills, such as progressive relaxation, cognitive renewal, communication, and mindfulness, which can often moderate suffering and move the individual toward restoration of physical and emotional health. Finally, Level Three interventions are professional interventions, such as nutritional counseling, biofeedback, psychotherapy, and guided imagery, managed by the professional but involving high levels of participation from the patient.

Pathways Principle: The Pathways Model addresses the continuum of health and disease and the role of both health risk behaviors and well behaviors in shaping the individual's overall health. The Pathways Model assesses where the individual is currently on the continuum and identifies current levels of health, insufficiency, deficiency, or disease. The Pathways Model advocates reducing any health risk behavior, such as smoking, overuse of caffeine, or sleep deprivation, that contributes to ill health. The Pathways Model also introduces a stepwise program for improving well behaviors, addressing body, mind, and spirit through Level One changes in everyday health behaviors, Level Two self-regulation skills, and Level Three professional interventions.

Rethinking Health and Disease

The Pathways Model challenges many assumptions that the average North American makes about health. Consider the assumption that it is normal for blood pressure to slowly increase with age and no action is necessary unless one's systolic blood pressure reaches 140 or the diastolic pressure reaches 90. The American Heart Association cautions that any blood pressure higher than 120/80 should be regarded as prehypertension—a caution intended to encourage illness prevention. Yet medical treatment is often delayed until the diagnostic criteria are met. The normalcy of this age-related increase in blood pressure is called into question by cross-cultural comparisons. Research by Joossens (1980) and MacGregor (1985) shows the familiar rise in BP with age, with the mean systolic BP in the 20–29 age range less than 120 mmHg, the average in the 30s at approximately 130 mmHg, and the average in the 60s at approximately 145 mmHg. They reports similar age-related increases for residents of Belgium, Portugal, Sweden, The United States, Wales, and even the Bahamas. But their research also shows a striking contrast with residents of Botswana, New Guinea, the Solomon Islands, and West Malaysia, all of whom show relatively level BP over the life cycle. The discriminating variable seems to be sodium. Those nations whose standard diet involves adding salt show problematic increases in BP, and those nations with low-sodium diets show blood pressures which are both lower and level.

This example shows that the pathway to illness need not be individual. If an entire culture adopts a lifestyle element which is adverse for health, the consequent disease will be shared widely.

The Geography of Illness: Exporting Western Health Risks

Is this problem of disorders of lifestyle, stress, and emotional maladaptation merely a problem in the affluent societies of North America and Western Europe? The short answer is NO! The globalization of the Western dietary pattern, along with Western lifestyles, is rapidly exporting Western patterns of disease as well. The nations of the developing world are not yet done with the old diseases. Public health, an expensive undertaking, has lagged in the developing world. Clean water for drinking and cooking is widely unavailable and public sanitation nonexistent. UNICEF estimates that 884 million people still lack access to safe drinking water and 2.5 billion to adequate sanitation (UNICEF, 2009). The United Nations included improvements in sustainable access to an improved water source among its Millennium Development Goals, minimal goals for improving the human condition by the year 2015. Given the lack of sanitation and clean water, the old scourges continue to plague developing countries, with cholera, malaria, and typhoid outbreaks common throughout the developing world, and polio still endemic in Pakistan, India, Afghanistan, and Nigeria.

Even while the nations of the developing world struggle to provide sanitation, build water systems, eradicate mosquitoes, immunize children, and treat the old infectious diseases, the new diseases of the West are also spreading at an alarming rate. This is the dark side of economic and cultural "globalization." The health systems of Africa, Asia, and much of South America are struggling to cope with the old diseases and the new simultaneously.

One recent study sampled participants in 52 countries and compared the health effects of three dietary patterns, the Western diet (high in fried foods, salty snacks, eggs, and meat), the Oriental diet (high intake of tofu, soy, and other sauces), and the so-called Prudent diet (high in fruits and vegetables) (Iqbal et al., 2008). Those individuals in the highest quartile for the Western diet, eating the most fried foods, salty snacks, and meat and eggs, showed a 92% increased risk for myocardial infarction (MI), compared to those in the lowest quartile. The Prudent diet, in contrast, served to lower the risk for MIs, and the Oriental diet neither raised nor lowered the risk.

The dangers for health are clear, yet the move toward the Western diet, smoking, and lifestyle continues. Western foods and tobacco are widely advertised—marketed by multinational corporations to the poor—and at the same time the broad cultural aspirations toward Western ways reinforce Western dietary and lifestyle choices.

A report on the call centers of India provides a case study on the health risks of Western influences. Presently approximately 1.6 million Indians work in call centers and other jobs outsourced from the USA (Mahapatra, 2007). Call center employees, mostly in their 20s and 30s, typically develop poor diet; excessive smoking and drinking of alcohol; sedentary lifestyle; weight gain; disturbed sleep cycle, partly due to shift work; and loneliness. These employees show increasing incidence of sleep disorders, heart disease, digestive problems, depression, and family discord. In 2005, heart disease, strokes, and diabetes cost India $9 billion in lost productivity. The current estimates by the Indian Council for Research on International Economic Relations project an annual cost of $200 billion within 10 years (Mahapatra, 2007).

Neither the economies nor the health systems of the developing world can afford this new wave of Western diseases.

There are a number of pathways for this new wave of Western-style illness, along with the Western diet. Other significant factors are urbanization and industrialization; the health effects of technological change and stress; the decline of traditional communities, family supports, and values; increase in sedentary lifestyles, with the automobile, television, and the cyber world; and increase in Western habits such as smoking and alcohol consumption. The young Indian, Kenyan, or Brazilian, who leaves the village for the city, also leaves behind restrictive traditional mores, close family and communal relationships, and the typical foods and physical work of rural life. Instead he or she turns to the lifestyle visible in Western television and movies, without the restraints of elders to caution about the risks inherent in these choices.

Extensive research has explored the interrelationships among worksite conditions, job stress, and health. The classic "Whitehall" studies of British civil servant found a clear relationship between work status, control, and coronary heart disease. Social class affected self-reported health status in a direct relationship (lower class, poorer health) (Johnson, 2009). A large Swedish study investigated styles of leadership and sickness at the worksite. Workers reporting to an inspirational type leader had fewer sick days in contrast to workers in a dictatorial or autocratic environment (Nyberg, Westerlund, Magnusson Hanson, & Theorell, 2008). Workplace stress not only affects risk for physical illness but is also significantly correlated with incidence of depressive and anxious symptoms in addition to mood and anxiety disorders (Dobson & Schnall, 2009). The current common practice of downsizing is assumed to affect the displaced worker; however, studies of the workers who kept their jobs highlighted the deleterious effects of remaining in a company that has lost one third of the workforce. The remaining employees must increase their workload and face potential elimination of their own positions while functioning in a tense and unhappy environment. Predictably, the remaining workers were at higher risk for cardiovascular disease and poorer mental health (Gordon & Schnall, 2009). Although more detailed discussions of the influence of the worksite on health and wellness are beyond the scope of this chapter, awareness of job stress as a potential mediator of illness and effective coping as a component of the pathway to health are directly relevant. Health-care systems are now challenged to develop and communicate new practical pathways to health and recovery that consider the social environment, including neighborhood, worksite, and family.

Wellness Is an Option

The Pathways Model challenges both individuals and communities to review past choices and turning points and commit to positive choices and lifestyles. Community effort is important, because it is challenging at best for individuals to swim upstream, to adopt and sustain positive wellness practices when the surrounding community embraces high-risk lifestyles. Community-wide campaigns accompanied by public education can facilitate more extensive changes in lifestyle.

There is a basis for hopefulness about achieving better health through well lifestyles. Deaths from heart disease fell by 25.8% over a recent 6-year period in the USA (1999–2005), while deaths from stroke declined by 24.4% in the same period (American Heart Association, 2008; Science Daily, 2008). Further progress, however, will require additional changes in health risk behaviors. Individuals eating healthier, reducing smoking, and increasing exercise will make the difference.

Individuals, whether they are well or ill, have increasingly sought complementary and alternative therapies, such as energy therapies, herbal remedies, and manipulation and mind–body therapies. Strong research evidence supports some of these interventions, while others are considered to be experimental (Trindle, Davis, Phillips, & Eisenberg, 2005). Despite a great deal of controversy about effectiveness and safety of the complementary therapies, this much is clear. Many individuals want to be active partners in their health care; they seek holistic interventions; and they want to change dysfunctional habits in favor of moving toward health, if no cures are possible.

The concepts of positive psychology, focused on well-being, positive qualities, and happiness, were introduced in a seminal article by Seligman and Csikszentmihalyi (2000). Since then the positive psychology model has triggered an abundance of practical research studies focused on how ordinary people can optimize their well-being and quality of life. Understanding and treating illness has been the mainstay of medicine and psychology for centuries and is ignored neither in the concepts of positive psychology nor in the Pathways Model. However, emphasizing quality of life, prevention of illness, and personal satisfaction has strongly influenced the development of the Pathways Model.

Pathways Principle: The Pathways Model depends on individuals' understanding of their paths toward illness and their motivation to change. Emphasis is placed on reestablishing normal biological processes or rhythms before moving on to more complicated interventions. A positive, health- enhancing focus is maintained throughout all the levels of therapy. Complementary and alternative therapies are incorporated as appropriate.

Conclusion: Pathways to Health

The Pathways Model of illness and health is framed in a basic understanding of physiology and psychology and developed through years of clinical experience. Caring for patients with stress-related disorders highlighted the need for a multitier model of intervention, beginning with reestablishment of normal physiological rhythms and learning basic psychophysiological skills, followed by more complex therapies. Patients want to understand their illness and how they became ill; many seek to identify the decision points where they turned toward illness so that they can begin to progress toward health. In the Pathways Model, Level One interventions involve the discovery of maladaptive basic rhythms such as disrupted sleep, eating, and breathing. The exploration of the effects of maladaptive basic rhythms on the development and maintenance of illness provides patients a logical starting point in therapy. The Level Two interventions build on the reestablished normal biological rhythms and add the skills of relaxation, communication, cognitive renewal, and exercise. It is important for patients to gain a sense of competence or self-efficacy during this stage. For example, learning the difference between the experience of muscle tension and that of muscle relaxation builds personal control. Identification of negative thoughts and putting them to the test of realism reconnects patients with real life and decreases catastrophic thought patterns.

Level Three interventions consist of those more complex modalities such as psychotherapy, biofeedback, guided imagery, and medical management, all of which rest on the platforms of Level One and Level Two. In-depth analysis of dysfunctional emotional reactions, aberrant physiological responses to stress, and self-defeating behaviors is followed by instruction in strategies to foster emotional stability, healthy thinking, and timely biological recovery from stressful situations. At the end of treatment, patients feel empowered to continue on their own because they understand their own pathway to illness, their decision points along the way, and their pathway to current and continued health.

References

American Heart Association. (2008, Jan. 22). *Heart and stroke death rates steadily decline; risks still too high.* American Heart Association. Public release. Available at http://www.eurekalert.org/pub_releases/2008-01/aha-has012208.php.

Centers for Disease Control and Prevention. (2005). *Chronic disease overview.* Website on Chronic Disease Prevention and Health Promotion. Retrieved November 12, 2008, from http://www.cdc.gov/nccdphp/overview.html.

Davidson, K. W., Kupfer, D. J., Bigger, J. T., Califf, R. M., Carney, R. M., Coyne, J. C., et al. (2006). Assessment and treatment of depression in patients with cardiovascular disease: National Heart, Lung, and Blood Institute working group report. *Annals of Behavioral Medicine, 32*(2), 121–126.

Dean, S. (2009). *Macrobenefits of micronutrients. Presentation to the Food as Medicine Conference.* San Francisco, CA: Center for Mind-Body Medicine.

Dobson, M., & Schnall, P. L. (2009). From stress to distress. In P. L. Schall, M. Dobson, & E. Rosskam (Eds.), *Unhealthy work: Causes, consequences, cures* (pp. 115–134). Amityville, NY: Baywood Publishing Company, Inc.

Flegal, K. M., Carroll, M. D., Ogden, C. L., & Curtin, L. R. (2010). Prevalence and trends in obesity among US adults, 1999–2008. *Journal of the American Medical Association, 303*(3), 235–241.

Fleishman, M. (2002). Issues in psychopharmacosocioeconomics. *Psychiatric Services, 53*, 1532–1534.

Fleishman, M. (2003). Economic grand rounds: Psychopharmacosocioeconomics and the global burden of disease. *Psychiatric Services, 54*, 142–144.

Fisher, E. B., Thorpe, C. T., DeVellis, C. M., & DeVellis, R. F. (2007). Healthy coping, negative emotions and diabetes management. *The Diabetes Educator, 33*(6), 1090–1103.

Gordon, D. R., & Schnall, P. L. (2009). Beyond the individual: Connecting work environment and health. In P. L. Schall, M. Dobson, & E. Rosskam (Eds.), *Unhealthy work: Causes, consequences, cures* (pp. 1–15). Amityville, NY: Baywood Publishing Company, Inc.

Iqbal, R., Anand, S., Ounpuu, S., Islam, S., Zhang, X., Rangarajan, S., et al. (2008). Dietary patterns and the risk of acute myocardial infarction in 52 countries. Results of the INTERHEART study. *Circulation, 118*, 1911–1912.

Johnson, J. V. (2009). The growing imbalance: Class, work and health in an era of increasing inequality. In P. L. Schall, M. Dobson, & E. Rosskam (Eds.), *Unhealthy work: Causes, consequences, cures* (pp. 37–60). Amityville, NY: Baywood Publishing Company.

Joossens, J. V. (1980). Dietary salt restriction: The case in favor. In J. I. S. Robertson, G. W. Pickering, & A. D. S. Caldwell (Eds.), *The therapeutics of hypertension. Congress and Symposium Series, Number 26* (pp. 243–250). United Kingdom: Academic Press and the Royal Society of Medicine.

Kessler, R. C., Berglund, P., Demler, O., Jin, R., & Walters, E. E. (2005). Lifetime prevalence and age-of-onset distributions of DSM-IV disorders in the national co-morbidity survey replication. *Archives of General Psychiatry, 62*, 593–627.

Levy, A. G., Maselko, J., Bauer, M., Richman, L., & Kubzansky, L. (2007). Why do people with an anxiety disorders utilize more non-mental health care than those without? *Health Psychology, 26*(5), 545–553.

Lynn, J. (2004). *Sick to death and not going to take it anymore: Reforming health care for the last years of life*. Berkeley/Los Angeles: University of California Press.

MacGregor, G. A. (1985). Sodium is more important than calcium in essential hypertension. *Hypertension, 7*, 628–640.

Mahapatra, R. (2007, Dec. 25). *India's outsourcing industry faces growing health problems, from obesity to depression*. Associated Press Archive. Retrieved January 5, 2012, from http://nl.newsbank.com/nl-search/we/Archives?p_product=APAB&p_theme=apab&p_action=search&p_maxdocs=200&s_dispstring=india's%20outsourcing%20industry%20faces&p_field_advanced-0=&p_text_advanced-0=(%22india's%20outsourcing%20industry%20faces%22)&xcal_numdocs=20&p_perpage=10& p_sort=YMD_date:D&xcal_useweights=no.

McEwen, B. S., & Lasley, E. N. (2003). Allostatic load: When protection gives way to damage. *Advances in Mind–Body Medicine, 19*(1), 28–33.

McGrady, A., & McGinnis, R. (2005). Psychiatric disorders in patients with syncope. In B. Grubb & B. Olshansky (Eds.), *Syncope: Mechanisms and management* (pp. 214–224). Malden, MA: Blackwell Futura.

Minino, A. M., Heron, M. P., Murphy, S. L., & Kochanek, K. D. (2007). Deaths: Final data for 2004. *National Vital Statistics Reports, 55*(19), 1–119.

Mokdad, A. H., Marks, J. S., Stroup, D. F., & Gerberding, J. L. (2004). Actual causes of death in the United States, 2000. *Journal of the American Medical Association, 291*, 1238–1245.

Murry, C. J. L., & Lopez, A. D. (Eds.). (1996). *The global burden of disease: A comprehensive assessment of mortality and disability from diseases, injuries, and risk factors in 1990 and projected to 2020*. Cambridge, MA: Harvard University Press.

Newcomer, J. W., & Hennekens, C. H. (2007). Severe mental illness and risk of cardiovascular disease. *Journal of the American Medical Association, 298*, 1794–1796.

Nyberg, A., Westerlund, H., Magnusson Hanson, L., & Theorell, T. (2008). Managerial leadership is associated with self reported sickness absence and sickness presenteeism among Swedish men and women. *Scandinavian Journal of Public Health, 36*, 803–811.

Office for Minority Health. (2009). *Obesity and African Americans*. Web site of the Office of Minority Health. Retrieved January 14, 2009, from http://www/omhrc.gov/templates/content.aspx?ID-6456.

PSC Prospective Collaborative Group. (2009). Body-mass index and cause-specific mortality in 900 000 adults: Collaborative analyses of 57 prospective studies. *The Lancet, 273*, 1083–1096.

Science Daily. (2008, Jan. 24). Heart and stroke death rates steadily decline: Risks still too high. *Science Daily*. Available at http://www.sciencedaily.com/releases/2008/01/080122165630.html.

Seligman, M. E. P., & Csikszentmihalyi, M. (2000). Positive psychology: An introduction. *American Psychologist, 55*(91), 5–14.

Thorpe, K., Florence, C., Howard, D., & Joski, P. (2004). The impact of obesity in rising health spending. *Health Affairs, Suppl Web Exclusives*, W4-480-6.

Todaro, J. F., Biing-Jiun, S., Niaura, R., & Tilemeier, P. L. (2005). Prevalence of depressive disorders in men and women enrolled in cardiac rehabilitation. *Journal of Cardiopulmonary Rehabilitation, 25*, 71–75.

References

Trindle, H. A., Davis, R. B., Phillips, R. S., & Eisenberg, D. M. (2005). Trends in use of complementary and alternative medicine by US adults: 1997–2002. *Alternative Therapies in Health and Medicine, 11*(1), 42–49.

UNICEF. (2009). *Water, environment, and sanitation*. UNICEF web site. Retrieved January 6, 2009, from http://www.unicef.org/wes/index.html.

Wang, P. S., Lane, M., Olfson, M., Pincus, H. A., Wells, K. B., & Kessler, R. C. (2005). Twelve-month use of mental health services in the United States. *Archives of General Psychiatry, 62*(6), 629–640.

WHO. (2009). Ten facts on the global burden of disease. Web site of the World Health Organization. Retrieved January 12, 2009, from http://www/who.int/features/factfiles/globalburden/en/index.html.

Chapter 2
Genetic Etiology of Illness

Abstract This chapter begins with definitions of important concepts in genetics and continues with summaries of genetic influences on personality and behavior. Interactions between heredity and environment are described within the context of the Pathways Model. Genetic factors that create necessary and/or sufficient contributions to the physical and psychiatric disorders that are the focus of this text are emphasized.

Keywords Genetics and illness • Heredity and environment • Genotype • Phenotype

Definitions

Genes are units of inheritance positioned at locations on a chromosome. A gene is a segment of DNA that contains the coding information for a set of protein molecules, made up of linear chains of amino acids. Alleles are alternate forms of a gene. The alleles for a trait occupy the same locus or position on homologous chromosomes and govern the same trait. Traits that are hereditary, such as eye color or blood type, depend entirely on the particular genes that a person inherits. In contrast, traits that are acquired depend on nongenetic factors such as the person's tendency to wear their hair short. Genotype is the associated gene carried by a person; phenotype is the observable feature. In twin studies, when identical or monozygotic twins show the same trait or feature and dizygotic or fraternal twins do not, then genetic influences are implicated. Concordance refers to the similarity between a pair of twins in a particular trait or specific disease. Phenotypes may appear as blends or intermediate expressions determined by multiple genes. For example, skin and hair color are polygenetic (determined by genes at two or more positions on the chromosome), but these genes are also influenced by environmental factors, in addition to observation and learning (Bazzett, 2008). The heritability coefficient is defined as "the proportion of the observable differences measure within a sample of people that are directly attributable to the genetic differences between them" (Jang, 2005).

Race is often considered as a key determinant of health based on the observations that certain diseases occur more frequently in persons from certain parts of the world. But genetic ancestry is more closely correlated with geographic ancestry than with that of racial ancestry, due to immigration and intermarriage (Bamshad, 2005). It is important to remember that studies of "racial" factors rarely have included genetic analysis but instead rely on participants' self-report of ancestry.

In summary, the genotype (G) plus environment (E) plus GE interactions determines the phenotype (P) (Bazzett, 2008). Epigenetics refers to inherited changes in gene expression associated with mechanisms other than changes in the DNA sequence. Personality, behavior, and most medical and psychiatric disorders result from complicated interactions among multiple genes and environments. A useful way of understanding the interaction between heredity and environment is that the genotype determines the range of possible phenotypes. The phenotype emerges during development and maturation when genes interact with all the environmental factors to which the person is exposed (Rutter, 2006).

Genetics and Personality

The personality traits that a person exhibits result from a complex blend of genetic and environmental factors that are further sculpted by learning and cultural influences (Yong-Kyu, 2009). Determining the association between a specific polymorphism, such as the variable length of the serotonin transporter gene, and a personality trait is extremely difficult, even with large populations and extensive genetic analysis (Saffron et al., 2005). However, it is instructive to focus on genetic influences on one or two aspects of personality, since enduring characteristics impact behavioral choices, which in turn affect risk for medical and psychiatric illness.

Fear as an inherited trait can serve as a model system to explore inheritance patterns, modification of responses during development, and emergence of anxiety disorders. All animals are born with instinctive fears that are important for survival in their natural environments. The sight and smell of a predator sets into motion certain actions which increase the animal's chances of survival; these actions are not learned, but are available to the animal as soon as it is physically capable of enacting them (Panksepp, 1998). Similarly, the specific fears that human infants have at birth are necessary to protect them during the early years of life, but the adaptive significance of these fears changes with age (Eaves & Silberg, 2008). The core fears (confinement, isolation, pain) are modified over time as the child experiences different situations without adverse effects. For example, fear of the dark gradually declines during early and middle childhood, as the child's brain is able to distinguish darkness that is pleasant or comfortable in contrast to unsafe and potentially dangerous darkness. Rates of changes in fear intensity are variable by gender and age. Male adolescents with a greater predisposition to be frightened of strangers and darkness tended to maintain fear responses longer compared to those who had smaller genetic loading (Goldsmith & Lemery, 2000).

Neuroticism is a personality trait characterized by experience of negative emotions, such as anxiety, sad mood, and hostility. There is a significant heritable component to neuroticism, specifically in BDNF (brain-derived neurotrophic factor). A common variant of BDNF is the substitution of the amino acid valine (val) for methionine (met). In a study by Sen et al. (2003), persons who were homozygotes for the met allele had the lowest neuroticism scores, as indicated by the NEO Personality Inventory (Costa & McCrae, 1997). In contrast, the homozygotes for the val allele had the highest scores and the heterozygotes were in between. (If both alleles are the same, the individual is homozygotic, and if the alleles are different, he or she is heterozygotic.) BDNF gene variants may mediate not only the tendency for neurotic personality but also the pathophysiology of the clinical syndrome of depression (Sen et al., 2003). Furthermore, the neuroticism trait has been associated not only with psychological distress but an increased risk of a physical disorder, ulcerative colitis (Charles, Kato, Gatz, & Pedersen, 2008).

Genetics and Risk

Heredity can increase or decrease risk for pain sensitivity. Finan et al. (2010) studied the experience of pain in women with fibromyalgia. The pain experience and the effects of pain on mood were partially controlled by the catecholamine and opioid neurotransmitter systems and the catechol-o-methyltransferase (COMT) and the mu-opioid receptor (OPRM1) genes. Genetic and psychological analyses showed that women with the met/met genotype had worse mood and more functional impairment on days when pain was severe compared to those women with the val/met variant or the val/val genotype. Similar analyses were conducted on the asp (aspartate) or asn (asparagine) genotype. Patients with the asn/asn allele were less able to focus on any other experience other than their suffering compared to women with at least one asp allele. Diatchenko et al. (2005) also reported on genetic influences on pain sensitivity, by studying variants of genes that control COMT, an enzyme that regulates levels of catecholamines and enkephalins. A high probability of acute jaw pain becoming chronic temporomandibular joint disorder was partially determined by low COMT levels (i.e., relatively high catecholamines in the synapse). McLean (2011) analyzed the contribution of genetically induced pain sensitivity (COMT), the HPA axis, stress, and physical injury. Some, but not all, individuals who sustain a motor vehicle accident and a whiplash injury continue to suffer pain months after the event. Those who report chronic regional or widespread pain were more likely to demonstrate excessive physiological stress responses and the high-risk genetic variant. A summary of research associating candidate genes with variations in perception of experimental pain can be found in Fillingim (2010).

Using a behavior genetic model, temperamental fearfulness, as described earlier, is a moderately strong predictor of later anxiety. When the normal fear responses do not habituate over time during development and instead become exaggerated, the stress hormone cortisol remains elevated, providing a tentative physiological explanation for the behavioral responses. Fearful, shy children develop into adolescents with frequent social anxiety. These teens overreact to common stressors at school and with their peers. Later, as adults, their risk for generalized anxiety disorder and other anxiety disorders is increased (Goldsmith & Lemery, 2000).

The risk for a physical illness, such as hypertension, is also influenced by inheritance and modified by behavior. A group of 500 undergraduate students had their heart rate and blood pressure measured before, during, and after a test in mathematics. Those students who still had elevated blood pressures at the end of the test and were slower to return to baseline BP were those who had two parents with essential hypertension. So these students seemingly were unable to shut off the stress-mediated increases in sympathetic nervous system activity at the end of a stressful situation (Gerin & Pickering, 1995). Thus, the delay in recovery from stress increases the risk for essential hypertension later in life.

Plasminogen activator inhibitor (PAI-1) is a primary inhibitor of the fibrinolytic system, involved in clotting. When this fibrinolytic system is not inhibited to a sufficient extent, then the individual is more likely to demonstrate excessive clotting, increasing the risk for stroke (Yamamoto et al., 2002). Stress-induced changes were found in the expression of the gene responsible for plasminogen activator inhibitor type 1 (PAI-1), linking genetics and risk for a serious cardiovascular event.

Genetics and Environment

Life experiences and the environment can change the expression of a gene by coding the DNA that controls the function of that gene, not the genetic code itself (Mill & Petronis, 2007). Important studies on mother rats and pups showed that nurturing behavior by the mother increased the resilience of the pups by boosting the expression of the genes that modify release of corticosterone, the stress hormone. This is a good example of epigenetics. When the pups who had been well cared for by their mothers were exposed to restraint stress, they were less agitated. In contrast, the pups who received less licking and grooming by their mothers had fewer corticosterone receptors in the hypothalamus, resulting in deficient feedback and inability to deactivate the stress responses (Rutter, 2006). In human infants, the same principles apply. Neglect and lack of positive attachment figures impairs brain development, leading to lower intelligence, developmental delays, and later difficulties in socioemotional functioning (Perry, 2002).

A more complex interaction between genes and environment is demonstrated by the research that integrated parenting of difficult children with genetic influences, called evocative-environmental correlations (Eaves, Chen, Neale, Maes, & Silberg, 2005). A study of 473 preschool-aged children and their parents showed that children with the A1 allele of the dopamine D2 receptor gene were more likely to develop early-emerging anxious and depressive symptoms. These children also received less positive parenting, which has its own negative effects on mood and behavior (Hayden et al., 2010; Reiss et al., 1995). Further, the A1 allele and its emotional effects appear to elicit less positive parenting.

Caspi et al. (2003) reported that situational stress can lead to depression in some people but not in others, depending on the length of alleles in the serotonin transporter gene. Serotonin is a major neurotransmitter involved in regulation of mood. Individuals with the short allele in the serotonin transporter gene were more likely to become depressed after stressful life experiences. In another study of the transporter gene, medical students were tested for the short/long variant in the same serotonin transporter gene. Those students who experienced multiple stressors and had the two short alleles were the most likely to develop depressive symptoms (Rosen et al., 2010). However, the relationship between genes and environment is likely to be more complicated than a single gene can explain. Meta-analysis of several studies of the serotonin transporter gene and stress (that did not include the medical student study) found no evidence that a single gene variant was responsible for the stress–depression link (Risch et al., 2009).

The controversy about the link between stressful life circumstances and the serotonin transporter gene was further explored by Mueller, Armbruster, Moser, Canli, and Lesch (2011). These authors postulated that age may be the most important modifying variable and indeed showed that the relationships only occurred in younger adults and only when the primary stressful events had occurred during the first years of life.

Some environmental factors, such as physical activity, would seem to be protective against illness, but genetic factors may nullify the potential benefits of the positive behavior. A thought-provoking study of physical exercise in teenaged girls delineated two groups: some teens demonstrated positive effects of exercise on mood, while others did not. The girls who had a BDNF met allele benefited from activity, while girls with the val/val polymorphism gained little advantage with exercise to enhance positive mood. BDNF levels were abnormally low in the blood of depressed teens; the potential for successful treatment was highlighted in the study by Mata, Thompson, and Gotlib (2010). Treatment of teenagers suffering with clinical depression with antidepressants brought the levels of BDNF back to normal and returned mood to euthymia.

Genetics and Psychiatric Illness

Most of the psychiatric illnesses that have been studied suggest some degree of genetic influence, but even those with high heritability, like bipolar disorder and schizophrenia, are also influenced by the environment. Bipolar disorder is a chronic illness whose prevalence in the general population is about 1%. The hereditability of the disorder is approximately 0.8, meaning that 80% of the variance in transmission can be attributed to heredity (Mansour, Monk, & Nimgaonkar, 2005). In identical twins, there is a 50% concordance for schizophrenia, indicating a significant nongenetic contribution. As discussed above, genes linked to disorders may heighten sensitivity to environmental occurrences like stress, suggesting that genetic loading may be a necessary but not sufficient condition for a psychiatric disorder. Overlap also exists between certain disorders (bipolar disorder and schizophrenia) leading to hypotheses about shared susceptibility (Green et al., 2005). Although schizophrenia and bipolar disorder have been classified as distinct disorders through many revisions of the DSM, molecular genetic studies have highlighted overlapping risk for the psychotic, schizoaffective, and bipolar diagnoses (Craddock & Forty, 2006). In time, probably all emotional disorders will be shown to be polygenic, with each gene contributing only a small percentage to the disordered phenotype.

Studies of the actions of antidepressants are instructive in understanding the molecular pathways mediating unipolar depression, where the genetic contribution is estimated at about 40%. Candidate-associated proteins implicated in mood disorders include the serotonin transporter protein (Ogilvie et al., 1996), the norepinephrine transporter protein, c-AMP responsive element-binding protein (observed in depressed women), and cadherin, a fat-like protein affected by treatment with lithium (Bazzett, 2008). Chronic stress is a significant contributor to worsening mood, implicating the hypothalamic–pituitary–adrenal axis in depression (Bornstein, Schuppenies, Wong, & Licinio, 2006). Further, the expression of BDNF in the hippocampus is reduced by severe and prolonged stress, while in animal studies antidepressants increase BDNF levels (as mentioned earlier) as well as resistance to stress (Lee, Jeong, Kwak, & Park, 2010).

A large-scale study of 2,111 same-sex twins identified four coherent genetic factors: Axis I disorders, Axis II disorders, internalizing disorders, and externalizing disorders (Kendler, Aggen, Knudsen, Roysamb, & Neale, 2011). Distinguishing between Axis I and II disorders relies on differences between problems that are largely episodic and transient in contrast to disorders labeled as "enduring, pervasive, and stable over time" (Sadock & Sadock, 2003). Estimated proportion of the variance attributed to genetic effects (heritability) ranged from a high of 0.60 for agoraphobia to a low of 0.28 for dysthymia in these common Axis I disorders. For the Axis II personality disorders, the highest heritability was 0.50 for antisocial and the lowest was 0.29 for paranoid personality disorder. Support was evidenced, based on genetic analyses for separation of Axis I and Axis II disorders. However, the separation was far from perfect. Two Axis I disorders were in the Axis II internalizing cluster (dysthymia and social phobia), and from a solely genetic viewpoint, social phobia belonged with avoidant personality disorder and dysthymia in an unspecified personality disorder (Kendler et al., 2011).

Genetics and Physical Illness

Autonomic disorders are debilitating dysfunctions of the sympathetic or parasympathetic nervous systems. One such problem, postural orthostatic tachycardia (POTS), is characterized by increased heart rate upon assuming upright position. Instead of the normal increase in blood pressure and heart rate when these individuals stand up, parasympathetic dominance ensues, dropping the pressure, leading to syncope. Ten percent of individuals are born with low autonomic nervous system tone. The etiology of POTS can be partially explained by a gene defect in the norepinephrine transporter gene, causing reduced clearance at the synapse. More than normal amounts of norepinephrine leak out of the synapse, and there is reduced reuptake back into the synapse. Sympathetic activation decreases during attempts at changing position from sitting or lying to the upright stance (Shannon et al., 2000). Persons with POTS often experience significant functional impairments in the work, school, and social settings, so the comorbidity with anxiety and mood disorders is not surprising (McGrady & McGinnis, 2005).

The metabolic syndrome consists of the primary disorders: essential hypertension, type 2 diabetes, obesity, and hyperlipidemia. Markers for the syndrome include C-reactive protein (CRP), circulating inflammatory markers, tumor necrosis factor, interleukin-6 (IL-6), PAI-1, or reduced levels of anti-inflammatory substances such as adiponectin (Zimmet, Magliano, Matsuzawa, Shaw, & Shaw, 2005). In a study of Caribbean Hispanic families, the heritability for the metabolic syndrome was 24%; factor analysis yielded two independent factors: the first was lipids, glucose, and obesity, and the second factor was blood pressure. The heritability for factor 1 was 44% and that for factor 2 was 20% (Lin et al., 2005). Although familial aggregation was smaller in European families, all showed heritability (Freeman, Mansfield, Barrett, & Grant, 2002). Family history of diabetes evidenced genetic heterogeneity with linkages to at least four chromosomes (Cheng et al., 2010). Ghrelin is a circulating peptide which stimulates appetite. An association between the ghrelin gene and obesity in adults was identified (Pulkkinen, Ukkola, Kolehmainen, & Uusitupa, 2010). There is also significant overlap among the factors comprising the metabolic syndrome and abnormal autonomic tone, in particular lower heart rate variability (Gehi et al., 2009). Nonetheless, the practitioner should recall that the metabolic syndrome results from genetic predisposition, *in addition to* environmental, personality, and behavioral factors (Maury, Ramsey, & Bass, 2010).

Genetic Factors in Coexisting Disorders

Reviewing the literature on the role of heredity on mental and physical illnesses immediately draws attention to the multiplicity of interactions among emotional and medical disorders. A few examples highlight this observation. Circadian clock genes are implicated not only in sleep disorders (Cuninkova & Brown, 2008) but in major depression and bipolar disorder (Mansour et al., 2005) and seasonal affective disorder (Hampp et al., 2008). Depressed patients report poorer sleep efficiency, early morning awakenings, and non-restorative sleep (Lamont, Legault-Coutu, Cermakian, & Boivin, 2007). Another common comorbidity is the association between elements of the metabolic syndrome (specifically obesity and diabetes), sleep cycle, and depression (Scott, Carter, & Grant, 2008). Sleep deprivation has been correlated with eating habits, increased appetite, and the current epidemic of overweight American adults (Hamet & Tremblay, 2006). Further, it is postulated that the circadian regulatory system in the hypothalamus and in peripheral tissues is closely aligned with eating behavior, activity schedule, and ultimately with the metabolic networks (Marcheva, Ramsey, Afinati, & Bass, 2009).

Summary

Knowledge of genetic influences on disease is important, but should not necessarily lead to drastic changes in treatment models. The isolation of a pathogenic gene points to "the beginning of a chain of events leading to the disease." In mental disorders, this chain of events is likely to be highly complex: not related to a single gene and lengthy in terms of how soon the phenotype will be expressed. Development, aging, and stress in addition to many other environmental influences continuously modify the observable phenotype and the risk for medical and emotional illnesses.

References

Bamshad, M. (2005). Genetic influences on health. *Journal of the American Medical Association, 294*, 937–946.
Bazzett, T. J. (2008). *An introduction to behavior genetics.* Sunderland, MA: Sinauer Associates, Inc.
Bornstein, S. R., Schuppenies, A., Wong, M. L., & Licinio, J. (2006). Approaching the shared biology of obesity and depression: The stress axis as the locus of gene-environment interactions. *Molecular Psychiatry, 11*, 892–902.
Caspi, A., Sugden, K., Moffitt, T. E., Taylor, A., Craig, I. W., Harrington, H., et al. (2003). Influence of life stress on depression: Moderation by a polymorphism in the 5-HTT gene. *Science, 301*, 386–389.
Charles, S. T., Kato, K., Gatz, M., & Pedersen, N. L. (2008). Physical health 25 years later: The predictive ability of neuroticism. *Health Psychology, 27*(3), 369–378.
Cheng, C.-Y., Lee, K. E., Duggal, P., Moore, E. L., Wilson, A. F., Klein, R., et al. (2010). Genone-side linkage analysis of multiple metabolic factors: Evidence of genetic heterogeneity. *Obesity, 18*(1), 146–152.
Costa, P. T., Jr., & McCrae, R. R. (1997). Stability and change in personality assessment: The Revised NEO Personality Inventory in the Year 2000. *Journal of Personality Assessment, 68*, 86–94.
Craddock, N., & Forty, L. (2006). Genetics of affective (mood) disorders. *European Journal of Human Genetics, 14*, 660–668.
Cuninkova, L., & Brown, S. A. (2008). Peripheral circadian oscillators: Interesting mechanisms, and powerful tools. *Annals of the New York Academy of Science, 1120*, 358–370.
Diatchenko, L., Slade, G. D., Nackley, A. G., Bhalang, K., Sigurdsson, A., Belfer, I., et al. (2005). Genetic basis for individual variations in pain perception and the development of a chronic pain condition. *Human Molecular Genetics, 14*(1), 135–143.
Eaves, L. J., & Silberg, J. L. (2008). Developmental-genetics effects on level and change in childhood fears of twins during adolescence. *Journal of Child Psychology and Psychiatry, 49*(11), 1201–1210.
Eaves, L., Chen, S., Neale, M., Maes, H. H., & Silberg, J. (2005). Questions, models and methods in psychiatric genetics. In K. Kendler & L. Eaves (Eds.), *Psychiatric genetics* (pp. 19–94). Washington, DC: American Psychiatric Publishing, Inc.
Fillingim, R. B. (2010). Individual differences in pain: The roles of gender, ethnicity, and genetics. In S. Fishman, J. Balantyne, & J. Rathmell (Eds.), *Bonica* (pp. 86–98). Philadelphia: Wolters Kluwer Lippincott Williams & Wilkins.
Finan, P. H., Zautra, A. J., Davis, M. C., Covault, J., Tennen, H., & Lemergy-Chalfant, K. (2010). Genetic influences on the dynamics of pain and affect in fibromyalgia. *Health Psychology, 29*(2), 134–142.

Freeman, M. S., Mansfield, M. W., Barrett, J. H., & Grant, P. J. (2002). Heritability of features of the insulin resistance syndrome in a community-based study of health families. *Diabetes Medicine, 19*, 994–999.

Gehi, A., Lampert, R., Veledar, E., Lee, F., Goldberg, J., Jones, L., et al. (2009). A twin study of metabolic syndrome and autonomic tone. *Journal of Cardiovascular Electrophysiology, 20*(4), 422–428.

Gerin, W., & Pickering, T. G. (1995). Association between delayed recovery of blood pressure after acute mental stress and parental history of hypertension. *Journal of Hypertension, 13*, 603–610.

Goldsmith, H. H., & Lemery, K. S. (2000). Linking temperamental fearfulness and anxiety symptoms: A behavior-genetic perspective. *Biological Psychiatry, 48*, 1199–1209.

Green, E. K., Raybould, R., Macgregor, S., Gordon-Smith, K., Heron, J., & Craddock, N. (2005). Operation of the schizophrenia susceptibility gene, neuregulin 1, across traditional diagnostic boundaries to increase risk for bipolar disorder. *Archives of General Psychiatry, 62*, 642–648.

Hamet, P., & Tremblay, J. (2006). Genetics of the sleep-wake cycle and its disorders. *Metabolism, 10*(Suppl 2), S7–S12.

Hampp, G., Ripperger, J. A., Houben, T., Schmutz, I., Blex, C., Perrau-Lenz, I., et al. (2008). Regulation of monoamine oxidase A by circadian-clock components implies clock influence on mood. *Current Biology, 18*, 678–683.

Hayden, E. P., Klein, D. N., Dougherty, L. R., Olino, T. M., Laptook, R. S., Dyson, M. W., et al. (2010). The dopamine D2 receptor gene and depressive and anxious symptoms in childhood: Associations and evidence for gene-environment correlation and gene-environment interaction. *Psychiatric Genetics, 20*, 304–310.

Jang, K. L. (2005). *The behavioral genetics of psychopathology*. Mahwah, NJ: Lawrence Erlbaum Associates, Publishers.

Kendler, K. S., Aggen, S. H., Knudsen, G. P., Roysamb, E., & Neale, M. C. (2011). The structure of genetic and environmental risk factors for syndromal and subsyndromal common DSM-IV Axis 1 and all Axis II disorders. *The American Journal of Psychiatry, 168*(1), 29–39.

Lamont, E. W., Legault-Coutu, D., Cermakian, N., & Boivin, D. B. (2007). The role of circadian clock genes in mental disorders. *Dialogues in Clinical Neuroscience, 9*(3), 333–342.

Lee, S., Jeong, J., Kwak, Y., & Park, S. K. (2010). Depression research: Where are we now? *Molecular Brain, 3*(8), 3–8.

Lin, H. F., Boden-Albala, S. H., Juo, N., Park, N., Rundek, T., & Sacco, R. L. (2005). Heritabilities of the metabolic syndrome and its components in the northern Manhattan family study. *Diabetologia, 48*(10), 2006–2012.

Mansour, H. A., Monk, T. H., & Nimgaonkar, V. L. (2005). Circadian genes and bipolar disorder. *Annals of Internal Medicine, 37*(3), 196–205.

Marcheva, B., Ramsey, K. M., Afinati, A., & Bass, J. (2009). Clock genes and metabolic disease. *Journal of Applied Physiology, 107*(5), 1638–1646.

Mata, J., Thompson, R. J., & Gotlib, I. H. (2010). BDNF genotype moderates the relation between physical activity and depressive symptoms. *Health Psychology, 29*(2), 130–133.

Maury, E. R., Ramsey, K. M., & Bass, J. (2010). Circadian rhythms and metabolic syndrome: From experimental genetics to human disease. *Circulation Research, 106*(3), 447–462.

McGrady, A., & McGinnis, R. (2005). Psychiatric disorders in patients with syncope. In B. Grubb (Ed.), *Syncope mechanisms and management* (2nd ed., pp. 214–224). Masschusetts: Olshansky Blackwell Futura.

McLean, S. A. (2011). The potential contributions of stress systems to the transition to chronic whiplash-associated disorders. *Spine, 36*, 226–232.

Mill, J., & Petronis, A. (2007). Molecular studies of major depressive disorder: The epigenetic perspective. *Molecular Psychiatry, 12*, 799–814.

Mueller, A., Armbruster, D., Moser, D. A., Canli, T., & Lesch, K.-P. (2011). Interaction of serotonin transporter gene-linked polymorphic region and stressful life events predicts cortisol stress response. *Neuropsychopharmacology, 36*, 1332–1339.

Ogilvie, A. D., Battersby, S., Bubb, V. J., Fink, G., Harmar, A. J., Goodwim, G. M., et al. (1996). Polymorphism in serotonin transporter gene associated with susceptibility to major depression. *Lancet, 347*, 731–733.

Panksepp, J. (1998). *Affective neuroscience. The foundations of human and animal emotions.* New York: Oxford University Press.

Perry, B. D. (2002). Childhood experience and the expression of genetic potential: What childhood neglect tells us about nature and nurture. *Brain and Mind, 3,* 79–100.

Pulkkinen, L., Ukkola, O., Kolehmainen, M., & Uusitupa, M. (2010). Ghrelin in diabetes and metabolic syndrome. *International Journal of Peptides, 10*(M.), 1155–1163.

Reiss, D., Hetherington, M., Plomin, R., Howe, G. W., Simmens, S. J., Henderson, S. H., et al. (1995). Genetic questions for environmental studies. *Archives of General Psychiatry, 52,* 925–936.

Risch, N., Herrell, R., Lehner, T., Liang, K. Y., Eaves, L., Hoh, J., et al. (2009). Interaction between the serotonin transporter gene (5-httlpr), stressful life events, and risk of depression: A meta-analysis. *Journal of the American Medical Association, 301,* 2462–2471.

Rosen, D., Mascaro, N., Arnau, R., Escamilla, M., Tai-Seale, M., Ficht, A., et al. (2010). Depression in medical students: Gene-environment interaction. *Annals of Behavioral Science and Medical Education, 16,* 8–14.

Rutter, M. (2006). *Genes and behavior: Nature-nurture interplay explained.* New York: Blackwell Publishing.

Sadock, B. J., & Sadock, V. A. (2003). *Kaplan and Sadock's synopsis of psychiatry* (9th ed.). Philadelphia: Lippincott Williams & Wilkins.

Saffron, A. G., Turri, M. G., Munafo, M. R., Surtees, P. G., Wainwright, N. W. J., Brixey, R. D., et al. (2005). The serotonin transporter length polymorphism, neuroticism, and depression; a comprehensive assessment of association. *Biological Psychiatry, 58,* 451–456.

Scott, E. M., Carter, A. M., & Grant, P. J. (2008). Association between polymorphisms in the clock gene, obesity and the metabolic syndrome in man. *International Journal of Obesity, 32,* 658–662.

Sen, S., Nesse, R. M., Stoltenberg, S. F., Li, S., Gleiberman, L., Chakravarti, A., et al. (2003). A BDNF coding variant is associated with the NEO Personality Inventory domain neuroticism, a risk factor for depression. *Neuropsychopharmacology, 28,* 397–401.

Shannon, J. R., Flattern, N. L., Jordan, J., Jacob, G., Black, B. K., Biaggioni, I., et al. (2000). Orthostatic intolerance and tachycardia associated with norepinephrine transporter deficiency. *The New England Journal of Medicine, 342,* 541–549.

Yong-Kyu, K. (2009). *Handbook of behavior genetics.* New York: Springer Science Business Media, LLC.

Yamamoto, K., Takeshita, K., Shimokawa, T., Hong, Y., Kenichi, I., Loskutoff, D., et al. (2002). Plasminogen activator inhibitor-1 is a major stress-regulated gene: Implications for stress-induced thrombosis in aged individuals. *The National Academy of Sciences, 99,* 890–895.

Zimmet, P., Magliano, D., Matsuzawa, Y., Shaw, A. B., & Shaw, J. (2005). The metabolic syndrome: A global public health problem and a new definition. *Journal of Atherosclerosis and Thrombosis, 12,* 195–300.

Chapter 3
Psychosocial Etiology of Illness

Abstract Psychosocial factors contribute to the onset of illness and the recovery of health. Careful attention to the person's life history (or "psychosomatic history") discloses individual patterns of illness onset and recovery and times of exacerbations and clinical improvement. Stressful life events trigger illness, as do experiences of separation and loss. Traumatic experiences predispose the individual to develop more health problems and to display increased pain from health problems. Health risk behaviors raise the individual's vulnerability for illness. Social supports buffer individuals against illness, as do positive coping, healthy lifestyles, and wellness-oriented behaviors.

Keywords Psychosocial • Life events and illness • Separation and loss • Trauma and illness • Health risk behaviors • Social supports • Healthy behaviors

Introduction

The present chapter overviews what current research tells us about psychosocial dimensions of health and illness. Negative psychosocial events can become a pathway to illness, and conversely positive psychosocial events can become a pathway to health. There are several ways in which psychosocial elements can contribute to illness: the role of life events, including separation and loss, in the timing of illness; the relationship between early trauma and later illness; and the contributions of maladaptive and health risk behaviors to illness. Here the term illness is used most broadly, to refer to medical illness, psychiatric and emotional disorders, and personal troubles and distress. Next the chapter will examine how psychosocial interventions can enhance health, which includes the role of social supports in buffering against illness and empowering health-enhancing states, and the power of well lifestyles and positive habits in diminishing illness and promoting wellness. A brief case history illustrates how dramatically a simple psychosocial intervention can alleviate illness and human suffering.

Life Events, Trauma, and Health

The Psychosomatic History

In 1943 Flanders Dunbar published one of the classic texts in the newly emerging field of psychosomatic medicine—*psychosomatic diagnosis* (Dunbar, 1948, fifth printing). She devoted the entire first chapter to an interview process, which she labeled "The Psychosomatic History." She drew on a 5-year study of serial admissions to Presbyterian University Medical Center in New York, in coordination with Columbia University Medical School. The chapter was comprehensive and detailed and contains many useful guidelines for clinical assessment. In this context, however, I want to highlight the basic format of her clinical history taking.

Dunbar set out to supplement the traditional medical history, which she found omitted most of the psychosocial elements that played critical roles in the onset of many illnesses. She also undertook at the same time to develop clinical approaches and procedures, which could undo the Cartesian split, to guide the physician's attention back to mind and body simultaneously, as an intertwined unitary process. The first principle of modern psychosomatic illness is that every illness is both physical and emotional. The relative contributions of genetics, physiological malfunctions, and psychosocial events may vary from one condition to another and even from one episode of an illness to another in the same individual. Later, Elmer Green reworded this principle as the "psychophysiological principle": "Every change in the physiological state is accompanied by an appropriate change in the mental emotional state, conscious or unconscious; conversely, every change in the mental emotional state, conscious or unconscious, is accompanied by an appropriate change in the physiological state" (Green, Green, & Walters, 1970, p. 3).

Dunbar developed the psychosomatic history technique to answer the question: "Under what circumstances do normal physiologic reactions to emotional situations become pathogenic?" (Dunbar, 1948, p. 30). In parallel columns, she recorded the "Events in Life Situation" and the "Patient's Response," the latter including the onset of medical or emotional complaints. Her focus was on patterns of behavior, habitual responses to stress, areas of adjustment, and injuries from the environment. Implicit is the recognition that even individuals suffering from a recognized medical disorder, with known genetic loading and biological mechanisms, are not equally sick all of the time. Rather, their conditions wax and wane with life events and emotional processes. If we wish to understand the full significance of illness for this individual, we must identify factors which *predispose* toward illness, those which *trigger* illness, and those which *buffer* against illness (Wickramasekera, 1988, 1993).

Dunbar emphasized the intertwining influences of character (personality and coping styles), somatic makeup (constitution and typical physiological stress response), and life events. For example, a child might experience onset of diabetes, initially learn solid self-management using diet and oral medication, yet suffer a series of episodes of unregulated blood sugar in adolescence and early adulthood, precipitated by the loss of critical support systems (moving out of the home, graduating from college, and the breakup of a marriage). Identification of such psychosocial influences on illness is critical in each area of medical care—in primary practice and throughout the specialties—and equally critical throughout mental health care.

The psychosomatic history illustrates the intertwining of personality, life events, and the onset and course of illness. As detailed in the Assessment chapter, juxtaposing significant life events with medical history facilitates a pathways assessment of recurrent health problems.

Stressful Life Events and Health

In the 1960s, Thomas Holmes and Richard Rahe reviewed the medical records of over 5,000 individuals. They developed the Social Readjustment Rating Scale, commonly known as the Holmes–Rahe Life Events scale (Holmes & Rahe, 1967). The scale includes 43 common life events, ranging from change in residence to divorce, and assigns a numerical value to each life event. A series of subsequent studies showed that subjects' scores on the life events ratings were predictive of the onset of illness and declines in functioning (Rahe, 1990; Rahe & Arthur, 1978; Rahe et al., 1972; Rahe, Mahan, & Arthur, 1970).

More recent studies continue to show a significant correlation between stressful life events and increased risk of illness and explored this relationship in special populations. Coker et al. (2011) found that children with more family stressful life events had impaired scores on the "Health Related Quality of Life Inventory." Lietzén et al. (2011) followed 16.881 adults (ages 20–54), with no previous episodes of asthma, and found that high total exposure to stressful life events was predictive of the onset of asthma. The effect was robust, even when statistical corrections were made for demographics, smoking, and having a cat or dog in the home.

Additional research has also refined the understanding of the role of life events in causing illness. For example, Lin, Ensel, Simeone, and Kuo (1979) used a Chinese–American sample and corroborated that stressful life events predict the initiation of psychiatric illness, but social supports mitigated against this onset. The relative contribution of social supports in predicting illness onset was greater than the weight of stressful events.

Life Events Including Separation and Loss. Six of the top eight items in the Holmes Rahe Social Readjustment Rating Scale include life events that involve separation from or loss of significant others or job: "death of spouse," "divorce," "marital separation," "death of close family member," and "fired at work." As Dunbar's early work indicated, researchers have long recognized that life events involving separation and loss are powerful in producing distress and dysfunction in the human organism. James Lynch, in his *The Broken Heart: The Medical Consequences of Loneliness* (1977), and later publications (Lynch, 1998; Lynch & Convey, 1979) highlighted the importance of separation, loss, and loneliness in triggering cardiovascular illness and other forms of medical and psychiatric illness. Both morbidity and mortality increase following significant losses.

More recent research has introduced some nuances, showing that not all losses are equivalent in their effects. Michael and Ben-Zur (2007) studied 130 individuals who had been widowed or divorced. The participants completed questionnaires assessing current well-being and adjustment and life satisfaction before and after the loss. Widowed persons generally showed greater life satisfaction before than after the loss, while divorced individuals showed greater life satisfaction after the loss. The widowed group also showed less problem-focused coping and less emotion-focused coping than the divorced sample. Dating, living with a new partner, and problem-focused coping were all predictive of higher well-being in both groups.

Stressful life events are a potential pathway to illness, and the course of the "psychosomatic history" often tells the tale of illness as well. Separation and loss provide especially potent triggers for the onset of medical and emotional illness. Other factors, such as social supports, may mitigate the negative impact of stressful life events.

The Role of Trauma in Later Illness

Some stressful life events cross a severity threshold and earn the designation "traumatic." Clinicians have long observed that patients seen in medical clinics seem to include a disproportionate number of persons who have suffered trauma or abuse in childhood. Trauma history seems to predispose patients to develop more medical and psychiatric complaints, to show more preoccupation with their illness, and to utilize medical services more heavily. Recent medical epidemiological research, involving several large population and clinical studies, consistently supports this clinical observation. Research evidence documents that human beings who suffer significant emotional trauma or abuse in childhood are more vulnerable to the onset of many medical and psychiatric conditions. In this section we will sample a selection of research establishing this early trauma—adult illness connection.

Felitti et al. (1998) reported that four kinds of adverse childhood events (ACEs) predicted adult medical illness: (1) psychological abuse, (2) physical abuse, (3) sexual abuse, and/or (4) exposure to parental substance abuse, mental illness, partner abuse, or criminal behavior. For the individuals who suffered more of these ACEs than average, the following medical problems showed elevated rates: ischemic heart disease, cancer, stroke, chronic bronchitis, emphysema, diabetes, skeletal fractures, and hepatitis.

Batten, Aslan, Maciejewski, and Mazure (2004), drawing on findings from the National Co-morbidity Survey, reported on individuals who suffered traumatic childhood maltreatment (defined as sexual abuse, physical abuse, or neglect). Their study found that women who were maltreated as children showed a ninefold increase in heart disease compared to women not maltreated as children. Individuals of both genders with childhood maltreatment showed a significance increase in depression incidence in their lifetime.

Rosenberg et al. (2000) focused specifically on individuals with a history of physical abuse or sexual abuse. Their study included 48 gynecological outpatients, 35 inpatients with seizure, and 24 psychiatric admissions. Ninety-six patients reported a trauma history. Of these patients, 66 reported past abuse, and 45 qualified for PTSD diagnoses. The total number of traumatic events, including episodes of physical and sexual abuse, correlated significantly with medical utilization. The five highest utilizers of medical services received PTSD diagnoses.

Spitzer et al. (2009) conducted a study of 3,171 individuals residing in the community. They adjusted their results statistically to account for the contributions of sociodemographic factors, smoking, body mass index (BMI), blood pressure, depression, and alcohol use disorders. Even after the effects of these diverse factors were subtracted, their study showed that subjects with a trauma history had significantly higher odds ratios for developing angina pectoris and heart failure, stroke, bronchitis, asthma, renal disease, and polyarthritis. The authors concluded that there is a strong association between trauma history and cardiovascular and pulmonary diseases.

Sareen et al. (2007) undertook a survey of 36,984 individuals in the Canadian Community Health Survey. They found that respondents with PTSD showed higher rates of cardiovascular disease, respiratory disease, chronic pain syndrome, gastrointestinal illness, and cancer. PTSD was also associated with chronic fatigue syndrome and multiple chemical sensitivities.

Sansone, Wiederman, and Sansone (2001) applied a "path analytic" statistical model to establish childhood precursors for adult preoccupation with physical symptoms. Their study showed substantial relationships among childhood trauma, borderline personality functioning, current depression, worry, and physical preoccupation. The authors concluded that childhood trauma predicts adult preoccupation with physical symptoms.

Zatzick, Russo, and Katon (2003) studied 73 trauma surgery inpatients during the initial hospitalization and again at 12 months post-injury. They found that female gender and the severity of combined PTSD and depression predicted the magnitude of symptoms at 1 year. In this study neither PTSD nor depression severity alone was predictive of somatic symptoms.

Sachs-Erickson, Kendall-Tackett, and Hernandez (2007) reported on data obtained in the National Co-morbidity Study, a nationally representative sample. Patients with history of childhood physical abuse or sexual abuse report more current health problems than those without trauma. In the group that did report a current health problem, those participants with a trauma history reported more pain complaints when describing current health symptoms, than respondents with no trauma history. Childhood abuse predicted these pain reports independently of the presence of depression. With regard to one type of pain, migraine headache, adults with a prior history of abuse in childhood were more likely to develop chronic (or transformed) migraine and the age of onset was younger (Tietjen et al., 2010b). Outpatients with migraine were more likely to have experienced any form of maltreatment in their younger years, compared to general outpatients without headache (Tietjen et al., 2010a).

Van Houdenhove, Luyten, and Egle (2009) studied the role of trauma in individuals with chronic pain and fatigue. They found that 64 % of patients with fibromyalgia and chronic fatigue syndrome reported either childhood or adult trauma, and 39 % of these patients reported both childhood and adult trauma. Their research supports the conclusion that trauma in either childhood or adult years is a predisposing factor for both fibromyalgia and chronic fatigue syndrome.

Mulvihill (2005) conducted an integrative review of the literature published from 1997 to 2003. The research reviewed supports a strong impact of childhood trauma on psychological health, and an even greater impact on physical health. Childhood trauma has been shown to increase the prevalence for eating disorders, substance abuse, phobias, multiple personality disorders, irritable bowel syndrome, rheumatoid arthritis, and autoimmune disorders.

Mechanisms for the Role of Trauma in Health. Mulvihill (2005) also identified probable mechanisms by which childhood trauma negatively impacts later health. Children faced with threat initially show hyperarousal—an alarm response. With increased threat, the child's body eventually releases endogenous opioids, and dissociation begins. Under acute stress, cortisol enhances survival—with greater alertness, activity level, and subjective well-being. With prolonged elevation in cortisol, however, the child shows withdrawal, dysphoria, and fatigue. Chronic secretion of cortisol depresses immune function and leads to hypocortisolism. The thymus, an immune system organ, is smaller in abused and neglected children, with ongoing health consequences. Hypocortisolism contributes to chronic fatigue syndrome, fibromyalgia, rheumatoid arthritis, and asthma. With chronic stress, homeostatic mechanisms break down. This topic is discussed in detail in the chapter on Psychophysiological Pathways to Illness.

Other research has shown that patients suffering with posttraumatic stress disorder show decreased heart rate variability (HRV) (Zucker, Samuelson, Muench, Greenberg, & Gevirtz, 2011). HRV is a marker for resilience and positive health. Higher HRV is associated with autonomic homeostasis and the ability to self-regulate emotions (Porges, Doussard-Roosevelt, & Maiti, 1994). Low HRV is a predictor for morbidity and cardiovascular illness, especially in persons with a past history of cardiovascular disorders (Kleiger, Miller, Bigger, & Moss, 1987). Lowered HRV is an indication of autonomic nervous system dysregulation, which plays a role in many chronic medical conditions. In this fashion, both HRV and autonomic nervous dysregulation may serve as mechanisms for the effects of trauma on physical health.

In addition, Kendall-Tackett (2009) has proposed that prior trauma "primes" the inflammatory response system, so that it "reacts more rapidly" to later stressors. She suggests that increases in inflammation contribute to the onset of a variety of chronic illnesses. She reviewed the research evidence to support this hypothesis. She also suggests that a variety of therapies that decrease inflammation might be used to "halt the progress" toward chronic illness (2009, p. 35).

Early traumatic experiences, including childhood physical abuse, sexual abuse, and neglect, are pathways to illness, increasing the incidence and severity of illness and distress in adult life. Several mechanisms have been identified as mediating the impact of trauma on later health: the effects of a chronically prolonged stress response, suppressed immune function, long term hypocortisolism, lowered HRV, autonomic dysregulation, and a priming of the inflammatory response system by trauma.

Negative Coping, Health Risk Behaviors, and Risky Lifestyles

When I ask my patients what they do to cope with stress, they sometimes comment, "Nothing, nothing. I don't know what to do." Yet upon closer examination, we usually discover that human beings always do something under stress. They may become immersed in negative or maladaptive emotion-focused coping, becoming immersed in *negative affectivity*, such as chronic anger or depression, with demonstrably negative effects on physiology. Cohen, Tyrell, and Smith (1993) exposed 394 health subjects to the common cold and showed that the level of negative affectivity was a predictor of susceptibility to infection, independent of other factors, such as the magnitude of stressful life events.

Unfortunately, many human responses to stress involve *health risk behaviors*, which increase the individual's risk for increase medical and mental health problems. Under stress, some individuals increase alcohol consumption; others smoke more cigarettes or increase the use of street drugs or prescription medications. Some may argue with family or self-isolate, while others gamble, over spend, or become promiscuous. The occasional multitalented individual will do several of the above at once and escalate a moderately stressful situation into a crisis. Baban and Craciun (2007) point out that individual health risk behaviors cluster together to form a *risky lifestyle*, more dramatically disposing the individual to both medical illness and psychiatric disturbance.

Gray (1993) identified the following health risk behaviors as major factors undermining health globally: tobacco use, alcohol abuse, physical inactivity, unhealthy dietary habits, risky sexual practices, and non-adherence to effective medication regimens and to screening programs. Half of the premature deaths from the ten leading causes of death in developed countries relate to these health risk behaviors (Gray, 1993). Numerous research studies have demonstrated that reducing health risk behaviors reduced morbidity and mortality. The costs of illness related to health risk behaviors are of such magnitude that international health organizations spend substantial portions of their budget attempting to reduce the frequency of health risk behaviors (Rutter & Quine, 2004).

Negative coping, health risk behaviors, and risky lifestyles are pathways to illness. Negative affect renders the individual susceptible to illness. Health risk behaviors introduce elements overtly disposing to illness. In the case of cigarette smoking, individuals introduce known carcinogens into their system. Sedentary life style and the abuse of fast food unleash metabolic factors leading to systemic dysregulation and later disease. Risky lifestyles cluster together multiple risk behaviors, compounding adverse effects.

Psychosocial Pathways to Health

Social Supports

Social support consists of regular contact and involvements with others. During illness, social supports increase one's access to health care and assist the individual in coping with disease. In well times, social supports and social activity are critical in eliciting and maintaining positive mood and self-esteem. Individuals differ vastly in their usual frequency of interactions with others, their feelings of connection to others, and their satisfaction with social contacts. The presence of adequate social supports diminishes the impact of threatening events on our health, and restoration of social supports is a frequent trigger for a recovery of emotional and physical health.

A still growing empirical literature has documented the presence of social supports as a factor reducing mortality and morbidity in a variety of populations and in the face of many illnesses and health threats. Numerous studies showed that "human beings with spouses, friends, and family members who provide psychological and material resources are in better health than those with fewer supportive social contacts" (Cohen & Wills, 1985).

Cassel (1975) and Cohen and Wills (1985) developed the stress-buffering hypothesis, suggesting that the presence of adequate social supports can buffer individuals against the adverse health effects of stress. Cohen and Wills' research showed that social supports in fact had a buffering effect, providing protection against adverse effects during stressful times, and an additional main effect, that is, that social supports produce more positive health directly, even in the absence of stress.

Holt-Lunstad, Smith, and Layton (2010) conducted a meta-analytical review of the 148 studies covering over 300,000 participants and examining the impact of social relationships on mental health, morbidity, and mortality. Their conclusion was that the influence of social relationships on mortality was comparable to well-established risk factors for mortality, such as smoking, and exceeded the impact of well-known risk factors for mortality, such as obesity and physical inactivity. Their research emphasizes the power of social supports to buffer human beings against illness, in spite of the presence of many risk factors for illness.

In recent years, research has moved from a simple demonstration that social support enhances health to more complex models that can guide more strategic interventions utilizing psychosocial support. Current studies develop complex research designs to detect interactions among social support, self-esteem, focus for the social support, objective measures of health status, and physiological indices, increasing understanding of how—by what pathways and mechanisms—social support causes improved health.

Carcone, Ellis, Weisz, and Naar-King (2011) conducted a study examining the social support variable in adolescents with diabetes. The distinguished four types of social support in these situations are the following: support for the adolescent from family, support for the adolescent from friends, support for the caregiver from another adult, and support for the family from the health care provider. One hundred forty-one adolescents and their adult caregivers participated in the study, completing questionnaires and monitoring blood glucose and hemoglobin A1c levels. A structural equation model was developed, and the research showed that support for the caregiver from another adult was directly related to support to the adolescent from family, and indirectly related to better illness management. Support to the family from health care providers was not related to support for the adolescent, and support to the adolescent from friends was not related to better illness management. In summary, intervention programs should include components focusing on providing social supports to parental caregivers, with the dual hopes of enhancing parental support for adolescents and of improving illness management.

An experimental study by Cosley, McCoy, Saslow, and Epel (2010) studied the interaction of compassion for others with social support in buffering the adverse physiological effects of stress. When provided with social support during the task, those participants who were higher in compassion for others showed lower blood pressure reactivity, lower cortisol reactivity, and higher high-frequency HRV reactivity, during a social stress task. They also reported liking the supportive evaluators more. Compassion for others appears to increase one's ability to accept social support, thus leading to more benign reactions to stress. Symister and Friend (2003) undertook a complex study of 86 end-stage renal disease patients, who were by the necessities of their illness, increasingly dependent on family and friends for assistance and support. In their study, they asked, for example, whether social support can elicit positive emotional states, as well as reduce negative states. They assessed the effects of several categories of positive social support (appraisal support, tangible support, self-esteem support, and belonging support) as well as of problematic support (negative social interactions). They also included a measure of optimism, to determine whether social support increases positive expectations about the future. Their results showed that self-esteem was a mediating variable, such that individuals with higher self-esteem gained more benefit from social supports in reducing depression and increasing optimism.

Mallinckrodt, Armer, and Heppner (2012) conducted a study of 203 women with breast cancer, in order to delineate more specifically the relationship of social support with adjustment and distress. They hypothesized a curvilinear threshold-based model, such that having "enough" social support would reduce adverse effects and increase positive effects. Their findings supported a threshold model. Most of the correlation between social support and the outcomes was found in women in the bottom quartile for social support. Among these women, social support correlated significantly with both positive adjustment and distress. In the top three quartiles, social support was unrelated or marginally related to adjustment and distress.

Social supports provide an effective pathway to health. Social supports serve to buffer individuals from the adverse health effects of stress and produce additional positive health-enhancing effects, even in the absence of stress. Social supports elicit positive emotional states and optimism and reduce negative states such as depression. Social supports interact with other factors such as self-esteem and compassion for others, producing aggregated effects. Social supports may moderate the illness or disease process or enhance the individual's adjustment to living with illness.

Positive Coping, Health Supportive Behaviors, and Well Lifestyles

There are several kinds of coping skills, all of which serve as buffers against the effects of stress on the individual. Problem-focused coping acts on the environment to remove or modify threatening events. Emotion-focused coping involves actions to control distressing feelings. Some studies include a third form of coping, relationship-focused coping, which involves modes of coping aimed at managing, regulating, or preserving relationships during stressful periods (O'Brien & Delongis, 1996). Persons with strong coping skills cope more adequately with stressful events and develop fewer medical and emotional symptoms.

A number of studies have found relative advantages for certain kinds of coping in the face of illness, often problem-focused coping or relationship-focused coping. A British study by Whitmarsh, Koutantji, and Sidell (2003) studied 93 patients with cardiac disease and examined the patients' perceptions of their illness, their mood, and the favored coping strategies, to assess which factors disposed them to better attendance in cardiac rehabilitation. Patients with better attendance in rehabilitation tended not to attribute the cause of their illness to a germ or virus and were more likely to attribute their illness to lifestyle. Those who attended tended to suffer more anxiety and depression than poor attenders and nonattenders. As hypothesized, the attenders tended more than nonattenders to utilize problem-focused coping. However, they also made more coping efforts overall and tended to use all forms of coping—problem-focused, emotion-focused, and maladaptive coping—than nonattenders.

The Ways of Coping Scale (WOCS), developed by Folkman and Lazarus (1980) and later revised (Folkman & Lazarus, 1985), identified a total of eight coping strategies: confrontive coping, distancing, self-controlling, seeking social support, accepting responsibility, escape/avoidance, planful problem solving, and positive reappraisal. An abundance of research has applied the WOCS to human beings with illness, and here too, some coping strategies seem to be more optimal than others. Yi, Smith, and Vitaliano (2005) studied 404 high school age athletes, examining profiles associated with better resilience in the face of stress. They assessed the participants initially on levels of negative life events and coping strategies, and during the athletic season, the participants kept daily logs of illness activity. The researchers labeled as resilient those participants who were exposed to high levels of life stress yet remained healthy, with minimal absenteeism from sports. The resilient participants relied extensively on problem-focused coping (planful problem solving) and seeking social support, while the non-resilient participants tended to rely on blaming others and escape/avoidance. This is a valuable study, drawing on a population of athletes at the higher level of health and functioning and exploring factors supporting resilience in the face of stress in this group.

Just as there are health risk behaviors, we can identify health supportive behaviors ("healthy behaviors") and well lifestyles. In some cases, the healthy behaviors are the absence of a health risk behavior, as in "the absence of smoking." A number of popularized lists have been published, identifying seven or ten habits that will support higher level health. For our purposes, we will refer to the "preventative practices" identified in Healthy People 2010 (HP2010), which have the advantage of being a national consensus-based list, supported by extensive research evidence. The HP 2010 goals were further operationalized by the Centers for Disease Control for their "Behavioral Risk Factor Surveillance System," as follows:

1. Consume five servings or more of fruit and vegetables per day.
2. Engage in moderate physical exercise (brisk walking bicycling, gardening), on at least 5 days per week, for at least 30 min per day, or vigorous aerobic exercise (running, aerobics, heavy yard work) on 3 or more days per week for at least 20 min.
3. Avoid cigarette smoking.
4. Avoid binge drinking, defined for men as having at least five or more drinks and for women as having at least four or more drinks, on at least one occasion in the last 30 days.
5. Avoid heavy drinking, defined for men as having more than two drinks per day for the last 30 days and for women as having more than one drink per day for the last 30 days.
6. Engage in regular leisure time physical activity, as defined by an absence of recreational exercise (such as running, calisthenics, golf, gardening, or walking for exercise), other than their regular job, during the past month.
7. Maintain weight within healthy limits. Overweight is defined by a BMI greater than 25.0 kg/m^2. Obesity is defined by a BMI greater than 30.0 kg/m^2.
8. Obtain adequate hours of rest or sleep on a regular basis. Insufficient sleep is defined by failure to get "enough" sleep on at least 14 nights during the preceding month (Li et al., 2011).

Persons wishing to optimize their personal health would do well to cultivate the habits reflected in these eight HP 2010 goals.

Positive, adaptive coping and health supportive behaviors are pathways to health. Positive coping sustains better adjustment and optimal medical and emotional health. Problem-focused coping may have some advantages overall, especially in the face of illness. Nevertheless, positive coping of all kinds can reduce distress and support wellness. Healthy behaviors and well lifestyles support optimal health. Individuals desiring optimal health should consume adequate quantities of fruits and vegetables, engage in frequent aerobic exercise, avoid cigarette smoking, avoid binge and heavy drinking, maintain weight below a BMI of 25 kg/m^2, and obtain adequate hours of sleep and rest on a regular basis.

Pathways Interventions: The Case of Esther

The following case illustrates that psychosocially based interventions deserve a central place in the pathways Model, along with the spectrum of lifestyle and habit changes, self-regulation skills, and mind–body therapies.

Initial Visit and Assessment

Esther was a 76-year-old widowed woman, referred by her internist for a chronic pain problem and clinical depression. Esther was recommended specifically for a group-based chronic pain program in a general hospital setting. Her physician made clear that her depression was a greater concern for him, but that Esther was more open to a medical referral for pain treatment than for psychotherapy for depression.

Esther arrived for her initial evaluation, dressed elegantly in a grey-boiled wool jacket, a blouse with a laced collar, and pearls. Her hair was beautifully groomed. As Esther began to talk, however, a very different picture emerged. Esther lived alone, in a high-rise subsidized apartment, in a neighborhood riddled with crime in a Midwestern city. She rarely left the apartment. Wednesdays she took a bus to a supermarket for groceries, and once every 4–8 weeks she took a bus to her internist's office.

Esther had been married to Bernard, a bank officer who died suddenly at age 48 of undiagnosed heart disease. Her adult children—a physician daughter and a son in financial services—lived on the East Coast. Both were busy with career and families and rarely visited Esther. She saw herself as a burden to them, as they assisted her occasionally with expenses. She received a pension from her husband's employment, but her assets had been exhausted in the children's education. Her only remaining family member in proximity was a sister, who Esther rarely saw. The sister was affluent, and Esther was embarrassed visiting her.

Esther described herself as a socially active woman in her early adult years. She participated in parent organizations for her children's school and was active in her synagogue. After her spouse's death, she gradually disengaged, feeling like a "fifth wheel" and embarrassed when she could not afford the activities her one-time friends shared.

Esther suffered the onset of mild arthritis pain in her hands and wrists in her forties. The pain escalated when her spouse died, and she decreased activities. When her children completed their educations and accepted positions in Boston and New York, she was proud, but increasingly isolated and housebound. At this time, she became severely depressed and she began to suffer severe low back and knee pain, and activity became increasingly painful. She was diagnosed with severe progressive osteoarthritis and degenerative disk disease. For her, the concept that her condition was progressive and degenerative frightened her, as she visualized herself alone in her apartment, unable to care for herself.

Esther's physician treated her conservatively, with antidepressant medication and non-steroidal anti-inflammatory medication. But, as she emphasized, her life was empty and depressing, and the antidepressant medication helped her sleep but did not lift her mood.

Esther's initial evaluation showed severe clinical depression and severe anxiety, warranting the diagnoses of major affective disorder, with recurrent depressive episodes, and generalized anxiety disorder. Her Beck Depression Inventory (BDI) score was 39, severe, and her Beck Self-Rating Anxiety Scale score was 32, moderate. On the BDI, she endorsed an item stating that she had thoughts of killing herself, but would not carry them out. On questioning, she admitted that her suicidal thoughts were recurrent, but insisted that she had neither intent nor any plan to harm herself. Her initial psychometric testing also included a Tellegen Absorption Scale, which suggested that she was highly susceptible to absorption, and probably a good candidate for hypnotic pain treatment.

An initial brief biofeedback assessment/demonstration was undertaken, to show her that her musculature might be contributing to her pain problems. This assessment showed elevated muscular tension in the trapezius muscles of the upper back and shoulders and an asymmetry, with higher elevations of muscle tension on the left side, after she was asked to stand and reach. There was a very poor recovery, when she was asked to sit and relax, and the asymmetry persisted.

Esther was pleasant and cooperative in the interview, but evasive about continuing treatment. She verbally committed to attend a group-based pain management program, but inserted several "ifs" as scheduling of future sessions was discussed. She emphasized the Medicare co-pays, the burden of leaving her apartment, the fears of being assaulted in her neighborhood, and the difficulty of traveling by bus to the hospital setting. She seemed interested in the biofeedback and stated that she might want to learn how to relax her musculature if it could help her pain.

Pathways Assessment: Relevant Pathways. Esther's family history was positive for osteoarthritis and for clinical depression. The onset of the osteoarthritic symptoms seemed unremarkable, with mild and manageable symptomatology uncomplicated by emotional stress. The early loss of her spouse and the later separation from her adult children seemed to be triggers for exacerbation of her pain, depression, and anxiety. Her response to pain consisted largely of avoidance of activity, which exacerbated her immobility over time. Her emotional vigilance and apprehensions about her finances and health contributed, along with the inactivity, to a chronically over-activated musculature and postural distortion, which was assumed to aggravate the arthritic pain.

Social isolation and inactivity contributed to a near-complete lack of social rewards. Esther's life had degenerated to low-level maintenance activities with few joys. Phone calls on Sunday evening with her children were the high point of each week, although she cried herself to sleep after the calls.

Pathways Assessment: Readiness for Change. The interview with Esther suggested that she was at the pre-contemplation stage (Prochaska et al., 1994). She could see little hope for relief from her pain and could not imagine a return of joy to her life. Her avoidant coping strategies were not serving her well, but she had little experience with actively solving a problem. She knew only the difficulty of living with pain, and the hope that something done at the hospital might moderate her pain.

Initial Pathway Interventions

Esther attended the first session in the group-based pain program, along with seven other men and women. The first module in the program included the idea of making small commitments to personal changes—changing long-term habits, setting small but manageable goals, and practicing new coping skills at home. Esther became flustered as some other group members set fairly demanding goals. I suggested that for her a single small Level One goal might be best, so she would not create a failure situation for herself. She nevertheless decided to set two Level One goals.

Level One: Social Activity. One of the group members reached out to Esther, trying to help her feel more at home in the group. Learning that Esther was Jewish, she asked her about the upcoming Passover holiday, which would occur later in the week. She asked Esther about the Seder meal, and Esther disclosed that she had not attended a Seder celebration in over 10 years. The group member persisted in the discussion, and Esther mentioned that her sister always invited her, and her brother-in-law offered to drive her, but she refused, not wishing to be a burden. After some uncomfortable silence and a moment of tearing, Esther talked about her childhood Seder experiences and the Seders her husband led until his death. She reluctantly agreed to consider accepting her sister's invitation, if her sister called again that week.

Level One: Soothing. Esther also committed herself to playing some of her favorite classical music, in the afternoon, when her joint pain became more severe. She disclosed that she was a music lover, and concerts by the local symphonic orchestra had been one of her favorite outings with her husband. She committed to sitting and rocking, while she absorbed herself in the music, as a way to give herself some pleasure and diversion, as well as something to look forward to. She set the goal of engaging in this self-soothing three to four times in the first week.

Progress in Level One. Esther missed the second group session in Week One. She attended the first session in Week Two. Esther was excited about her Seder meal experience. She had reconnected with two nieces at the Seder and expressed regret at not seeing them sooner. She also had agreed to visit her sister more often. Esther was animated and talkative, and barely mentioned her pain. When asked, she was apologetic about her self-soothing goal. She had engaged in the self-soothing with music twice, playing the same Brahms violin concerto each time. She found this surprisingly pleasant and distracting from her pain, but had not met her three to four times goal, and felt disappointed in herself. She was encouraged to accept and celebrate her progress on both goals, which impressed other group members as significant. She reset the goal to use music for self-soothing two to four times per week. She also set a new goal to see her sister or one of her nieces at least weekly.

Esther did not return to the pain management program, ever, and did not return messages left at her apartment by the support staff. The clinical team concluded that she was not ready for change and sent her a supportive letter, commending her initial progress on Level One goals of social activity and self-soothing. She was also encouraged to return for more group-based or individual services in the future.

Esther surprised the entire clinical team. The following December, a lengthy holiday letter arrived, wishing each individual member of the clinical team a joyous holiday. Esther described her life as transformed and explained that she had not needed any further services, because she was much happier. She had continued to visit and engage herself with her sister and nieces and their families and began to attend her synagogue again with her sister. She acknowledged that she still had her pain daily, but that this was less a factor in her life now. Esther continued to send annual holiday letters with news and gratitude for an additional 6 years.

Summary

The case of Esther serves as an example that progress on Level One or Level Two can sometimes produce enough meaningful change and that no specific therapeutic services are needed. Human beings are resourceful, and once they begin making changes and solving problems, they often continue to draw on their strengths with minimal or no assistance. Esther's depression and sense of isolation resolved rapidly with family support, and her emotional health and activity level improved.

References

Baban, A., & Craciun, C. (2007). Changing health risk behaviors: A review of theory and evidence-based interventions in health psychology. *Journal of Cognitive and Behavioral Psychotherapies, 7*(1), 45–67.

Batten, S. V., Aslan, M., Maciejewski, P. K., & Mazure, C. M. (2004). Childhood maltreatment as a risk factor for adult cardiovascular disease and depression. *The Journal of Clinical Psychiatry, 65*, 249–254.

Carcone, A., Ellis, D. A., Weisz, A., & Naar-King, S. (2011). Social support for diabetes illness management: Supporting adolescents and caregivers. *Journal of Developmental and Behavioral Pediatrics, 32*(8), 581–590. doi:10.1097/DBP.0b013e31822c1a27.

Cassel, J. C. (1975). Social sciences in epidemiology: Psychosocial processes and stress—theoretical formulation. In F. L. Struening & M. Guttentag (Eds.), *Handbook of evaluation research* (pp. 537–549). Beverly Hills, CA: Sage Publication.

Cohen, S., Tyrell, D. A. J., & Smith, A. P. (1993). Negative life events, perceived stress, negative affectivity, and susceptibility to the common cold. *Journal of Personality and Social Psychology, 64*(1), 131–140.

Cohen, S., & Wills, T. A. (1985). Stress, social support and the buffering hypothesis. *Psychological Bulletin, 98*, 310–357.

Coker, T. R., Elliott, M. N., Wallander, J. L., Cuccaro, P., Grunbaum, J. A., Corona, R., et al. (2011). Association of family stressful life change events and health related quality of life in fifth grade children. *Archives of Pediatric and Adolescent Medicine, 165*(4), 354–359.

Cosley, B. J., McCoy, S. K., Saslow, L. R., & Epel, E. S. (2010). Is compassion for others stress buffering? Consequences of compassion and social support for physiological reactivity to stress. *Journal of Experimental Social Psychology, 46*(5), 816–823. doi:10.1016/j.jesp. 2010.04.008.

Dunbar, F. (1948). *Psychosomatic diagnosis* (5th ed.). New York: P. B. Hoeber.

Felitti, V. J., Anda, R. F., Nordenberg, D., Williamson, D. F., Spitz, A. M., Edwards, V., et al. (1998). Relationship of childhood abuse and household dysfunction to many of the leading causes of death in adults. The Adverse Childhood Experiences (ACE) study. *American Journal of Preventive Medicine, 14*, 245–258.

Folkman, S., & Lazarus, R. S. (1980). An analysis of coping in a middle-aged community sample. *Journal of Health and Social Behavior, 21*, 219–239.

Folkman, S., & Lazarus, R. S. (1985). If it changes, it must be a process: A study of coping during three stages of a college examination. *Journal of Personality and Social Psychology, 48*, 150–170.

Gray, A. (1993). *World health and disease*. Buckingham, UK: Open University Press.

Green, E., Green, A., & Walters, E. D. (1970). Voluntary control of internal states: Psychological and physiological. *Journal of Transpersonal Psychology, 2*, 1–26.

Holmes, T. H., & Rahe, R. H. (1967). The social readjustment rating scale. *Journal of Psychosomatic Research, 11*(2), 213–218. doi:10.1016/0022-3999(67)90010-4.PMID 6059863.

Holt-Lunstad, J., Smith, T. B., & Layton, J. B. (2010). Social relationships and mortality risk: A meta-analytic review. *PLoS Medicine, 7*(7), e1000316. doi:10.1371/journal.pmed.1000316.

Kendall-Tackett, K. A. (2009). Psychological trauma and physical health: A psychoneuroimmunology approach to etiology of negative health effects and possible interventions. *Psychological Trauma: Theory, Research, Practice, and Policy, 1*(1), 35–48. doi:10.1037/a0015128.

Kleiger, R. E., Miller, J. P., Bigger, J. T., & Moss, A. J. (1987). Decreased heart rate variability and its association with increased mortality after acute myocardial infarction. *The American Journal of Cardiology, 59*, 256–262.

Li, C., Balluz, L. S., Okoro, C. A., Strine, T. W., Lin, J. M., Town, M., et al. (2011). *Surveillance of certain health behaviors and conditions among states and selected local areas—Behavioral Risk Factor Surveillance System, United States, 2009*. Surveillance Summaries: Morbidity And Mortality Weekly Report. Surveillance Summaries/CDC [MMWR Surveill Summ]. Atlanta, GA: Centers for Disease Control and Prevention.

Lietzén, R., Virtanen, P., Kivimäki, M., Sillanmäki, L., Vahtera, J., & Koskenvuo, M. (2011). Stressful life events and the onset of asthma. *The European Respiratory Journal, 37*(6), 1360–1365.

Lin, N., Ensel, W. M., Simeone, R. S., & Kuo, W. (1979). Social supports, stressful life events, and illness: A model and an empirical test. *Journal of Health and Social Behavior, 20*(2), 108–119.

Lynch, J. J. (1977). *The broken heart: The medical consequences of loneliness*. New York, NY: Basic Books.

Lynch, J. J. (1998). Decoding the language of the heart: Developing a physiology of inclusion. *Integrative Physiological and Behavioral Science, 33*(2), 130–136.

Lynch, J. J., & Convey, W. H. (1979). Loneliness, disease, and death: Alternative approaches. *Psychosomatics, 20*(10), 702–708.

Mallinckrodt, B., Armer, J. M., & Heppner, P. P. (2012). A threshold model of social support, adjustment, and support after breast cancer treatment. *Journal of Counseling Psychology, 59*(1), 150–160.

Michael, K., & Ben-Zur, H. (2007). Stressful life events: Coping and adjustment to separation or loss of a spouse. *Illness, Crisis & Loss, 15*(1), 53–67.

Mulvihill, D. (2005). The health impact of childhood trauma: An interdisciplinary review, 1997–2003. *Issues in Comprehensive Pediatric Nursing, 28*(2), 115–136.

O'Brien, T. B., & Delongis, A. (1996). The interactional context of problem-, emotion-, and relationship-focused coping: The role of the big five personality factors. *Journal of Personality, 64*(4), 775–813.

Porges, S. W., Doussard-Roosevelt, J. A., & Maiti, A. K. (1994). Vagal tone and the physiological regulation of emotion. *Monographs of the Society for Research in Child Development, 59*(2/3), 167–186.

Prochaska, J. O., Velicer, W. F., Rossi, J. S., Goldstein, M. G., Marcus, B. H., & Rakowski, W. (1994). Stages of change and decisional balance for twelve problem behaviors. *Health Psychology, 12*, 39–46.

Rahe, R. H., & Arthur, R. J. (1978). Life change and illness studies: Past history and future directions. *Journal of Human Stress, 4*(1), 3–15. doi:10.1080/0097840X.1978.9934972. PMID 346993.

Rahe, R. H., Mahan, J. L., & Arthur, R. J. (1970). Prediction of near-future health change from subjects' preceding life changes. *Journal of Psychosomatic Research, 14*(4), 401–406. doi:10.1016/0022-3999(70)90008-5. PMID 5495261.

Rahe, R. H., Biersner, R. J., Ryman, D. H., & Arthur, R. J. (1972). Psychosocial predictors of illness behavior and failure in stressful training. *Journal of Health and Social Behavior, 13*(4), 393–397. doi:10.2307/2136831. JSTOR 2136831. PMID 4648894.

Rahe, R. H. (1990). Life change, stress responsivity, and captivity research. *Psychosomatic Medicine, 52*(4), 373–396.

Rosenberg, H. J., Rosenberg, S. D., Wolford, G. L., Manganiello, P. D., Brunette, M. F., & Boynton, R. A. (2000). The relationship between trauma, PTSD, and medical utilization in three high risk medical populations. *International Journal of Psychiatry in Medicine, 30*(3), 247–259.

Rutter, D., & Quine, L. (2004). *Changing health behavior*. Buckingham, UK: Open University Press.

References

Sachs-Erickson, N., Kendall-Tackett, K., & Hernandez, A. (2007). Childhood abuse, chronic pain, and depression in the National Comorbidity Survey. *Child Abuse & Neglect, 31*, 531–547.

Sansone, R. A., Wiederman, M. W., & Sansone, L. A. (2001). Somatic preoccupation and its relationship to childhood trauma. *Violence and Victims, 16*(1), 39–47.

Sareen, J., Cox, B. J., Stein, M. B., Afifi, T. O., Fleet, C., & Asmundson, G. J. G. (2007). Physical and mental comorbidity, disability, and suicidal behavior associated with posttraumatic stress disorder in a large community sample. *Psychosomatic Medicine, 69*, 242–248.

Spitzer, C., Barnow, S., Volzke, H., John, U., Freyburger, H. J., & Grabe, H. J. (2009). Trauma, posttraumatic stress disorder, and physical illness: Findings from the general population. *Psychosomatic Medicine, 71*, 1012–1017.

Symister, P., & Friend, R. (2003). The influence of social support and problematic support on optimism and depression in chronic illness: A prospective study evaluating self-esteem as a mediator. *Health Psychology, 22*(2), 123–129.

Tietjen, G. E., Brandes, J. L., Peterlin, B. L., Eloff, A., Dafer, R. M., Steint, M. R., et al. (2010a). Childhood maltreatment and migraine (Part 1). Prevalence and adult revictimization: A multicenter headache clinic survey. *Headache, 50*, 20–31.

Tietjen, G. E., Brandes, J. L., Peterlin, B. L., Eloff, A., Dafer, R. M., Steint, M. R., et al. (2010b). Childhood maltreatment and migraine (Part II). Emotional abuse as a risk factor for headache chronification. *Headache, 50*, 32–41.

Van Houdenhove, B., Luyten, P., & Egle, U. T. (2009). The role of childhood trauma in chronic pain and fatigue. In V. L. Banyard, V. E. Edwards, & K. A. Kendall-Tackett (Eds.), *Trauma and physical health: Understanding the effects of extreme stress and of psychological harm* (pp. 37–64). London: Routledge.

Whitmarsh, A., Koutantji, M., & Sidell, A. (2003). Illness perception, mood and coping in predicting attendance at cardiac rehabilitation. *British Journal of Health Psychology, 8*, 209–221.

Wickramasekera, I. (1988). *Clinical behavioral medicine*. New York, NY: Plenum.

Wickramasekera, I. (1993). Assessment and treatment of somatization disorders: The high risk model of threat perception. In J. W. Rhue, S. J. Lynn, & I. Kirsch (Eds.), *Handbook of clinical hypnosis* (pp. 587–621). Washington, DC: American Psychological Association.

Yi, L. P., Smith, R. E., & Vitaliano, P. P. (2005). Stress-resilience, illness, and coping: A person-focused investigation of young women athletes. *Journal of Behavioral Medicine, 28*(3), 257–265.

Zatzick, D. F., Russo, J. E., & Katon, W. (2003). Somatic, posttraumatic stress, and depressive symptoms among injured patients treated in trauma surgery. *Psychosomatics, 44*(6), 479–484.

Zucker, T. L., Samuelson, K. W., Muench, F., Greenberg, M. A., & Gevirtz, R. N. (2011). The effects of Respiratory Sinus Arrhythmia biofeedback on heart rate variability and posttraumatic stress disorder symptoms: A pilot study. *Applied Psychophysiology and Biofeedback, 34*(2), 135–143.

Chapter 4
Psychophysiological Etiology of Illness

Abstract Research has documented multiple examples of linkages between psychological states and physical conditions in chronic pain, cardiovascular disease, sleep disorders, metabolic diseases, and respiratory illnesses. The target systems or tissues are partially determined by heredity, lifestyle choices, and environment in various proportions. This chapter will describe several paradigms that were developed to explain the general psychophysiological pathways to illness, while later chapters will provide examples of specific disorders. Although this is not an exhaustive list, the models chosen for discussion here will facilitate understanding of stress-related, frequently observed pathways to illness and lay the foundation for the later chapters on pathways to health.

Keywords Psychophysiology of stress • Somatization • Acute stress • Chronic stress • Physiological mechanisms

Introduction

Research has documented multiple examples of linkages between psychological states and physical conditions in chronic pain, cardiovascular disease, sleep disorders, metabolic diseases, and respiratory illnesses. The target systems or tissues are partially determined by heredity, lifestyle choices, and environment in various proportions. This chapter will describe several paradigms that were developed to explain the general psychophysiological pathways to illness, while later chapters will provide examples of specific disorders. Although this is not an exhaustive list, the models chosen for discussion here will facilitate understanding of stress-related, frequently observed pathways to illness and lay the foundation for the later chapters on pathways to health.

The General Adaptation Syndrome, described by Hans Selye, provided a framework for understanding physical responses to stress. As summarized in McGrady (2007), the presumption was that any stress produced the same, lock step response, organized by the endocrine system. The critical role of the brain in processing stimuli, reappraisal of potentially distressing situations, resulting in different responses to the same stressor, was recognized later (Lazarus, 1984). The acknowledgement that "only humans can become stressed out from things that exist in idea only" (McEwen, 2002, p. 34) created a new avenue for research in the stress-related disorders and emergence of therapies directed towards cognitive change.

A tool for assessment of the cumulative effects of situational stress on risk for physical illness was developed in 1967 and later revised to include more current items. The Social Readjustment Scale, commonly known as the Life Events Scale (Hobson & Kamen, 1998; Holmes & Rahe, 1967), tallies the number of negative and positive life events and assigns a weight to each item, depending on the extent of adaptation needed. A weighted score above 300 was posited to increase the risk for illness. Any change in circumstances, whether a happy occasion or the loss of a job, creates demands for adaptation on the part of that person. This model of linking life events to stress-related illnesses remains useful today, particularly as a starting point for clinicians to explain mind–body interactions to patients with unexplained symptoms. However, it does not account for individual perception of those life events.

Cohen and Rodriguez (1995) described pathways linking psychological (termed affective) distress with illness and illness behaviors (how people act when they are sick). They acknowledged that it was not necessary to limit the conversation to the effects of psychiatric "disorders," but that negative affect and subclinical symptoms also influenced behavior and physical conditions. Several pathways to illness and determinants of illness behavior were defined, including biological, cognitive, social, emotional, and behavioral. Although appraisal was not specifically mentioned in the model, it is implied as a causative factor of affective distress. Of further importance in this model is Cohen and Rodriguez' discussion about physical illness and illness behaviors feeding back and potentially worsening psychological states.

The High Risk Model of Threat Perception, elucidated by Wickramasekera (1995), was originally applied to a population of psychiatric patients. Both negative and positive modifying factors were identified. This model highlights the concept of risk and resilience factors that may *predispose* patients to somatize distress, *trigger* such distress, or help to *buffer* the individuals against somatization. *Somatize* and *somatization* here refers to the processes by which emotional conflict, physiological tension, or stress are transduced into physical symptoms and illness. McGrady, Lynch, Nagel, and Wahl (2003) utilized the High Risk Model in a group of family practice patients. Negative affect, accumulated life events, and avoidance coping increased the risk for physical symptoms (as measured by the PRIME-MD somatizing subscale) as well as for chronic illnesses. In contrast, social support and approach coping increased resilience and lowered the risk for somatic symptoms.

The concept of allostatic load (wear and tear on the body) (McEwen, 2002) posits that physiological systems can anticipate what may happen, in contrast to the idea of homeostasis where the system only reacts to change. There are four ways by which allostatic load develops in response to stress. First, frequent activation of stress response systems; for example, the recurrence of a variety of stressors may increase blood pressure and heart rate, which predisposes to cardiovascular problems (McEwen, 2004). The second scenario is the inability to adjust or adapt to change, so that the stress response occurs to repeated similar stimuli that should have become routine. Thirdly, at the end of a stressful event, some people continue to respond and physiological systems do not return to baseline; this can be conceptualized as a failure of recovery processes. Fourth, the stress response is hyporeactive, so the release of cortisol and catecholamine is insufficient, permitting over-activation of other systems. For example, the normal regulation of the immune system depends on sufficient cortisol; without it, exaggerated immune responses such as those in allergic reactions can occur (McEwen & Lasley, 2003).

Models of Mind–Body Interactions

Association Between Psychological Stress and Illness

There are multiple mechanisms that underlie the somatization of emotional conflicts, stress, and illness. The major mediators are the neural, endocrine, and immune systems. These systems interrelate in timed, sequential patterns influenced by conscious prefrontal lobe-driven decisions about behavior, superimposed on instinctual or unconscious reactions governed by lower brain centers.

In the nervous system, neurotransmitters signal excitation or inhibition, or balance the two. There are two broad categories of neurotransmitters: the small molecule, rapidly acting type and the slowly acting larger molecule neuropeptides. GABA and glycine, the major inhibitory neurotransmitters, modify the activity of the central nervous system by decreasing the frequency of nerve impulses and/or increasing reuptake of the neurotransmitters, thereby limiting their effects in the neuronal synapse, thus inhibiting neural responses to signals from other neurons. Norepinephrine, epinephrine, and dopamine are excitatory transmitters, which constitute the catecholamine family. Norepinephrine is found in both the central and the autonomic nervous systems, while epinephrine is released only from the adrenal medulla, and dopamine resides only in the brain. Cholinergic neurons release acetylcholine and modulate the balance between excitation and inhibition in the brain and stimulate activity in the parasympathetic nervous system. The major excitatory neurotransmitter in the central nervous system is glutamate. Serotonin also has excitatory properties, as demonstrated by the correlation between low levels of serotonin and depression.

The neuropeptide/growth factor class is excitatory or inhibitory and consists of hypothalamic releasing hormones (example: thyrotropin-releasing hormone), pituitary peptides (example: b-endorphin), peptides that act on the gastrointestinal system and the brain (example: substance P), and those from other tissues (example:

angiotensin II). The reader is referred to a neuroscience text for additional detail (Purves et al., 2004) or to a psychiatric text for examples of insufficient or excessive transmitters and psychopathology (Sadock & Sadock, 2007).

Somatization and Medically Unexplained Symptoms

The somatoform class of disorders listed in the DSM IV-TR includes somatization disorder, hypochondriasis, pain disorder, body dysmorphic disorder, conversion disorder, and factitious and malingering disorders (APA, 2000). Common to this entire class of disorders is the variance between the reported symptoms or patient experience and the medical evidence. The symptoms are not validated by physical exam or standardized medical and other testing. Patients' reported distress is out of proportion to the existing objective pathology, or there is an excessive concern about what most people would categorize as normal fluctuations in tension, heart rate, and intestinal motility (Neimark, Caroff, & Stinnett, 2005).

Despite the relevance of somatization, hypochondriasis, and pain disorder to the cases presented in other chapters, there are many instances where medically unexplained symptoms do not meet the formal criteria for a disorder in this DSM class (APA, 2000). The prevalence of somatization disorder meeting all DSM IV-TR criteria is very low, even in psychiatric populations. A study of patients with medically unexplained symptoms showed that only 23% had a DSM-validated somatoform diagnosis (Smith et al., 2005). Multiple definitions of somatization have also been suggested, particularly useful in primary care practices, where most physicians follow the International Classification System (ICD) rather than the DSM (Lynch, McGrady, Nagel, & Zsembik, 1999). Therefore, a broader working concept of somatization is necessary. The concept of medically unexplained symptoms (MUPS) may present a better paradigm to understand mind–body connections and the pathways to illness described in this chapter. MUPS can be thought of as distress signals, ways of drawing attention to negative psychophysiological states. Further exploration of MUPS in persons of all ages often leads to findings of clinical anxiety or depression (Neimark et al., 2005). Both the mood and anxiety disorders are characterized by somatic complaints such as tension, difficulty sleeping, or heart palpitations (anxiety) and fatigue, weight loss, or declining sexual interest (depression).

Somatization is not limited to the adult or elderly populations but also occurs in children and adolescents, with implications for later emergence of emotional sequelae. Based on the study by Hofflich, Hughes, and Kendall (2006), the presence of an anxiety disorder in children increased the number of reported somatic complaints, compared to children without anxiety; children with both anxiety and depression had statistically more complaints than those with anxiety alone. The most commonly reported somatic symptoms were shaky, sick to the stomach, sense of unreality, dizzy, tense, and "can't catch breath." Adolescents who consistently reported multiple somatic symptoms without clear evidence of disease also had increased risk for major depression as adults (Egger, Costello, Erkanli, & Angold, 1999). It is clear that the tendency to internalize stress and distress into physical symptoms often begins early in life and is further magnified in adulthood. The underlying mechanisms are not fully understood; no single factor, even a powerful one, reliably produces a physical illness. The anxiety disorders and the medical problems emerge from a psychophysiological process involving genetics, environment, autonomic, endocrine functions and behavior.

Postulated Mechanism: Hyperexcitability. A recurrent theme that helps one to understand the links between emotion and physical ills is hyperexcitability, as illustrated in the following examples of posttraumatic stress disorder (PTSD) and migraine headaches. In PTSD, the criteria for diagnosis include hyperarousal, in addition to avoidance and reexperiencing (DSM IV-TR). The major brain regions involved in the processing of fearful stimuli are the hippocampus, the amygdala, and the cortex. The hippocampus is a brain structure important in learning and memory; the amygdala mediates fear responses, whereas the prefrontal cortex is responsible for executive functions. The orbitofrontal cortex is designed to "show a flexible response in stressful contexts of uncertainty," creating the neural basis by which instinctual emotional responses are controlled through cognitive processes (Purves et al., 2004).

In a study of cerebral blood flow changes in response to unpleasant and pleasant stimuli, the former produced increased blood flow in the subcortical limbic regions, whereas pleasant stimuli produced increased cerebral blood flow, primarily in the prefrontal cortex (Paradiso & Johnson, 1999; Rahko et al., 2010). The hyperadrenergic state after trauma is responsible for over-consolidation of memory of the event in the hippocampus, which is very resistant to extinction. Recalling and reexperiencing the event is similar to the same stress reoccurring, releasing additional catecholamines, which created the hyperadrenergic state in the first place.

It seems that the processing of a traumatic event resides in lower brain centers, in preference to rational appraisal and eventual lessened emotionality. In PTSD, instead of a flexible response, sufferers demonstrate amplification of fear responses and generalization of event memories to neutral objects and show invariable reactions to stimuli (Schore, 2002). In contrast, amnesia may occur for the entire or certain aspects of the trauma in some people, either soon after the traumatic event (acute stress disorder) or for longer periods (PTSD) (Pittman, 1989). Autonomic blunting and dissociation, a less common but documented response to trauma, reminiscent of the somatic freeze reaction (fight, flight, freeze), may explain the memory deficits and subsequent difficulties paying attention that may be long lasting (Simeon, Guralnik, Knutelska, Yehuda, & Schmeidler, 2003).

Hyperexcitability of the brain has been identified as a major contributor to the pathophysiology of migraine (Goadsby, Lipton, & Ferrari, 2002; Lee, Zambreanu, Menon, & Tracey, 2008). Clinicians are well aware that patients with migraine often are sensitive to triggers from both the external physical environment (smells, foods, weather changes) and the so-called emotional environment (stress, conflict, loss) (Burstein & Jakubowski, 2005). The nucleus cuneiformis (NCF) of the brainstem in migraine subjects sustains lower than normal descending inhibition or increased descending facilitation. The NCF can facilitate nociception (the neural processing and transmission of pain and noxious stimuli) through cholinergic and glutamatergic mechanisms, or the NCF can produce opioid-mediated analgesia. Expectation of pain, as experienced by chronic migraineurs who have suffered severely for years, lowers the threshold for both perception of pain and responses to noxious stimuli. In addition, abnormal functioning of the nervous system is not limited to the times of pain but exists during the interictal state (Moulton et al., 2008) (the interictal state is the time period between migraine episodes).

Mechanism: Loss of Balance in Regulatory Systems. A second major mechanism linking psychological factors to physical illness is the disrupted balance in regulatory systems. The role of inflammatory processes in mental and physical illness will be used as an example of this concept. Inflammation is necessary to resolve acute infections and to prevent localized infections from spreading throughout the body. Healing consists of an orderly sequence of events that begins with an inflammatory state, followed by proliferative and remodeling phases that restore tissue structure and function (Widmaier, Raff, & Strang, 2006). However, excessively aggressive mobilization of the immune system or under-responsiveness to antigens represents loss of balance with maladaptive consequences.

Patients with medically unexplained symptoms report malaise and feelings of being unwell (Chapman, 2010). This "sickness response" is partially mediated by cytokines that act on the vagus nerve, the hypothalamus, and other central nervous system sites. In the short term, this behavioral response is adaptive, similarly to the inflammatory response. Basically, people who don't feel well tend to minimize social interactions, rest, and recuperate. However, over the long term, when the feelings of being sick do not resolve, people feel isolated, unproductive, and unmotivated, often depressed. Indeed, the sickness response shares multiple factors with clinical depression, including a proinflammatory immune response (Anisman, 2009). Chronic low level inflammation may represent the underlying link between depression, particularly its neurovegetative features, and the metabolic syndrome (diabetes, hypertension, and obesity). In a study of this potential association, depressive symptoms were measured with the Beck Depression Inventory, and the extent of the inflammatory response was assessed by CRP (C-reactive protein) and interleukin-6 (IL-6). Inflammation correlated positively with BDI-II scores (Capuron et al., 2008).

Multiple lines of evidence support the hypothesis that stress affects the immune system in both acute and chronic conditions, but the relationships are complex (Kiecolt-Glaser, 2009). Performance stress, that is, speaking in front of others or math tasks, produced a transient but significant increases in cortisol and proinflammatory cytokines (Altemus, Rao, Dhabhar, Ding, & Granstein, 2001). Longer term stress, such as caring for a spouse with dementia, sustained the increased serum IL-6 that was originally seen acutely after the spouse was diagnosed with dementia. Former caregivers (after the spouse had died) continued to manifest the elevated levels of IL-6, also suggesting that stress effects are long lasting (Kiecolt-Glaser et al., 2003). Immune system dysregulation can also result from different types of relationship stress such as hostile conflict with partners, between parents and children, and with workplace peers (Kiecolt-Glaser et al., 2005). However, subtleties in communication styles also modulate the effects of conflict on the immune system. Use of cognitive words such as "think, because, consider" in conflict discussion between spouses showed a lesser response in IL-6 and tumor necrosis factor (TNF) compared to those who used more name calling and emotionally charged words. Healthy communication between spouses during conflict prevented the exaggerated immune response (Graham et al., 2009).

Regulation of the immune response is maintained in part by the nervous system, via the vagus nerve, which can inhibit cytokine release and prevent chronic inflammation, a pathway termed: the cholinergic anti-inflammatory pathway (Tracey, 2007). Signals of inflammation activate the motor response in the vagus nerve, i.e., acetylcholine release, to inhibit cytokine production and thereby the extent of the immune response. The role of the vagus nerve is well known in vegetative, low-stress conditions, as it facilitates digestion and other restorative functions. The branch of the vagus nerve that originates in the nucleus ambiguous acts like a brake, decreasing the excitability of the sinoatrial node and modulating heart rate variability (Porges, 2007).

Individuals' sleep quality and quantity interacts with mood state to influence the immune system. The sleep of depressed individuals is also disturbed; in particular, they display insufficient restorative, slow-wave sleep. Hypothalamic–pituitary–adrenal dysregulation, combined with poor-quality sleep, further affects the immune system in psychiatrically ill individuals (Irwin, 2008). Balance in regulatory systems is crucial to physiological responses to every stressor, whether it be a skin wound or a difficult interpersonal conflict. For example, the efficiency of healing of experimentally induced skin wounds (punch biopsy) decreased in a normal population of stressed students. In dental students during examinations, every subject healed more slowly during exams than during vacations. Glucocorticoids, stress-activated information transducers, can suppress the proinflammatory cytokines that are necessary for resolution of wounds, slowing the rate of healing (Christian, Graham, Padgett, Glaser, & Kiecolt-Glaser, 2006). In summary, acute inflammation in response to a pathogen or skin injury is therapeutic and part of healing. Stress interferes with normal healing through the HPA axis' effects on the immune system. Conversely, during psychological stress, as described above, mobilization of the immune system occurs without physical cause or injury, leading to chronic inflammation with its associated long term harmful effects in the body (Irwin, 2008).

Over-activation of the Hypothalamic–Pituitary–Adrenal Axis (HPA). The hypothalamus occupies a key position in regulation of vegetative and endocrine functions and behavioral responses. Cardiovascular, gastrointestinal activities, body temperature, and fluid balance are important systems controlled by the HPA axis. Stimulation of specific areas of the hypothalamus causes the anterior pituitary gland to secrete hormones. The adrenal gland (cortical portion) releases cortisol and aldosterone, while the medullary portion secretes epinephrine and a small amount of norepinephrine (Widmaier et al., 2006). It is important to remember that once these mediators are released and have produced their effect in the stress response, they must be turned off. Under normal conditions, cortisol is part of a pathway in which there is feedback and regulation so that when the stressful situation is complete, cortisol and catecholamine levels return to baseline. However, damaging effects are observed over time if the system is dysregulated by producing too much of these substances, or the system fails to recover at the end of stress (McEwen, 2002, p. 190). Kudielka and Kirschbaum (2005) reviewed the literature on gender differences in HPA responses to stress. It is clear that men and women do not share identical risks for physical and psychiatric disorders. Women are more likely to demonstrate symptoms of anxiety, mood, and somatization disorders, whereas the risk for schizophrenia is not gender dependent and men have higher rates of substance abuse and dependence disorders. The authors summarized the research in part by suggesting that adult men, when exposed to cognitive psychological stress, showed greater increases in cortisol and greater reactivity, patterns that have been linked to cardiovascular disease. The relatively hypoactive reactions to cognitive stress in women may be linked to autoimmune diseases, whereas the exaggerated HPA responses observed in women in interpersonal conflict may be associated with the higher rates of depression.

Interrelationships between the neural and immune systems are evidenced by the involvement of the neurotransmitters described above in many functions of the immune system, including direct contacts between sympathetic, parasympathetic terminals, and immune cells (Smythies, 2011). Chronic stress affects both the HPA axis and the inflammatory process. Levels of the proinflammatory cytokines (interleukin-6 which stimulates C-reactive protein, an acute phase marker of systemic inflammation) are increased after stress (Papanicolaou, Wilder, Manolagas, & Chrousos, 1998). Persons who self-identify as lonely show an under-expression of genes bearing anti-inflammatory glucocorticoid response elements and overexpression of genes involved in activation of proinflammatory NK cells (Cacioppo & Hawkley, 2009). Social isolation and loneliness have also been correlated with a larger cortisol increase upon awakening and higher cortisol during waking hours. Chronicity of stress and inflammation is particularly damaging, since many physical disorders, for example the metabolic syndrome, are now understood to be mediated at least in part by chronic low-level inflammation.

Overactivity of the sympathetic nervous system and increased release of both epinephrine and cortisol into the bloodstream are strongly implicated in the development of essential hypertension and cardiovascular disease. For example, in men studied under stress conditions, systolic blood pressure was slower to recover after a challenging task (Grant, Hamer, & Steptoe, 2009). Rumination, repeatedly attending and mentally repeating the negative aspects of a stressful interaction or situation, was shown to elicit increased salivary cortisol. Personal insults or neglect by a significant other, stressors not traumatic in severity, lead to fear or excessive worry, which is difficult to control. Rumination over past events or about possible future negative situations reverberates through the person's mind, leading to fear, which in turn has physiological consequences, i.e., increased cortisol and catecholamines (McCullough, Orsulak, Brandon, & Akers, 2007).

Depressed individuals demonstrate rapid heart rates, high levels of stress hormones, and a state of physiological hyperarousal, despite the passivity and immobility that is their apparent superficial demeanor. Heart rate variability is lower in severe depression but also in individuals with milder symptoms; both groups have increased mortality from coronary heart disease (Stein et al., 2000). The regulatory advantage conferred by the baroreflex system that monitors and partially controls blood pressure is muted in depressed persons, and platelet reactivity (related to clotting) is increased, suggesting increased risk for heart disease. "Depression is a disorder that affects the function of the whole body including the cardiovascular, metabolic and immune systems" (Lett et al., 2004).

The stress hormone cortisol renders nerve cells more sensitive to the excitatory neurotransmitter glutamate. In conditions of acute stress, the ability of the brain to remember and react quickly is critical for successful defense. However, when glutamate release is elevated for long periods of time, neuronal toxicity occurs resulting in memory impairment, commonly observed in stressed psychiatric and nonpsychiatric populations (McEwen, 2002, p. 131). Memory for emotionally arousing experiences is over-consolidated through the effects of cortisol, facilitating the adaptive avoidance of similar situations. When defense reactions are maintained long term, such as occurs in PTSD, functional impairments occur which are maladaptive. Memory retrieval, working memory, and declarative memory are more likely to be impaired by chronic exposure to stress hormones, particularly the glucocorticoids (de Quervain, Aerni, Schelling, & Roozendaal, 2009; Marin, Pilgrim, & Lupien, 2010).

Mechanism: Disruption in Circadian Rhythms. The fourth postulated mechanism is disruption in circadian rhythms. The master timekeeping switches are located in the suprachiasmatic nuclei of the anterior hypothalamus (SCN) in the brain, while other clocks reside in peripheral tissues. The sleep/wake rhythm is entrained primarily by sunlight in addition to food consumption and activity. The SCN dictates pacing of body temperature, rest/activity, and appetite/satiety, all of which normally show diurnal patterns. Food intake and metabolism feed back to influence the biological clocks and releases of insulin and leptin. Studies of shift workers have shown that some cannot adjust to the changes in timing of sleep, food intake, and activity, resulting in adiposity and malaise. Cortisol release shows a diurnal pattern and a within day pattern; stress disrupts the timing of the clocks and the timed release of cortisol, interfering with metabolism (release of insulin and leptin) (Froy, 2007; McEwen & Lasley, 2003).

Frequent sleep disruption eventually leads to chronic sleep deprivation and becomes a chronic stressor, an example of allostatic load (McEwen & Lasley, 2003). Lack of restorative sleep decreases the resources that the person has to deal with stress, so metabolic and psychological consequences occur. Fewer hours of sleep have been correlated with higher basal metabolic index, a predictor of later obesity (Bose, Olivan, & Laerere, 2009). In a study of fibromyalgia, patients were hypersensitive to negative events. The number of hours of sleep and the quality of sleep, particularly slow-wave deep sleep, were related to experiences of fatigue and negative affect. Shorter, poor-quality sleep increased patients' reports of negative mood and slowed recovery from experiences of negative events (Hamilton et al., 2008). Persons who have chronic negative mood and also have frequent disruption of sleep are most vulnerable to physical health problems (Wrosch, Miller, Lupien, & Pruessner, 2008).

Risk and Resilience Factors

Can we describe those persons who are more likely to somatize trauma, conflict, or negative affect into physical symptoms? The previous sections suggest that those individuals who feel too much, who are isolated, who retain memories in too vivid detail, and who cannot reappraise stressful situations are at risk. In contrast, persons who have social support, whose sleep–wake–eat cycle is in balance, who exercise regularly, and who demonstrate flexible coping styles are able to deflect the effects of stress.

People Who Feel Too Much Are at Risk. Humans read emotions by recognizing the configuration of underlying facial muscles; faces and postures convey social signals without a single word spoken. Understanding what others feel occurs by "action representation" mechanisms that shape emotional reactions. Inferior frontal and posterior parietal neurons (mirror neurons) fire during the execution as well as the observation of an action. Watching facial expressions indicating emotions activates multiple areas of the brain (premotor areas, frontotemporal, the amygdala, anterior insula), all of which increase signaling during imitation of emotional facial expression (Carr, Iacoboni, Dubeau, Mazziotta, & Lenzi, 2005). Activity in the mirror neurons permits the observer to understand the feelings of the observed person (Izzard, 2009). Under stressful conditions, corticoids facilitate activity of mirror neurons, an adaptive mechanism leading to specific survival behaviors (Yuen et al., 2011). When individuals are in a situation where they perceive threat from actions or facial expression, the amygdala and cortical regions are activated. Facial sets associated with threat activate classic fear responses, whereas facial expressions associated with disgust predict potential contamination (Anderson, Christoff, Panitz, DeRosa, & Bareieli, 2005). It is tempting to hypothesize that persons with an overabundance of mirror neurons are more sensitive to others and more empathetic and understanding. However, those who feel too much are at risk for absorbing negative emotions from others and sharing their suffering to an extreme extent.

Those Who Over-consolidate Memories Are at Risk. Memory for negative events and reliving them determines in part the severity and the chronicity of the stress response after a negative situation. Reexperiencing from memory a traumatic event produces the same psychophysiological responses, or perhaps greater responses, as did the original situation. Some individuals are so sensitive to memory-inducing stimuli, such as smell, sound, or picture that they will recall entire scenes, complete with images and dialogue, because of a very small trigger. For example, a particular smell can trigger a positive or negative memory and images; an odor associated with childhood recreates an entire story and the associated emotions (Dossey, 2001; Vial, 2009).

Interestingly, in conversation, the sense of smell is reserved to describe an object ("I smell the flower") or for negative judgment (that stinks). Never does it signify understanding, as in I smell (see) what you mean. Yet, seeing something that is reminiscent of the past is not more powerful than an odor in recreating negative memories. Prevention of consolidation of memories may also defer or minimize PTSD. Post deployment, after combat injury, soldiers who were given morphine (an opiate) had a lower risk of PTSD than those who were not given morphine. The authors postulated that the mechanisms are pain reduction (lessening the severity of the pain aftermath of the injury, which can intensify the trauma) and interference with consolidation of memories (mu receptors, beta adrenergic). Opiates decrease memory consolidation (Holbrook, Galarneau, Dye, Quinn, & Dougherty, 2010).

People with Low Support Are at Risk. Lower social support in adults has been associated with elevated cortisol levels, less efficient immune responses, and increased risk for illness. When energy is limited, immunosuppression is favored to conserve resources; but when a strong immune response is needed, isolated, lonely individuals mount an insufficient response (Segerstrom, 2008). Low socioeconomic status is a risk factor as well, because often, people of low education and income lack a variety of supports. For example, personal coping resources are constantly needed to manage acute and chronic stress—noise, discrimination, single parenthood, and financial hardship. Increased physiological activity and maladaptive behaviors (that the person is actually trying to use to adapt) are evident in persons of low economic status (Gallo & Matthews, 2003).

During the early years of a child's development, the social environment can shift patterns of gene expression (epigenetics), in particular DNA methylation and histone modification. Animal models provide good examples of positive and negative social influences on the developing brain. Rat mothers normally lick and groom their pups, keeping them close. The pups that were nurtured in this way became adults and tended to groom and lick their pups as they were themselves. In contrast, chronic social stress plays a major role in the development of distress and altered behavior in rats (Champagne, 2010a). Stress decreased grooming and licking behaviors shown by adult rats for their pups. Later, these pups which were not licked tended to demonstrate minimal licking and grooming of the next generation. Lack of nurturing behaviors is believed to affect the hippocampus, such that the stress response is exaggerated and prolonged. In human children, the social environment, particularly nurturing by the primary caregiver (or its absence) also affects brain development. However, chronicity is one of the keys to estimating the amount of damage incurred as a result of stress (Champagne, 2010b). The longer children spend in a socially poor environment, the more dramatic the increase observed in HPA activity and the greater the difficulty in establishing emotional attachment to caregivers. This relationship also holds in the animal models described above. The effects of deficient parenting behaviors are not permanent in rats nor in humans. It is important to note, however, that socially enriched environments are associated with more adaptive adjustment, normalization of HPA axis feedback loops, and improvement in cognitive functioning.

Social interaction can also modify the relationship between indicators of cardiac health and mood via personal behaviors and the HPA axis. Depressed individuals show lower heart rate variability and lower vagal tone, so that the cardiovascular system is overly reactive. Negative mood positively correlated with heart rate during the day, as measured by ambulatory monitoring, and there is some evidence that nighttime dipping in blood pressure does not occur as regularly in persons with negative mood (Stein et al., 2000). Schwerdtfeger and Friedrich-Mai (2009) explored social interactions in depressed people and their correlation with HRV. Short interactions and conversations did increase HRV, but only those interactions with close friends or family, where there was a secure relationship, had the beneficial effect. Dialogues with strangers had no effect on HRV.

Personal Mastery and Optimism Promote Resilience

Personal mastery is defined by a sense of control or power over situations that arise and a feeling of confidence that problems can be solved. Whereas mastery is a general term, self-efficacy is usually related to specific tasks. Both, however, are correlated with reappraisal of past stressful situations that created negative feelings. Strong emotional experiences also mobilize physiological responses in multiple systems; memory of even a portion of the event recreates the entire drama with the same context. In contrast, reappraisal of emotional experience as not currently threatening can modify or change the physiological reactions and behavior (Ochsner, Bunge, Gross, & Gabrieli, 2005).

In chronically stressful situations, such as caregiving for a spouse with dementia, the sense of mastery over the environment influences both physiological and psychological state. Not all caregivers develop psychiatric disorders. Mausbach et al. (2008) found that higher self-efficacy or personal mastery buffered the effects of stress on plasminogen activator inhibitor (PAI-1), minimizing the risk for intramural fibrin deposits and the formation of thrombi. In contrast, low mastery increased the likelihood of both cardiovascular disorders and psychiatric symptoms as measured by the Brief Symptom Inventory (Mausbach et al., 2006).

Optimism is also a predictor of positive health outcomes (Pressman & Cohen, 2005; Rasmussen, Scheier, & Greenhouse, 2009). Priming words affect response to task and tendency to fix mistakes. If students are primed with positive words (smart, competent) prior to starting a difficult task, they will not only perform better but will rectify mistakes. In contrast, students primed with negative words (stupid, incompetent) did not react to mistakes in the same way; correction was slower, and sometimes the same mistake was repeated (Segerstrom, 2007). The perceived support of others and a belief that one can cope with future situations increases resilience and facilitates both effective responses and recovery from stressful situations. Resilient individuals thrive despite potentially compromising life events (Schetter & Dolbier, 2011).

Summary

In summary, models have been suggested to explain the relationship between psychological factors, both positive and negative, and physical health. The neural, endocrine, and immune systems are the major mechanisms that underlie somatization of negative emotional variables into maladaptive physiological states. Risk and its counterpart resilience are influenced by the person's capacity for intense feelings and by the presence of nurturing in early development and social support later. Mastery and self-efficacy, optimism, and coping skills are positive factors that support psychological and physical well-being.

References

Altemus, M., Rao, B., Dhabhar, F. S., Ding, W., & Granstein, R. D. (2001). Stress-induced changes in skin barrier function in healthy women. *The Journal of Investigative Dermatology, 117*, 309–317.

American Psychiatric Association. (2000). *Diagnostic and statistical manual of mental disorders* (4th ed., text revision). Washington DC: American Psychiatric Association.

Anderson, A. K., Christoff, K., Panitz, D., DeRosa, E., & Bareieli, J. D. E. (2005). Neural correlates of the automatic processing of threat facial signals. In J. Cacioppo & G. Bernston (Eds.), *Social neuroscience: Key readings* (pp. 185–198). New York, NY: Psychology Press.

Anisman, H. (2009). Cascading effects of stressors and inflammatory immune system activation: Implications for major depressive disorder. *Journal of Psychiatry & Neuroscience, 34*(1), 4–20.

Bose, M., Olivan, B., & Laerere, B. (2009). Stress and obesity: The role of the hypothalamic-pituitary-adrenal axis in metabolic disease. *Current Opinion in Endocrinology, Diabetes, and Obesity, 16*(5), 340–346.

Burstein, R., & Jakubowski, M. (2005). Unitary hypothesis for multiple triggers of the pain and strain of migraine. *The Journal of Comparative Neurology, 493*, 9–14.

Cacioppo, J. T., & Hawkley, L. C. (2009). Perceived social isolation and cognition. *Trends in Cognitive Sciences, 13*(10), 447–454.

Capuron, L., Su, S., Miller, A. H., Bremner, J. D., Goldberg, J., Vogt, G. J., et al. (2008). Depressive symptoms and metabolic syndrome: Is inflammation the underlying link? *Biological Psychiatry, 64*(10), 896–900.

Carr, L., Iacoboni, M., Dubeau, M., Mazziotta, J. C., & Lenzi, G. L. (2005). Neural mechanisms of empathy in humans: A relay from neural systems for imitation to limbic areas. In J. T. Cacioppo & G. G. Berntson (Eds.), *Social neuroscience* (pp. 143–152). New York: Psychology Press.

Champagne, F. A. (2010a). Epigenetic influence of social experiences across the lifespan. *Developmental Psychobiology, 52*, 299–311.

Champagne, F. A. (2010b). Early adversity and developmental outcomes: Interaction between genetics, epigenetics, and social experiences across the life span. *Perspectives on Psychological Science, 5*(5), 564–574.

Chapman, C. R. (2010). The psychophysiology of pain. In S. M. Fishman, J. C. Ballantyne, & J. P. Rathmell (Eds.), *Bonica's management of pain* (pp. 375–388). Philadelphia: Wolters Kluwer/Lippincott Williams & Wilkins.

Christian, L. M., Graham, J. E., Padgett, D. A., Glaser, R., & Kiecolt-Glaser, J. K. (2006). Stress and wound healing. *Neuroimmunomodulation, 13*, 337–346.

Cohen, S., & Rodriguez, M. S. (1995). Pathways linking affective disturbances and physical disorders. *Health Psychology, 14*(5), 374–380.

De Quervain, D., Aerni, A., Schelling, G., & Roozendaal, B. (2009). Glucocorticoids and the regulation of memory in health and disease. *Frontiers in Neuroendocrinology, 30,* 358–370.

Dossey, L. (2001). Surfing the Odornet: Exploring the role of smell in life and healing. *Alternative Therapies in Health and Medicine, 7*(2), 12–16, 100–108.

Egger, H. L., Costello, E. J., Erkanli, A., & Angold, A. (1999). Somatic complaints and psychopathology in children and adolescents: Stomach aches, musculoskeletal pains, and headaches. *Journal of the American Academy of Child and Adolescent Psychiatry, 38,* 852–860.

Froy, O. (2007). The relationship between nutrition and circadian rhythms in mammals. *Frontiers in Neuoendocrinology, 28,* 61–71.

Gallo, L. C., & Matthews, K. A. (2003). Understanding the association between socioeconomic status and physical health: Do negative emotions play a role? *Psychological Bulletin, 129*(1), 10–51.

Goadsby, P. J., Lipton, R. B., & Ferrari, M. D. (2002). Migraine—current understanding and treatment. *The New England Journal of Medicine, 346*(4), 257–270.

Graham, J. E., Loving, T. J., Stowell, J. R., Glaser, R., Malarkey, W. B., & Kiecolt-Glaser, J. K. (2009). Cognitive word use during marital conflict and increases in proinflammatory cytokines. *Health Psychology, 28*(5), 621–630.

Grant, N., Hamer, M., & Steptoe, A. (2009). Social isolation and stress-related cardiovascular, lipid, and cortisol responses. *Annals of Behavioral Medicine, 37,* 29–37.

Hamilton, N. A., Affleck, G., Tenne, H., Karlson, C., Luxton, D., Preacher, K., et al. (2008). Fibromyalgia: The role of sleep in affect and in negative event reactivity and recovery. *Health Psychology, 27*(4), 490–494.

Hobson, C. J., & Kamen, J. (1998). Stressful life events: A revision and update of the social readjustment rating scale. *International Journal of Stress Management, 5*(1), 1–23.

Hofflich, S., Hughes, A. A., & Kendall, P. C. (2006). Somatic complains and childhood anxiety disorders. *International Journal of Clinical and Health Psychology, 6*(2), 229–242.

Holbrook, T. L., Galarneau, M. R., Dye, J. L., Quinn, K., & Dougherty, A. L. (2010). Morphine use after combat injury in Iraq and post-traumatic stress disorder. *The New England Journal of Medicine, 362,* 110–117.

Holmes, T. H., & Rahe, R. H. (1967). The social readjustment rating scale. *Journal of Psychosomatic Research, 11,* 213–218.

Irwin, M. R. (2008). Human psychoneuroimmunology: 20 years of discovery. *Brain, Behavior and Immunity, 22,* 129–139.

Izzard, C. E. (2009). Emotion, theory and research: Highlights, unanswered questions and emerging issues. *Annual Review of Psychology, 60,* 1–25.

Kiecolt-Glaser, J. K. (2009). Psychoneuroimmunology: Psychology's gateway to the biomedical future. *Perspectives on Psychological Science, 4*(4), 367–369.

Kiecolt-Glaser, J. K., Loving, T. J., Stowell, J. R., Malarkey, W. B., Lemeshow, S., Dickinson, S. L., et al. (2005). Hostile martial interactions, proinflammatory cytokine production and wound healing. *Archives of General Psychiatry, 62,* 1377–1384.

Kiecolt-Glaser, J. K., Preacher, K. J., MacCallum, R. C., Atkinson, C., Malarkey, W. B., & Glaser, R. (2003). Chronic stress and age-related increases in the proinflammatory cytokine IL-6. *Proceedings of the National Academy of Sciences, 100,* 9090–9095.

Kudielka, B. M., & Kirschbaum, C. (2005). Sex differences unite HPA axis responses to stress: A review. *Biological Psychology, 69,* 113–132.

Lazarus, R. S. (1984). On the primacy of cognition. *The American Psychologist, 39,* 124–129.

Lee, M. C., Zambreanu, L., Menon, D. K., & Tracey, I. (2008). Identifying brain activity specifically related to the maintenance and perceptual consequence of central sensitization in humans. *The Journal of Neuroscience, 28*(45), 11642–11649.

Lett, H. S., Blumenthal, J. A., Babyak, M. A., Sherwood, A., Strauman, T., Robbins, C., et al. (2004). Depression as a risk factor for coronary artery disease: Evidence, mechanisms, and treatment. *Psychosomatic Medicine, 66,* 305–315.

Lynch, D. L., McGrady, A., Nagel, R., & Zsembik, C. (1999). Somatization in family practice: Comparing 5 methods of classification. *Primary Care Companion Journal of Clinical Psychiatry, 1,* 85–89.

References

Marin, M. F., Pilgrim, K., & Lupien, S. J. (2010). Modulatory effects of stress on reactivated emotional memories. *Psychoneuroendocrinology, 35*(9), 1388–1396.

Mausbach, B. T., Patterson, T. L., von Kanel, R., Mills, P. J., Ancoli-Israel, S., Dimsdale, J. E., et al. (2006). Personal mastery attenuates the effect of caregiving stress on psychiatric morbidity. *The Journal of Nervous and Mental Disease, 194*(2), 132–134.

Mausbach, B. T., von Kanel, R., Patterson, T. L., Dimsdale, J. E., Depp, C. A., Aschbacher, K. A., et al. (2008). The moderating effect of personal mastery on the relations between stress and plasminogen activator inhibitor-1 (PAI-1) antigen. *Health Psychology, 27*(2 Suppl), S172–S179.

McCullough, M. E., Orsulak, P., Brandon, A., & Akers, L. (2007). Rumination, fear, and cortisol: An in vivo study of interpersonal transgressions. *Health Psychology, 26*(1), 126–132.

McEwen, B. (2002). *The end of stress as we know it*. Washington, DC: John Henry Press.

McEwen, B. S. (2004). Protection and damage from acute and chronic stress. *Annals of the New York Academy of Sciences, 1032*, 1–7.

McEwen, B. S., & Lasley, E. N. (2003). Allostatic load: When protection gives way to damage. *Advances in Mind–Body Medicine, 19*(1), 28–33.

McGrady, A. (2007). Psychophysiological mechanisms of stress. In P. M. Lehrer, R. L. Woolfolk, & W. E. Sime (Eds.), *Principles and practices of stress management* (3rd ed., pp. 16–37). New York: The Guilford Press.

McGrady, A., Lynch, D., Nagel, R., & Wahl, E. (2003). Application of the high risk model of threat perception to medical illness and service utilization in a family practice. *The Journal of Nervous and Mental Disease, 191*, 255–259.

Moulton, E. A., Burstein, R., Tully, S., Hargreaves, R., Becerra, L., & Borsook, D. (2008). Interictal dysfunction of a brainstem descending modulatory center in migraine patients. *PLoS One, 3*(11), e3799. doi:10.1371/journal.pone.0003799.

Neimark, G., Caroff, S. N., & Stinnett, J. L. (2005). Medically unexplained physical symptoms. *Psychiatric Annals, 35*, 298–305.

Ochsner, K. N., Bunge, S. A., Gross, J. J., & Gabrieli, J. D. E. (2005). Rethinking feelings: An fMRI study of the cognitive regulation of emotion. In J. Cacioppo & G. Bernston (Eds.), *Social neuroscience: Key reading* (pp. 253–270). New York: Psychology Press.

Papanicolaou, D. A., Wilder, R. L., Manolagas, S. C., & Chrousos, G. P. (1998). The pathophysiologic roles of interleukin-6 in human disease. *Annals of Internal Medicine, 128*, 127–137.

Paradiso, S., & Johnson, D. L. (1999). Cerebral blood flow changes associated with attribution of emotional valence to pleasant, unpleasant, and neutral visual stimuli in a PET study of normal subjects. *The American Journal of Psychiatry, 156*(10), 1618–1629.

Pittman, R. K. (1989). Post-traumatic stress disorder, hormones and memory. *Biological Psychiatry, 26*, 221–223.

Porges, S. W. (2007). The polyvagal perspective. *Biological Psychology, 74*, 116–143.

Pressman, S. D., & Cohen, S. (2005). Does positive affect influence health? *Psychological Bulletin, 131*, 925–971.

Purves, D., Augustine, G., Fitzpatrick, D., Hall, W. C., Lamaniia, A. S., & McNamara, J. O. (2004). *Neuroscience* (3rd ed.). Sunderland, MA: Sinauer Associates.

Rahko, J., Paakki, J. J., Starck, T., Nikkinen, J., Remes, J., Hurtig, T., et al. (2010). Functional mapping of dynamic happy and fearful facial expression processing in adolescents. *Brain Imaging and Behavior, 4*(2), 164–176.

Rasmussen, H. N., Scheier, M. F., & Greenhouse, J. B. (2009). Optimism and physical health: A meta-analytic review. *Annals of Behavioral Medicine, 37*, 239–256.

Sadock, B., & Sadock, V. (2007). *Synopsis of psychiatry: Behavioral sciences/clinical psychiatry* (10th ed.). Philadelphia, PA: Lippincott Williams & Wilkins.

Schetter, C. D., & Dolbier, C. (2011). Resilience in the context of chronic stress and health in adults. *Social and Personality Psychology Compass, 6*(9), 634–652.

Schore, A. N. (2002). Dysregulation of the right brain: A fundamental mechanism of traumatic attachment and the psychopathogenesis of post traumatic stress disorder. *The Australian and New Zealand Journal of Psychiatry, 36*, 9–30.

Schwerdtfeger, A., & Friedrich-Mai, P. (2009). Social interaction moderates the relationship between depressive mood and heart rate variability: Evidence from an ambulatory monitoring study. *Health Psychology, 28*(4), 501–509.

Segerstrom, S. (2007). Optimism and resources: Effects on each other and on health over 10 years. *Journal of Research in Personality, 41*, 772–786.

Segerstrom, S. (2008). Social networks and immunosuppression during stress: Relationship conflict or energy conservation? *Brain, Behavior and Immunity, 22*, 279–284.

Simeon, D., Guralnik, O., Knutelska, M., Yehuda, R., & Schmeidler, J. (2003). Basal norepinephrine in depersonalization disorder. *Psychiatry Research, 121*, 93–97.

Smith, R. C., Gardiner, J. C., Lyles, J. S., Sirbu, C., Dwamena, F. C., Hodges, A., et al. (2005). Exploration of DSM-IV criteria in primary care patients with medically unexplained symptoms. *Psychosomatic Medicine, 67*, 123–129.

Smythies, J. (2011). Some aspects of the normal role of neuromodulators in the immune system. *Neuroscience & Medicine, 2*, 274–280.

Stein, P. K., Carney, R. M., Freedland, K. E., Skala, J. A., Jaffe, A. S., Kleige, R. E., et al. (2000). Severe depression is associated with markedly reduced heart rate variability in patients with stable coronary heart disease. *Journal of Psychosomatic Research, 48*, 493–500.

Tracey, K. (2007). Physiology and immunology of the cholinergic anti-inflammatory pathway. *The Journal of Clinical Investigation, 117*(2), 289–296.

Vial, F. (2009). Extension of the theory of the unconscious in literature. In F. Vial (Ed.), *The unconscious in philosophy and French and European literature* (Value inquiry book series, p. 187). Amsterdam, NY: Editions Rodipi BV.

Wickramasekera, I. (1995). Somatization: Concepts, data, and predictions from the high-risk model of threat perception. *The Journal of Nervous and Mental Disease, 183*, 15–23.

Widmaier, E. P., Raff, H., & Strang, K. T. (2006). *Vander, Sherman & Luciano's human physiology* (10th ed.). New York: McGraw Hill.

Wrosch, C., Miller, G. E., Lupien, S., & Pruessner, J. C. (2008). Diurnal cortisol secretion and 2 year changes in older adults' physical symptoms: The moderating roles of negative affect and sleep. *Health Psychology, 27*(6), 685–693.

Yuen, E. Y., Liu, W., Karatsoreos, I. N., Ren, Y., Feng, J., McEwen, B. S., et al. (2011). Mechanisms for acute stress-induced enhancement of glutamatergic transmission and working memory. *Molecular Psychiatry, 16*(2), 156–170.

Chapter 5
Assessment in the Pathways Model

Abstract This chapter describes the process of assessment of clients according to the Pathways Model. Emphasis is placed on active participation of the client in identifying immediate concerns, major problems, and setting goals for treatment. Quotations from typical clients are utilized to highlight the importance of the therapeutic relationship. Examples of standardized testing are provided. Multilevel treatment recommendations using the Pathways Model derive from the self-report and professional evaluation.

Keywords Assessment • Self-assessment • Patient education • Stages of change

Goals of Assessment

Assessment is a complex process that begins with understanding why the client came to therapy and how the client chose a particular provider or practice. Self-assessment and professional assessment of proximate needs and longer term goals are discussed and prioritized. Motivation for therapy is estimated, based on clients' strengths and potential road blocks to completion. The goals of the assessment process itself are to arrive at a differential and final diagnosis and devise a preliminary treatment plan. However, the emergence of the therapeutic relationship at the end of the evaluation session (s) and maintaining an active role for the client in treatment are of major importance in the Pathways Model.

> My family got together and made this appointment for me.
> My doctor told me I had to come here or she wouldn't give me any more pain pills.
> My lifelong therapist retired and I had to come here.
> I should have made this phone call a long time ago.

Most initial appointments are made by clients themselves realizing that they need help or because of a recommendation by their physician. Encouragement by family or friends is sometimes the major factor that brings clients to a mental health provider.

In some cases, however, initial contact is not voluntary, but instead is the result of a formal intervention because the client has a substance abuse problem or the court has mandated assessment. In other cases, the referring physician refused to continue prescribing analgesics without proof that the client tried to manage pain in non-pharmacological ways. Sometimes, a relationship of many years between client and therapist has been broken because of therapist relocation, retirement, or illness, and the client has been forced to separate from someone who was considered a friend and confidante.

The self-reported history of present illness highlights the overt difficulties and the client's view of the main problem that brought them for help. Combined, these lead to problem identification and sometimes a clinical psychological diagnosis according to the Diagnostic and Statistical Manual of Mental Disorders (DSM IV-TR) (APA, 2000). The client often has an explanation in mind about what made him or her sick.

What I really think happened to me is this....
I wouldn't feel so bad if I had not done....
Depression runs in my family and I am catching it.
Since I lost my job, I don't know who I am anymore.
The first psychiatrist that I consulted said that my problems were minor and he didn't have time for me.

The client's model of illness is explored during the first or second session. This gives the provider a sense of how information is processed by the client, whether causation is based on logical or emotional reasoning and what the client believes can be changed (DeGruy, Dickinson, & Staton, 2002). Blaming the current situation completely on genetics raises questions about the client's motivation for psychological treatment. The client's story about what is believed to be the cause of illness reveals how much responsibility the client is willing to take and provides some indication of how much effort will be put into the path to wellness. Throughout the assessment process, the clinician listens with attention and empathy.

Self-Assessment

The client completes a health history, including the number of medical and psychiatric diagnoses (acute and chronic), the number of prescription medications and supplements, and herbal products that are used. The most recent appointment with a physician, a nurse practitioner, a physician assistant, or a DO for general medical care is indicated. If medical concerns are raised and the clinician is a nonphysician mental health provider, the client should be referred to his/her primary care physician.

Self-assessment includes data collection, for example, tracking the major symptom(s), whether it is mood, anxiety, pain, or physical problems like elevated blood pressure or body weight. Depending on the symptoms, this phase may require 1–2 weeks (for panic, depressed mood, pain, blood pressure, daily headache) or longer (for monthly migraine, insomnia, generalized anxiety). This information provides the therapist with information on daily variations in symptoms in addition to weekly averages. If the client identifies pain as a major issue, the daily log includes intensity, frequency, duration, and location.The sleep log contains spaces for the client to indicate the hours of sleep, the schedule, and the number of awakenings during the night and sleepiness during waking hours. The exercise log identifies the type of exercise, the length of the exercise, and the frequency of exercise. The self-assessment continues with the behavioral diary indicating smoking, alcohol consumption, and the use of caffeine and other stimulants. If obesity is the presenting problem, the client keeps a food diary and measures body weight. If hypertension or diabetes is the predominant disorder, the client is asked to self-monitor blood pressure or blood glucose.

> I did headache logs for weeks for my previous therapist, but he never looked at them.
> I am here for my high blood pressure; why are you asking me about anxiety?
> I take surveys on the Internet all the time and I found out that I am depressed.
> I am following instructions the best that I can, but my blood sugars go up and down.

Clear explanations for the requested data are important to build trust, to validate clients' narrative of their symptoms, and to increase client acceptance of therapy. When the client reveals actual data on suffering and the therapist acknowledges the implications of what it means to live with pain, the relationship solidifies. If the review of blood glucose values is met with tearfulness or defiance, positive affirmation of the client's efforts to maintain glycemic control conveys the intent of the therapist to be supportive while exploring other avenues of intervention.

Some clients are very computer literate and find a lot of useful information about common disorders on the Internet. Overall, use of digital health information is increasing and health-care providers in many hospital settings are required to use electronic medical records. Web resources are likely to become more widespread, as the currently younger population who grew up with computer games and social websites matures into adulthood and older age. Some clinical practices already use the Internet to communicate with clients. Email or secure message boards are used to provide clarifications about medications to clients or for clinicians to receive information from their clients (Caiata-Zufferey, Abraham, Sommerhalder, & Schultz, 2010; McMullan, 2006). What effect does the innovative digital health information technology have on assessment and treatment in the Pathways Model? The primary mode of communication remains face to face; Internet resources are best used as enhancements. For example, some practices maintain an online support group for clients with chronic headaches. A provider can refer to helpful websites and recommend audio or video materials so that clients can access these materials on their own (Lo & Parham, 2010). Relaxation "tapes" have been replaced by CDs and audio files that can be downloaded to electronic devices for easy access.

The self-assessment continues in a narrative form as the client is encouraged to write about the major sources of stress during the past year. The question can be asked as follows: "What are the major positive and negative factors that have impacted you in the past year? What are the minor sources of stress that occur on a daily or weekly basis? What situations or people in your life impact you very frequently both positive and negatively?"

> I'm here for my headaches; I didn't think it would be so complicated. Why are you asking about my family and friends?
> If I had the money for a divorce, everything would be ok again.

Professional Assessment

Standardized Tests. Standard questionnaires about the number of life events in the past year and the quantity of daily stressful circumstances expand the information from the written personal narrative. Insight derives from both of these sources regarding the clients' view of their worlds, how they live their lives, and the most important influences. For example, a client with chronic headaches who fills pages with incidents of conflict between herself and her mother will not repeat the question above ("Why are you asking about my family?"). The man with panic attacks who describes his anticipated loneliness when his wife is away will move away from a quick therapeutic solution and realize that divorce will not solve everything.

Next is the assessment of personal resources and resiliency. How does the client cope with the major stressors in their life and how do they cope with the more frequent but minor stressors in their life? What is the client's current ability to relax?

> Little things bother me much more than big things bother other people.
> I have never been able to relax… (unspoken – now you are going to try?).
> If you had been treated like I was as a kid, you would be sick too.

Obtaining the family, social, and relationship history flows naturally from the client's past history of illness. Questions can be directed to what it was like growing up in the client's family, interacting with parents, guardians, and siblings. Queries about the neighborhood, other families living nearby, and the safety of the area will identify factors that have influenced the client's view of the world. The therapist also asks how discipline was maintained and how the client and siblings were treated when they did something wrong.

At this point, the client is questioned about the use of substances, including which substance, quantity and frequency of consumption, and previous attempts to quit if any. Effects of substance consumption on work performance and interpersonal interactions are explored. The clinician listens for certain key phrases.

> I'm not here to talk about my drinking.
> I don't drink any more than other guys my age.
> My spouse thinks I drink too much, but she is wrong.

A critical question concerns the circumstances during which the client is using alcohol or other substances and what the client believes the effects of the substance to be (relaxing, energizing, soothing, sleep inducing, etc.). The therapist can use questionnaires to support the interview data regarding overuse, abuse, or dependence.

The intervention specialist needs to identify the support system, family, friends, support groups, and church activities. How does the client define the support system; what constitutes emotional support?

> I don't have anyone to talk to when I get down.
> I am always there for other people, but they are not there for me.

What are the effects of the symptoms and/or presenting problem on quality of life? Whatever the client's symptoms are, they may affect the person's ability to function in an occupation, at home, or in social settings.

> Everything is perfect in my life; I just have this chest pain.
> My pain is so bad that sometimes I don't want to live anymore.

Suicide potential, including thoughts, intent, and previous attempts, is critical to explore with clients with depression or pain. In addition to direct questioning, other queries will reveal a general state of hopelessness about the future. Overall risk (none, mild to significant) can be calculated using a standard format. Range and Knott (1997) reviewed 20 questionnaires for assessing suicidal risk and recommended the following 3 most highly: Beck's Scale for Suicide Ideation, Linehan's Reasons for Living Inventory, and Cole's self-scored version of Linehan's structured interview, called the Suicidal Behaviors Questionnaire.

Medical Assessment. The medical professional assessment consists of the basic physical exam and laboratory tests. Depending on the client's symptoms, EKG, blood glucose, peak flow, electrolytes, and immune function will be measured. Structured assessment by the mental health provider comprises standardized psychological testing and the mental status exam. Appropriate tools to assess quality of life, anxiety, depression, mania, attention, and psychopathology are chosen based on the clinician's expertise and need for specific information. Examples of standardized questionnaires are listed in Table 5.1 (Sadock and Sadock, 2008).

The spiritual assessment should also be part of the total assessment process. The clinician asks about the importance of organized religion, religious beliefs, and practices to the client, both in the past and currently. The effects of religious practice or the lack of a sense of spirituality on the client can also be addressed.

> My pastor told me to turn everything over to God.
> I raised my kids in a Christian home and now they treat me with such disrespect.
> Are your religious/spiritual practices or beliefs a source of distress or well-being?

Regular prayer, meditation, study, and attendance at worship services facilitate interactions with others who hold similar beliefs. The professional assessment for spiritual function can be conducted by a minister, a pastor, a rabbi, or a priest. Sometimes clients are comfortable with their own religious beliefs, but are troubled by perceived discrepancies between what was taught to them by religious leaders and actions of these same people. If clients express personal conflict regarding religious beliefs, such as believing that symptoms are punishment and that they have been abandoned by God, these beliefs must be discussed in the therapeutic context (Pargament, Koenig, Tarakeshwar, & Hahn, 2001). In summary, the clinician fosters spirituality in clients who find it helpful. In addition, similarities between religious meditation and relaxation-based mindfulness meditation can be explored and promoted as appropriate.

Table 5.1 Sample standardized psychological inventories

Anxiety

Beck, A.T. (1990). *Beck Anxiety Inventory*. San Antonio: Psychological Corporation, Harcourt Brace Jovanovich, Inc

Spielbreger C.D., Gorsuch, R.R., & Luchene, R.E. (1970). *State trait anxiety inventory*. Palo Alto: Consulting Psychologists Press

Anxiety, depression

Knight, R.G., Waal-Manning, J., & Spears, G.F. (1983). Some norms and reliability data for the state-trait anxiety inventory and the Zung self-rating depression scale. *British Journal of Clinical Psychology, 22*, 245–249

Snaith, R.P., & Zigmond, A.S. (1994). *The hospital anxiety and depression scale manual*. Windsor, Berkshire, England: Nfer-Nelson

Spitzer, R.L., WIlliams, J.B., Kroenke, K., Linzer, M., & DeGruy, F.V. (1994). Utility of a new procedure for diagnosing mental disorders in primary care. The PRIME-MD 1000 study. *JAMA, 272*, 1749–1756

Coping

Moos, R.H. (1993). *Coping resources inventory*. Odessa, FL: Psychological Assessment Resources, Inc

Depression

Beck, A.T., Steer R.A., & Brown, G.K. (2001). *Beck depression inventory II*. San Antonio: Psychological Corporation

Kroenke, K., Spitzer, R., & Williams, J. (2001). The PHQ-9: Validity of a brief depression severity measure. *Journal of General Internal Medicine, 16*, 606–613

Zung, W.W.R. (1965). A self-rating depression Scale. *Archives of General Psychiatry, 12*, 63–70

Hassles

Lazarus, R.S., & Folkman, S. (1989). *Manual: hassles and uplifts scale* (research ed.). Palo Alto, CA: Mind Garden

Life events

Hobson, C.J., Kamen, J., Szostek, J., Nethercut, C.M., Tiedman, J. W., & Wojnarowicz, S. (1998). Stressful life events: A revision and update of the social readjustment rating scale. *International Journal of Stress Management, 5*(1), 1–23

Miller, M.A., & Rahe, R.H. (1997). Life changes scaling for the 1990's. *Journal of Psychosomatic Research, 43*, 279–292

Mania

Altman, E.G., Hedeker, D.R., Janicak, P.G, Peterson, J.L., & Davis, J.M. (1994). The clinician administered rating scale for mania (*CARS-M*); Development, reliability, and validity. *Biology Psychiatry, 36*, 124–134

Mood

Hirschfeld, R.M.A. (2000). Development and validation of a screening instrument for bipolar spectrum disorder: The mood disorder questionnaire. *American Journal of Psychiatry, 157*(11), 1873–1875

Pain

Melzack, R. (1987). The short-form McGill questionnaire. *Pain, 30*, 191–197

Psychopathology

Greene, R.L. (1991). *MMPI/MMPI-2. An interpretive manual*. Boston: Allyn & Bacon

Quality of life

Damiano, A.M. (1996). *The sickness impact profile: User's manual interpretation guide*. Baltimore MD: John Hopkins University

Derogatis, LR. (1994). SCL-90-R. In M. Maruish (Ed.), *Brief system inventory, and matching clinical rating scales, in psychological testing, treatment planning, and outcome assessment*. New York: Erlbaum

(continued)

Table 5.1 (continued)

McHorney, C.A., Ware, J.E., Lu, J.F.R., & Sherbourne, C.D. (1994). The MOS SF-36 short-form health survey (*SF-36*), III: Tests of data quality, scaling assumptions, and reliability across diverse patient groups. *Medical Care, 32*(1), 40–66

Ware, J.E., & Sherbourne, C.D. (1992). The MOS 36 item short form health survey (SF-36). *Medical Care*, 30 (6), 473–483

Sleep

Johns, M.W. (1991). A new method of measuring daytime sleepiness: the Epworth sleepiness scale. *Sleep*, 14, 540–545

Substance abuse

Ewing, JA (1984). Detecting alcoholism: the CAGE questionnaire. JAMA, 25 (14), 1905–1907

Liskow, B., Campbell, J., Nickel, E.J., & Powell, B.J. (1995). Validity of the CAGE questionnaire in screening for alcohol dependence in a walk-in (*triage*) clinic. *Journal of Studies on Alcohol and Drugs*, 56, 277–281

Preparation for Intervention

Assessment of the Client's Readiness for Change

The last segment of the evaluation process consists of determining the client's readiness for change. The stages of change model consists of five levels or states: First, pre-contemplation where the person is not motivated and not interested in changing. Second is contemplation where the client is open to information but delays starting the change process. In the preparation stage, the client is ready to adopt new behaviors and is willing to put energy and effort into change. The action stage is when the client is actually performing the new behaviors, but being faithful to the new behaviors still requires effort on the part of the client. Lastly, the maintenance stage is defined as the stable period when the new behavior has become routine and part of the normal day's or week's activities (Prochaska & Velicer, 1997; Starr, Rogak, Kirsh, & Passik, 2010).

> My mother was this way (anxious) and us kids are this way and I don't think anything will change the way that we are.
> I am so afraid of moving around more because I couldn't stand it if the pain got worse.

The client who is unwilling to change is unlikely to be self-referred, but more often has been mandated to come to treatment. Building the therapeutic relationship in these cases relies on motivational interviewing (MI) (Rollnick, Miller, & Butler, 2008). MI is a client-centered process for enhancing or building intrinsic motivation. This occurs by exploring the client's motivation for change and resolving ambivalence. The assumption is that people want to feel better and, at the same time, they may resist change because of its novelty or because they fear failure. This approach evokes natural change on the part of the client. Nothing is imposed, but the client's own desire to get well is mobilized by the therapist. There are multiple connections between the stages of change model and MI. In the early stages the client and clinician discuss the pros and cons of the change, and the client moves toward taking responsibility for the situation that they are in at the present time. Later, the clinician and client anticipate barriers to change and identify sources of support. Part of the assessment process must include motivation and the sense of capability that the client has to make these changes.

> This sounds so simple now that you say it.
> I don't think I have any control over this problem.

Education. The first step in intervention is client education, which consists of appropriate lessons about basic principles of physiology and psychology, with relevance to the presenting problem (Widmaier, Raff, & Strang, 2004). Clients frequently ask about the effects of heredity and whether their problems were predestined, so it is important to educate clients about the role of the environment and learning. In particular, explanations about mind–body interactions, both negative and positive, are very useful. The therapist description of the effects of worry and anxiety on the body usually creates a way for clients to grasp the potential of relaxation practice. Clients begin to understand for the first time that despite heritage, they have a chance to make a difference in their lives. The basis of treatment is then explained to the client and emphasis is placed on becoming active partners in treatment. Written materials, CDs, and Internet resources are offered during treatment. The client's expectations of the therapist (availability off hours) and of the intervention are defined.

> My last therapist fell asleep during my session.
> If I can decrease my severe morning headaches, I can live with the lesser ones that are there all the time.
> My physician told me that when I lower my systolic blood pressure by 20 mm Hg, he will take away one medicine, the one with most of the side effects.
> I don't want to take any medicine; can biofeedback replace medicine?
> I only have 4 weeks; then I am going back to school.

Collaborative Goal Setting. The intervention is structured by collaborative goal setting (Locke & Lathan, 2002). Short-term (1–2 months) and long-term (6 months–1 year) goals are defined in detail. Emphasis should be placed both on end goals and process goals. Process goals are the ways that the client is going to reach those end goals, whether by relaxation therapy, by exploration of dysfunctional thinking patterns, by hypnosis, or by psychotherapy. Defining the primary process goals provides the client with a map of her therapy, where she is headed and how she is going to achieve that outcome. The approximate length of treatment is discussed at this time. Then the client's strengths and weaknesses are evaluated. For example, motivation, intelligence, and prior positive experience with therapy are strengths that also empower clients and build positive expectations (Bandura, 1997). Potential barriers to success include factors such as mandated treatment, prior negative experience with therapy, lack of social support, and crippling pain that sometimes prevents access to care. Patients with chronic pain are likely to require adjustments to appointment scheduling, better access to care, and ongoing conversations about motivation in order to eventually develop self-management skills (Dijkstra, 2005). A critical question that is often not asked is "how will you know that you are better?" Definition of short-term goals, sometimes only for each day or a few weeks, may be necessary for the client to continue commitment to therapy.

Ongoing Assessment. Assessment is ongoing during the intervention. The symptom log is kept by the client throughout treatment and the therapist then provides feedback. If applicable, physiological measurements are conducted at each session to provide feedback. Sometimes improvement is so gradual that calculating average pain scores for the past weeks is necessary to point out that indeed pain has lessened. In addition, changes in symptom pattern may be the first sign that treatment is effective. The client's motivation for continuing therapy should be assessed on a monthly basis, again going back to the principles of motivational interviewing to build the client's internal motivation for change. Progress toward goals is reinforced frequently so that the client anticipates further improvement. The Pathways Model begins with interventions designed to reestablish normal rhythms which have a high probability of success in generating a greater sense of well-being and personal control.

> I am so surprised to be feeling better.
> I actually look forward to these sessions.
> It's taken a long time, but I can see that my pain has decreased.

Final assessment, based on quantitative and qualitative data, takes place at the last session. Data from the logs, the physiological measurements, and psychological inventories is reviewed. The client's response to treatment from their perspective is also reviewed and discussed. Follow-up is planned as appropriate.

Summary

Assessment in the Pathways Model begins by the client's self-exploration followed by professional assessment as appropriate. The problem is then defined; the client's readiness for change is assessed and motivation for therapy is built from the desires of the client. The client's progress and the client's physiological and psychological reactions to the intervention are utilized on an ongoing basis to keep the client engaged in treatment. Final assessment also consists of a plan for the future, including how the clients will maintain the improvements that they have achieved during active treatment and a plan to prevent relapse. Sometimes, the client will recontact the clinician months or years after treatment was terminated if a relapse has occurred. This model should not assume criticism of clients because they have relapsed, but rather use the information about what triggered the relapse to assist clients in rebuilding their motivation and rebuilding their positive self-esteem so that future relapses have a lower probability of occurring. If the client has returned of her own volition after relapse, then the clinician should reenforce the importance of that behavior. Normalizing a relapse does not mean that it is of no importance, but rather that the relapse is not a death sentence for the intervention.

> Thanks, doc, you have helped me a lot. I can do this on my own from now on, but if I need you again, I'll be back.

References

Altman, E. G., Hedeker, D. R., Janicak, P. G., Peterson, J. L., & Davis, J. M. (1994). The clinician administered rating scale for mania (CARS-M); development, reliability, and validity. *Biology Psychiatry, 36*, 124–134.

American Psychiatric Association. (2000). *Diagnostic and statistical manual of mental disorders (4th ed., text rev.)*. Washington, DC: American Psychiatric Association.

Bandura, A. (1997). *Self-efficacy: The exercise of control*. New York: W.H. Freeman.

Beck, A. T. (1990). *Beck anxiety inventory*. San Antonio: Psychological Corporation.

Beck, A. T., Steer, R. A., & Brown, G. K. (2001). *Beck depression inventory II*. San Antonio: Psychological Corporation.

Caiata-Zufferey, M., Abraham, A., Sommerhalder, K., & Schultz, P. J. (2010). The impact of online health information seeking in the context of the medical consultation in Switzerland. *Qualitative Health Research, 20*(8), 1050–1061.

Damiano, A. M. (1996). *The sickness impact profile: User's manual interpretation guide*. Baltimore, MD: John Hopkins University.

DeGruy, F. V., Dickinson, W. P., & Staton, E. W. (2002). Mental symptoms. In F. V. DeGruy, W. P. Dickinson, & E. W. Staton (Eds.), *20 common problems in behavioral health* (pp. 441–459). New York: McGraw-Hill.

Derogatis, L. R. (1994). SCL-90-R. In M. Maruish (Ed.), *Brief system inventory, and matching clinical rating scales, in psychological testing, treatment planning, and outcome assessment*. New York: Erlbaum.

Dijkstra, A. (2005). The validity of the stages of change model in the adoption of the self-management approach in chronic pain. *The Clinical Journal of Pain, 21*(1), 27–37.

Ewing, J. A. (1984). Setecting alcoholism: The CAGE questionnaire. *JAMA, 25*(14), 1905–1907.

Greene, R. L. (1991). *MMPI/MMPI-2. An interpretive manual*. Boston: Allyn & Bacon.

Hirschfeld, R. M. A. (2000). Development and validation of a screening instrument for bipolar spectrum disorder: The mood disorder questionnaire. *The American Journal of Psychiatry, 157*(11), 1873–1875.

Hobson, C. J., Kamen, J., Szostek, J., Nethercut, C. M., Tiedman, J. W., & Wojnarowicz, S. (1998). Stressful life events: A revision and update of the social readjustment rating scale. *International Journal of Stress Management, 5*(1), 1–23.

Johns, M. W. (1991). A new method of measuring daytime sleepiness: The Epworth sleepiness scale. *Sleep, 14*, 540–545.

Kroenke, K., Spitzer, R., & Williams, J. (2001). The PHQ-9: Validity of a brief depression severity measure. *Journal of General Internal Medicine, 16*, 606–613.

Knight, R. G., Waal-Manning, J., & Spears, G. F. (1983). Some norms and reliability data for the state-trait anxiety inventory and the zung self-rating depression scale. *British Journal of Clinical Psychology, 22*, 245–249.

Lazarus, R. S., & Folkman, S. (1989). *Manual: Hassles and uplifts scale (research ed.)*. Palo Alto, CA: Mind Garden.

Liskow, B., Campbell, J., Nickel, E. J., & Powell, B. J. (1995). Validity of the CAGE questionnaire in screening for alcohol dependence in a walk-in (triage) clinic. *Journal of Studies on Alcohol and Drugs, 56*, 277–281.

Lo, B., & Parham, L. (2010). The impact of web 2.0 on the doctor-patient relationship. *The Journal of Law, Medicine & Ethics, 38*(1), 17–26.

Locke, E. A., & Lathan, G. P. (2002). Building a practically useful theory of goal setting and task motivation. *American Psychology, 57*(9), 705–717.

McHorney, C. A., Ware, J. E., Lu, J. F. R., & Sherbourne, C. D. (1994). The MOS SF-36 short-form health survey (SF-36), III: Tests of data quality, scaling assumptions, and reliability across diverse patient groups. *Medical Care, 32*(1), 40–66.

McMullan, M. (2006). Patients using the internet to obtain health information: How this affects the patient-health professional relationship. *Patient Education and Counseling, 63*, 24–28.

References

Melzack, R. (1987). The short-form McGill questionnaire. *Pain, 30*, 191–197.

Miller, M. A., & Rahe, R. H. (1997). Life changes scaling for the 1990's. *Journal of Psychosomatic Research, 43*, 279–292.

Moos, R. H. (1993). *Coping resources inventory*. Odessa, FL: Psychological Assessment Resources, Inc.

Pargament, K. I., Koenig, H. G., Tarakeshwar, N., & Hahn, J. (2001). Religious struggle as a predictor of mortality among medically ill elderly patients: A two year longitudinal study. *Archives of Internal Medicine, 161*, 1881–1885.

Prochaska, J. O., & Velicer, W. F. (1997). The transtheoretical model of health behavior change. *American Journal of Health Promotion, 12*, 38–48.

Range, L. M., & Knott, E. C. (1997). Twenty suicide assessment instruments: Evaluation and recommendations. *Death Studies, 21*, 25–58.

Rollnick, S., Miller, W. R., & Butler, C. C. (2008). *Motivational interviewing in health care*. New York: Guilford Press.

Sadock, B. J., & Sadock, V. A. (2008). Psychiatric history and mental status examination. In B. J. Sadock & V. A. Sadock (Eds.), *Concise textbook of clinical psychiatry* (3rd ed., pp. 1–9). Philadelphia: Lippincott Williams & Wilkins.

Snaith, R. P., & Zigmond, A. S. (1994). *The hospital anxiety and depression scale manual*. Windsor, Berkshire, England: Nfer-Nelson.

Spielbreger, C. D., Gorsuch, R. R., & Luchene, R. E. (1970). *State trait anxiety inventory*. Palo Alto: Consulting Psychologists Press.

Spitzer, R. L., WIlliams, J. B., Kroenke, K., Linzer, M., & De Gruy, F. V. (1994). Utility of a new procedure for diagnosing mental disorders in primary care. The PRIME-MD 1000 study. *Journal of the American Medical Association, 272*, 1749–1756.

Starr, T. D., Rogak, L. J., Kirsh, K. L., & Passik, S. D. (2010). Psychological and psychosocial evaluation. In S. M. Fishman, J. C. Ballantyne, & J. P. Rathmell (Eds.), *Bonica's management of pain* (pp. 270–278). Philadelphia: Wolters Kluwer/Lippincott Williams & Wilkins.

Ware, J. E., & Sherbourne, C. D. (1992). The MOS 36 item short form health survery (SF-36). *Medical Care, 30*(6), 473–483.

Widmaier, E. P., Raff, H., & Strang, K. (2004). *Vander, Sherman & Luciano's human physiology* (9th ed.). Boston: McGraw Hill.

Zung, W. W. R. (1965). A self-rating depression Scale. *Archives of General Psychiatry, 12*, 63–70.

Chapter 6
Interventions in the Pathways Model

Abstract This chapter details multilevel intervention plans based on the principles and concepts underlying the Pathways Model. The main focus of the Level One interventions is to reestablish normal biological rhythms that have been disrupted by conditioning, stress, or trauma. Skill building is the main objective of the Level Two interventions, for example, developing relaxation skills to calm the body, exercising to improve physical condition, and redirecting the mind towards positive thoughts. The Level Three interventions consist of more sophisticated psychophysiological and medical interventions.

Keywords Interventions • Stepped approach • Self-care • Self-management • Integrative care

Introduction

Interventions in the Pathways Model occur at three levels: (1) Level One—self-management changes that the person can design and implement on his or her own, (2) Level Two—changes carried out through the use of educational and community resources, and (3) Level Three—changes achieved through psychophysiological, medical, and psychological therapies, provided by professionals. An understanding of illness and health from a holistic, integrative perspective forms the foundation for implementation. Some of the interventions are utilized to build motivation or increase level of commitment to change in order to prepare the person for skill building, an integral part of the process of change. Behavioral, cognitive, emotional, and physiological change is possible because the brain continues to be capable of learning new behaviors and modifying previous habits into old age (Eriksen, Olff, Murison, & Ursine, 1999). The choice of one or more self-management strategies, the use of educational and community resources, and/or the referral for professional care are based on an understanding of how the person became ill. The overall

Pathways recovery plan emanates directly from the detailed Pathways assessment process described in the previous chapter. Often, if the person has been ill for some time or there is significant functional impairment, then professional intervention, i.e., medical, psychological, or psychophysiological care, will be necessary, and the professional may administer or assist the client in all three levels of intervention. Nonetheless, intervention in the Pathways Model always begins with the Level One platform and continues to Levels Two and Three as necessary.

Level One Interventions

According to the Pathways Model, Level One interventions involve those changes in behavior that are designed to reestablish normal body rhythms (McEwen, 2003).

Many people have disregarded signals that their body, mind, and spirit have been sending them for some time. Imposed daily schedules have the capacity to change the person's circadian (daily) rhythms to the detriment of overall health. Simply stated, many people forget how to take care of themselves. They have set aside the messages that their body is fatigued, needs rest, food, and water, or needs to be comforted. So, too, the mind has focused on many thoughts at once, or has been forced into patterns of thinking that may have originally been attempts at adaptation, but which over time have become maladaptive. So, the goals of the Level One interventions are to retrain the brain to reestablish normal body-mind circadian, natural rhythms (Sapolsky, 2003). Table 6.1 shows the basic Level One self-care interventions.

Mindful Breathing

The instinct to breathe is the most basic human instinct and appears at birth. The newborn inhales a deep breath and exhales with a loud scream or cry. From that moment, the breathing rhythm is established and continues throughout life. From a physiological viewpoint, the basic function of breathing is to bring air into the lungs, to provide oxygen dissolved in the blood to all of the tissues, and to expel carbon dioxide. The exchange of oxygen and carbon dioxide fulfills another critical function,

Table 6.1 Level One interventions in the Pathways Model

Breathe: abdominal breathing, resonant breathing, relaxing sign
Feed: calorie intake = energy expenditure, eating as fuel, mindful eating
Sleep: sufficient, rarely fragmented, restorative
Soothe: rocking, humming, praying
Move: muscular activity, motion, non-exertive actions

to maintain the acid–base balance, a function shared with the kidneys (Widmaier, Raff, & Strang, 2004). Basically, breathing ensures a fresh supply of oxygen and sustained optimal levels of carbon dioxide. In many cases, however, the normal breathing routine is disrupted by anxiety and by pathological processes in the lungs and respiratory system. In this case both oxygen and CO_2 can be depleted, with adverse effects on the body's self-regulation. The most basic need of the body has been warped into a maladaptive rhythm (Kabat-Zinn, 1994; Van Dixhoorn, 2007).

Relaxed abdominal *breathing* is the first intervention of Level One. The person is encouraged to learn, using scripted instructions, the technique of abdominal breathing. Because the breathing techniques are so basic to almost all forms of relaxation, a brief description, modified from Davis, Eshelman, and McKay (2008a), follows:

> The person places one hand on the abdomen and the other hand on the chest. The arms rest at the sides and neither the arms nor legs are crossed. The breath is drawn in through the nose for the count of 3 (1:1000, 2:1000, 3:1000) and exhaled for a longer time (1:1000; 2:1000... 6:1000) through the mouth. This pattern is repeated initially for a few minutes. The breathing should be relaxed and effortless. Effort undermines the relaxation effect. The mind focuses only on the breaths and where the breath is going after it is inhaled, as the most important activity of that moment. If during the few minutes of breathing the eyes become heavy and want to close, they can do that gently. Sometimes a client finds it easier to practice mindful, relaxed breathing with the eyes open and to use a focal point in the surrounding area, room, or outside to which to direct attention. After one week of daily practice of a few minutes of deep breathing per day, then the time can be increased to five minutes twice and then three times a day. During the second week in addition to five minutes of practicing three times a day, the relaxing sigh can be added. This is a single long inhalation and a noisy exhalation, letting go at the same time of sensations of tension in the muscles of the shoulder and the chest. The relaxing sign can be practiced multiple times during the day. Mindful, relaxed breathing is the cornerstone of relaxation. Many ancient traditions and other systems of medicine used breathing exercises as the primary source of relaxation and as an entry way to the internal state. For the Level One intervention, it is recommended that the focus be only on the breath. Shifting focus to the internal state is best left for later in the change process.

Nutrition and Feeding Behavior

The next Level One intervention is *feeding*. The second instinct that appears at birth, after breathing, is feeding. Reflexes are in place during gestation (ultrasounds show fetuses sucking their thumbs) so that the newborn can immediately obtain nourishment from the bottle or breast. Feeding is associated with comfort and satisfaction. Over time, the feeding instinct that began as a necessity for life and that was originally highly adaptive becomes warped by negative emotional states, such as anxiety, or through observation of others' behaviors. Much of what we learn about feeding and eating is based on what we have seen in our families, how food was prepared, and the role of eating in the life of the family. In the Pathways Model, feeding must be recast as a nourishing, comforting experience, instead of a rushed activity that is carried out with little regard to the foods' taste or its comforting qualities. Eating should be viewed as a part of self-care, not as something to be hurried through or associated with any type of punishment. The tendency to use food either as a reward or as punishment is deleterious to mental health (Gordon, 2008; Kabat-Zinn, 1994).

As a result of the self or professional assessment, the client already knows where the deficiencies reside in nutrition and perhaps most importantly in eating behaviors. Initially one needs to consciously practice the process of mindful eating. This process is begun by selecting one meal each day, for the practice. A single food or beverage is then chosen from whatever the meal offers. This single food is enjoyed mindfully, slowly, without rushing, and with great attentiveness. The foods or drinks that are chosen for this exercise are pleasant in taste, not empty calories; initially, the food may need to have a strong taste, particularly if food has been consistently consumed without tasting. Mindful eating is gradually expanded to one food at each meal and then to food that has a more subtle taste. Taking in nourishment with mindfulness sends a message to the brain that eating is part of self-care and thus worthy of this attention.

Sleep and Rest

The third instinct that appears at birth is the need to *sleep*—to rest and to refresh. So, maladaptive sleeping habits must be addressed early on in the pathway to change. As a result of the self-assessment or the professional assessment, the nature and severity of the sleep problem has been identified. There may be insufficient hours of sleep, delayed onset, fragmented sleep, nightmares, early awakening, insomnia, or morning fatigue (APA, 2000). The end results of these problems, too few hours of sleep and fragmented sleep, are the same. Upon awakening, the person complains of fatigue and sleepiness and does not feel ready to take on the challenges of the day. Instead, the main sensation upon awakening is one of dread and perhaps anxiety. Over time, people with difficulty falling asleep (or onset insomnia), very frequently fear bedtime because they anticipate being in bed for long periods of time without being able to go to sleep, which is an uncomfortable and anxiety-producing situation. If the sleep problem has been present for at least a month, then it is recommended that the relaxation techniques that are described in Level Two interventions be utilized to attempt to reestablish the normal pattern of sleep. If the problem is early morning awakening, this may signal a more serious problem such as clinical depression (APA, 2000). It is very common for people with clinical depression to have difficulty getting to sleep, staying asleep, and feeling rested in the morning. If the client is also suffering from persistent sadness, loss of interest in activities, and low motivation, in addition to sleep problems, professional intervention may be necessary (Buscemi et al., 2005; Dinges et al., 1997; Hamilton, Catley, & Karlson, 2007; Leproult, Copinschi, Buxton, & Van Cauter, 1997; Zohar, Tzischinsky, Epstein, & Lavie, 2005).

The Level One behavioral interventions for sleep disruptions are designed to reestablish the normal rhythm of sleeping and waking by identifying one sleep deficiency at a time and developing a plan to resolve it. Here are two examples. If sleep is too short, then the goal is to achieve increased restful sleep time. This may consist of decreasing time spent in other activities, such as watching television or playing computer games. If sleeping later is not an option, then an earlier bed time is implemented, but no more than 30 min earlier than usual. That change is continued for at least 10 days to 2 weeks before moving on to the second sleep problem. If, on the other hand, the hours in bed seem to be sufficient but the major problem is disrupted or fragmented sleep, then it is best to implement the sleep hygiene recommendations (detailed in Chapter 15), one or two at a time. Similarly to the recommendations for insufficient hours of sleep, allow 10 days to 2 weeks for each change to take effect.

Self-Soothing

Another basic need of the newborn is to be taken care of, nurtured, or comforted by the parent or caregiver. The infant needs to be *soothed* when she cries or demonstrates irritability and assisted in downregulating the nervous system to facilitate calm or to bring on sleep. Attachment between parent (caregiver) and child is a critical milestone in development and is correlated with later self-care. When the parent–child (caregiver) bond is well established, the child can test the boundaries of independence without undue fear. Secure attachment in childhood has been associated with increased resilience in stressful situations and more stable long-term relationships. In contrast, less secure attachment is more likely to predict anxious, avoidant interactions (Surcinelli, Rossi, Montebarocci, & Baldaro, 2010). For many reasons, including the disruption of the parent–child attachment process, many people never develop this capacity for self-soothing, or achieve it only in a fragile and ineffective way. When self-soothing is deficient, the developing individual is overwhelmed by increasing levels of irritability due to excess stimulation from other people or the environment. It follows then, that the recommendations for self-soothing are designed to decrease excessive physiological or emotional arousal, by repetitive simple behaviors. Without unduly complicating this discussion, it is known that physiological systems are not static and in fact oscillate according to complex neural programs. Oscillation fosters adaptability, while misguided attempts at stability can in fact lead to rigidity and depression (Giardino, Lehrer, & Feldman, 2000). These principles form the basis for this intervention. For example, if the person arrives home from work feeling tense, anxious, and overstimulated, it is recommended that she sits quietly, listens to music, rocks in a rocking chair, hums, or prays. Repetitive behaviors soothe the nervous system and decrease irritability. Rocking in a rocking chair or swinging the arms or feet in a mindful manner will help the individual to reestablish the beneficial effects of repetitive motion that are commonly used for babies and young children (Campbell, 1997; Neff, Kirkpatrick, & Rude, 2007). Repeating familiar words and phrases in a prayer format may also be helpful in quieting the mind. However, if it is determined that relationship issues, stemming originally from insecure or pathological attachments, are the main problem, Level Three interventions will be necessary (Schore, 2002).

Movement

The last intervention in the Level One tier is *movement*. The need to move and be active is another basic instinct. The newborn wants to move and to be active at certain times, whereas at other times there is a clear need for rest and quiet as discussed above. Unfortunately, many factors in contemporary lifestyles reduce activity and promote sedentary events over more active ones. Individuals ride in cars rather than walk, work at a desk rather than outdoors, and recreate by such means as computer games and television, rather than through sports or walking. Many of the physical and emotional illnesses that people deal with lead them to become even more sedentary. The vicious cycle continues as the inactivity itself then increases the severity of the illness. For example, persons who are gaining weight feel uncomfortable in social situations and begin to withdraw from these social situations; consequently, they do not leave the house as often as they did when they felt less self-conscious. While at home, the person tends to turn to food as comfort instead of using food for nutrition. Activity and movement are further compromised, thus increasing the tendency to gain weight (Sime, 2007).

From a psychological perspective, the person with symptoms of anxiety begins to fear previously neutral stimuli or situations. An avoidance of previous activities is one result; activity and movement decrease, and as the person becomes more isolated, anxiety increases further. Therefore, the person beginning this new self-care program needs to begin to move. As emphasized in this book, drastic changes are not recommended. The Level One intervention "movement" is not designed to build aerobic capacity but to reestablish the normal body rhythm of movement. The individual who has been inactive is *not* recommended to begin walking even one mile. Instead, we recommend that he or she begin to move for a very short distance and time. Then slowly increase time by up to 5–10 min, followed by increasing distance up to one quarter to one half mile.

Another basic Level One *movement* exercise has been promoted by James Gordon, a pioneer in the development of mind-body medicine. Gordon (2008, pp. 172–174) advocates a simple activity called "shaking and dancing." Almost every child, from the earliest age and regardless of culture, will show some tendency to move the body with music. "Shaking and dancing" provides an opportunity to recover this childlike awareness and comfort with the body's potential for rhythm and movement.

The exercise begins with the selection of two pieces of music to support the two phases of the exercise. The first piece should provide a fast driving rhythm with high energy, such as first segment of the "Kundalini" CD distributed by the

Osho International Foundation (http://www.osho.com). The second piece should provide a more melodic but still energetic dance rhythm, such as Jimmy Cliff's "You Can Get It if You Really Want." Instructions for the shaking and dancing exercise follow:

> Turn on the first musical segment. Position your body with your feet a shoulder width apart, the knees slightly bent, and your shoulders relaxed. Close your eyes to facilitate concentration. Begin to shake with the music, initially feeling the movement rise through your feet, knees, hips, and shoulders, until your entire body is involved. Allow your arms, legs, torso, and head – every portion of your body – to join in moving with the music. (If you sense pain, move more gently and set your own limits. Many individuals report a moderation of pain if they persist in the movement.) Relax your shoulders and allow yourself to bob and sway with the shaking. Shake vigorously and with enthusiasm. Allow your jaws to open, releasing any tension carried in the jaw. If you spontaneously feel like making any sound, allow it to emerge! Set aside any feelings of self-consciousness and allow yourself to enjoy the experience of your entire body shaking and becoming one with the music. Continue for about five minutes or until the music ends.
>
> Now silence the music and bring the shaking to an end. Breathe slowly and mindfully, relax, and enjoy experiencing the feelings throughout your body. Be aware of your body and of your breathing.
>
> Now switch on the second piece of music and begin to move with this music. Enjoy a kind of free-form dance movement, without the restraints of any "dance steps." Enjoy your body's movement and vitality. Again, set aside any self-consciousness and, for this moment in time, allow your body to enjoy its own dance. Stop after another four to five minutes.

Level Two Interventions

The Level Two interventions consist of basic relaxation techniques, physical exercise, identifying maladaptive thinking patterns, learning to pause, and beginning to communicate (Table 6.2). These interventions form the basic skills necessary to restore physical and emotional health. Skills stand on the platform that the client has developed through the daily use of the Level One interventions.

Educational and community resources can often provide all of the guidance needed to master Level Two skills. Relaxation training CDs, podcasts, educational DVDs, and books can provide instructions and encouragement. Community-based classes are often available to support new communication skills, exercise, meditation techniques, yoga, tai chi, and other self-management and self-regulation strategies. Reading material may also be available to provide additional instruction (McCall, 2007). However, if the person has long-standing emotional or physical

Table 6.2 Level Two interventions in the Pathways Model

Progressive relaxation	Communicate
Basic imagery	Exercise
Pause	Identifying thinking errors

problems or has little support from others, the professional can provide guidance and encouragement for the Level Two interventions.

Progressive Relaxation

Progressive Relaxation is a relatively simple relaxation technique that consists of alternating tension and relaxation in specific muscle groups of the body. This exercise is initiated by a few minutes of mindful breathing as described earlier in the chapter. The person begins relaxing the muscles of the upper body, then the neck and head and finally the lower body. Each muscle group is tensed for a few seconds and then relaxed for longer than the tension phase, while the individual attentively studies the contrast between the sensation of tension and relaxation. The first muscles to be tensed and relaxed are the right hand and arm, followed by the left hand and arm, the upper arms, the shoulders, the neck, the jaw, the mouth, the forehead, and eyelids. Slow breathing continues throughout the exercise. Benefits from this exercise include increased awareness of patterns of tension, earlier recognition of the onset of tension, and increased control over the body's tensing and relaxing. This exercise does not always have to include every muscle group but can be applied to particular areas of tension in the body (Davis, Eshelman, & McKay, 2008b; Lehrer & Carrington, 2003).

Physical Exercise

In Level Two, *movement*, now called *exercise*, increases in intensity and duration. Exercise begins with stretching or slow walking, as recommended earlier in the chapter, and then the distance is increased and then the speed of the walk. For example, if the individual has been engaging in movement for 5 min a day, the distance is increased to one quarter mile, and then the speed is increased. After 1 week, the distance is increased to one half mile, then the speed is increased, and so forth until the individual can walk one mile in 15–20 min. The Level Two goal is to walk two miles in 35 min three times a week (Norman & Mills, 2004; Sime, 2007).

Cognitive Renewal

The next Level Two intervention is *cognitive renewal*. The goal of cognitive renewal is to identify and transform negative and self-destructive thinking patterns that are interfering with physical and emotional health. Since the first step towards countering negative thoughts is to become aware of them, the process begins with observation of the self. The first goal is to become aware of and document in a notebook thoughts and self-talk in a nonjudgmental matter, similarly to what an observer would do. The individual cultivates the state of mind of a disinterested observer. This attitude is key to success, since there is a danger that he or she will begin to berate him or herself because of negative thinking, which in turn perpetuates negative thinking. For example, the individual identifies the presence of frequent self-criticism, such as "I am stupid, an idiot, a failure, and a loser." Acknowledgement, not approval of the negative thoughts, begins the process of change (Neff et al., 2007). Once people realize the types of thoughts that run through their minds and how frequently they occur, they are at risk for reacting in an extremely negatively way to this realization. Most human beings are already very hard on themselves and are in danger of making this an even more difficult exercise. The clinician is advised to caution each person in advance that these challenges can be expected in the first couple of experiences of monitoring thoughts.

When the observation phase has taken place for at least a week, then the negative thoughts should be countered in the following way. In the margin, next to the first negative self-statement, the individual should record ways to refute this particular statement. So, for example, he or she can considers this statement, "I can't do anything right." How can this statement be refuted? One of the ways to refute such a negative and overgeneralizing statement is to think of a recent situation in which the individual was correct in behavior and accomplished what he or she set out to do. This does not have to be a complicated, extensive task. The purpose is simply to refute the statement, to illustrate that the statement, "I can't do anything right," is not accurate and can be opposed by the statement "I got to work on time." Then, the individual continues with the second statement, for example, "I am a total failure." Now how can this statement be refuted? The individual need only remember a situation in which things were attempted and turned out well; he or she then writes a brief description of that event in the notebook (Gordon, 2008). Whenever the same negative statement recurs, the individual directs his or her memory to recall the situation with the positive outcome.

In this fashion, with repeated journaling of negative thoughts and repeated exercises in disputing the negative thoughts, it gradually becomes easier to spontaneously redirect one's awareness in more positive pathways. Self-compassion and self-understanding is encouraged during this sometimes difficult stage (Neff et al., 2007).This is the desired outcome of cognitive renewal.

Pause: Introducing a Moment of Awareness

The next Level Two intervention is called *pause*. A very frequent maladaptive behavior is reacting to stressful situations with little thought and planning. These rash reactions allow circumstances to run one's life and let outside events control and exert power over one's life. The ability to pause and consider one's options is critical in the process of regaining control over stressful situations. For example, the client considers how many times he/she has been in a situation where an acquaintance calls and requests assistance in a church project, and they have responded, "Of course I will do it," without any regard for their own health or well-being and without considering whether they are really able to complete the task. Now, this is something that the individual would like to do, because he or she is a regular church member and this event has been a good fund-raiser in the past. However, the date for which help is requested is also a date that this individual had planned another activity. So, the individual finds that he or she has responded, "of course," without actually considering the ramifications and the consequences.

The pause system recommends that one responds to the request by saying, "I will let you know tomorrow;. I have to check a couple of dates before I can give you an answer." Now, this may not sound like something really out of the ordinary and not difficult. However, human beings are inclined to respond with a resounding "Yes" to most requests from people that they respect and appreciate and in any situation where they are actually interested in the activity—whether or not this is actually something that they can accomplish. We recommend that all requests activate the "pause" button so that one learns to say, "I will have to get back to you." Now just the fact of utilizing the pause button begins to give the individual a sense of control that he or she didn't have before. The individual hasn't said "No," but has given him or herself time to think and consider other responsibilities, by making an assertive, not a hostile, statement. The *pause* and communicate recommendations set the stage for more detailed assertiveness training.

Mindfulness

Mindfulness is a particular way of directing attention and focusing on what is going on in the present moment, on purpose, and without judgment. It is not a religious practice or a set of beliefs, although the approach was developed from Eastern meditation practices. Mindfulness meditation is a Level Three intervention. It is a form of meditation that teaches the individual to notice and observe whatever comes into the stream of consciousness while suspending judgment and cultivating acceptance. Mindfulness-based Cognitive Behavioral Therapy (CBT) is also a Level Three intervention (Teasdale, Segal, & Williams, 1995). Mindfulness as a life skill is a Level Two practice, which teaches acceptance of each life experience and reduces the power of self-criticism and unrealistic expectations. Mindfulness brings the person's attention to the ongoing experience in order to fully appreciate it (Jevning, Anand, & Biedebach, 1996; Kabat-Zinn, 1994; Lazar et al. 2005). Mindfulness is a more advanced technique than most types of relaxation because it does not have the structure (such as a focusing on the muscles, on specific images, or on repetitive phrases) that facilitates the direction of attention in many other forms of relaxation (Baer, 2003).

Communication

The use of the pause technique leads into the last of the Level Two interventions, which is *communication*. Hurt feelings, anxiety, anger, depression, and insomnia frequently result from problems in communication and the sense of being misunderstood. Infants instinctively express their emotions and watch for reactions from their caregivers. If the infants' expressed emotion is noticed and acknowledged, there is a sense of validation. On the contrary, if expressed emotions are criticized, mocked, or minimized, the child later has no framework to understand her own feelings (Fruzzetti & Iverson, 2004). So, this Level Two intervention calls for an attempt to communicate in a more effective matter by first noticing the feelings that drive the communication. How can this begin? Healthier communication actually begins during the pause intervention, while the individual is repeating to a friend that he or she is not really sure about helping to decorate the church but has not made a decision. This is the beginning of learning to communicate in an assertive manner.

Another way to improve communication is by learning to make assertive statements about what one thinks and feels regarding neutral, noncontroversial issues. The reader may consider the following exercise: As you are reading this section of this chapter, make one of the following statements out loud if possible. "I understand this concept. I think that there is value here." Or "I'm finding this difficult to understand. I want to spend more time on this." Every day for a week, the individual should make at least one assertive statement about what he or she thinks and feels out loud, but in private. The second week, the individual makes one private assertive statement and then makes the same statement to another person. Initially, the individual should continue to use neutral topics for assertiveness practice to build self-confidence. In week three, the individual should expand his or her statements to less neutral topics. For example, while eating lunch with a coworker, he might say, "I really like the taste of this salad dressing; it's just right." Or "Sherie called to ask me to decorate the church on Saturday, but I have to tell her no." With practice the individual will be able to use assertive, non-aggressive statements to say "No" to requests that he or she either cannot or does not wish to accommodate, without losing the friendship (Alberti & Emmons, 2008).

Communication also includes the written word. In these times of e-mail and texting, most requests may actually not come in person or by phone, but electronically. These media pose the same or sometimes greater challenges, as the tendency is to respond immediately, without thinking. The same principles that were described above apply to e-mail and phone texts. The individual should practice pausing and taking a breath before responding. E-mail responses can be saved in the draft folder before sending. If thoughts and intent are not clear, journaling can be used to describe and clarify thoughts and feelings about the situation. Affective journaling has been associated with positive physiological and emotional outcomes (Pennebaker, 1999).

Social support and positive relationships are integral to mental and physical health (Dalgard, Bjork, & Tambs, 1995; Hughes et al., 2004; Olstad, Sexton, & Sogaard, 2001). Open, expressive, and assertive communication is critical to building and maintaining these positive relationships. With this in mind, learning to communicate in a positive way is critical to the success of Level Two interventions. Practice will be necessary to achieve communication that expresses one's own feelings and desires, without challenging others' beliefs. Facial expression and body language are major conveyors of emotion. Seeing another's distress in response to a statement or opinion can derail one's attempts at communication. As social psychologists have determined, "mirror neurons make emotions contagious." When seeing another's unpleasant facial expression, it is common to feel sad, disgusted, or anxious (Goleman, 2006). Therefore, expressions may have to be practiced with a mirror in order to match the body and face with the spoken word (Flack, Laird, & Cavallaro, 1999). In addition, awareness and understanding of the role of mirror neurons in social interactions will allow the person to override the tendency to capitulate to the disapproval signals from others.

Level Three Interventions

Level Three interventions consist of medication, psychotherapy, and specific mind-body modalities such as biofeedback, imagery, mindfulness meditation, and hypnosis most of which will be managed by a professional (Table 6.3). The Level One and Two behavioral changes are maintained and used as the background for professional intervention. The forthcoming clinical chapters contain sections on medication management appropriate to the clinical problem. Similarly, detailed descriptions of psychotherapy will be provided within the context of treatment of specific emotional and medical disorders. Definitions of the types of psychotherapy will be provided below, leaving the details until later. In contrast, biofeedback, imagery, and hypnosis will be described in the remainder of this chapter.

Psychotherapy

There are many different types of psychotherapy, but all share several characteristics, in particular a helping relationship and verbal communication between the person and the therapist (Brody et al., 2001; Duclos & Laird, 2001; Kandel, 1998). Some types of psychotherapy are better suited to mind-body problems, among them CBT, acceptance/commitment therapy (ACT), dialectical behavioral therapy (DBT), and brief psychodynamic therapy.

Table 6.3 Level Three interventions in the Pathways Model

Advanced relaxation	Biofeedback
Guided imagery	Hypnosis
Cognitive restructuring	Psychotherapy

Cognitive Behavioral Therapy (CBT). CBT is based on the premise that thoughts, attitudes, and the perception of events, not the situations themselves, determine one's feelings, physiological responses, and behavior (Beck, 1967). If the person consistently views the world and the self as negative, uncomfortable emotions, unhealthy behaviors, and stress-related physiological responses will occur. The basis of therapy is to assist the person to change thinking patterns in order to decrease symptoms and resolve underlying conflicts. When the patient presents illness and medical symptoms as the primary complaint, the cognitive behavioral therapist highlights the role of cognitive factors in determining how people cope with illness (Lau, Segal, & Zaretsky, 2003). Outcome studies have shown the effectiveness of CBT in treating such diverse medical problems as chronic pain, chronic fatigue syndromes, and irritable bowel syndrome as well as in changing such health-risk habits as cigarette smoking. Mindfulness training has been incorporated into CBT, particularly to address relapse issues after treatment for depression (Segal, Teasdale, & Williams, 2004).

Acceptance and Commitment Therapy (ACT). ACT is a form of psychotherapy developed by Hayes, Strosahl, & Wilson (2003), within the cognitive behavioral tradition, but integrating innovative paradigms for both explaining and remediating suffering. ACT begins by assuming that emotional suffering is typically caused by behavioral and experiential avoidance and psychological rigidity. This avoidance undermines coping and creates psychological disturbance. Through ACT, patients learn to "just notice," accept, and even embrace their moment to moment experiences, especially those they have previously avoided. ACT utilizes several key therapeutic strategies, such as metaphors, experiential exercises, and logical paradox to enable the patient to produce more contact with the immediate flow of experience (Hayes & Pierson, 2005). Acceptance of this immediate reality of the flow of experience and commitment to goals reflecting personal values are critical therapeutic processes in ACT.

Dialectical Behavioral Therapy (DBT). DBT is a form of behavioral therapy originally developed by Linehan et al. (1999) for the treatment of persons with a severe personality disturbance, called "borderline personality disorder." DBT combines the techniques of CBT, with mindfulness awareness, "distress tolerance" skills, emotion regulation skills, and interpersonal effectiveness training. The word dialectical in the name refers to Linehan's accomplishment in providing the patient with two seemingly contradictory messages within one communication, first that the patient will only reach healing through accepting himself or herself completely and, second, that the patient will only attain a better life through eliminating current destructive coping patterns and learning new life skills. Like Hegelian philosophy, Linehan's system of therapy emphasizes that only by reconciling contradictions will progress be achieved. The patient achieves a new life by embracing acceptance and change in each moment.

Brief Dynamic Psychotherapy. Brief dynamic psychotherapy is a form of verbal psychotherapy, which assists the patient to identify core emotional experiences playing out in each new life problem (Holmes, 1994). The patient learns to recognize the role of specific early life experiences in sensitizing the individual to this key, repetitive emotional experience. The individual with chronic or recurrent medical illness will come to recognize that the times in life when the illness recurs correspond to chapters of life in which he or she once again replays the central relationship scripts or dramas of early life—such as moments of rejection, loss, or personal inadequacy. As the individual comes to understand the key emotional conflicts or experiences and gains a new sense of mastery over them, he or she becomes better able to live life in the present, without the residue of past trauma and wounds. The mastery of the early conflicts unfolds within the "corrective emotional experience" of psychotherapy, centered on encountering acceptance and not rejection within the therapist-patient relationship.

Applied Psychophysiological Therapy

Biofeedback

Biofeedback is a therapy in which the person receives information ("feedback") about a particular physiological process with the goal of increasing both awareness and control of that process (Schwartz & Schwartz, 2003). The biofeedback instrument measures one or more physiological signals, transduces these raw signals into useful information, and presents the biofeedback trainee with immediate visual and auditory feedback. The individual uses the feedback to gain control over the physiological process, lowering muscle tension, warming peripheral temperature, and increasing the variability of heart rate. These physiological changes impact on the physiological mechanisms for the presenting illness or disorder and reduce symptom severity, and the individual gains self-efficacy—confidence in his or her power for having an impact on body and illness (Shaffer & Moss, 2006).

Major types of biofeedback are muscle or electromyographic biofeedback (EMG), skin temperature or thermal biofeedback, electrodermal biofeedback, brain wave or electroencephalographic (EEG), and heart rate variability biofeedback (based on paced breathing and regulation of heart rate changes). Biofeedback has been shown to be an effective treatment for a variety of medical conditions and emotional disorders. The research is strongest for the therapeutic efficacy of biofeedback for urinary incontinence, attention deficit hyperactivity disorder, chronic pain, seizure disorders, Raynaud's disease, temporomandibular disorders, and adult headache (Yucha & Montgomery, 2008). Biofeedback is frequently coupled with mindful breathing, progressive muscle relaxation, autogenic training, passive relaxation, imagery, and other Level Two and Three interventions. The treatment for headache, for example, may include muscle and temperature biofeedback, occasionally EEG biofeedback, along with autogenic training, progressive muscle relaxation training, CBT for negative emotions and worry, and stress management for current life problems.

Guided Imagery

Imagery is a process of creating or recreating an experience as a mental image, which involves one or more of the sensory modalities (Murphy, 2005; Watanabe et al., 2006). There are many applications of imagery from simple relaxing images to the use of imagery for behavioral rehearsal and problem-solving. Pleasant mental images involving the visual, auditory, olfactory, and kinesthetic senses are mobilized to help the person relax. The images bring about pleasant emotions and a sense of calm and peacefulness. Images can also be used for rehearsal and problem-solving. Students who are engaged in skill-based professions can enhance the learning process by adding visualization to practice. The repeated imagined completion of the skillful activity speeds the learning process. When a client is directed to form specific images or images are interpreted by a professional, the intervention is termed Guided Imagery. The use of imagery within psychotherapy is a powerful tool to assist the client in understanding painful images from the past and creating positive images of the present and future. The patient's imagery of his or her illness can provide diagnostic clues about the patient's prognosis for recovery (Achterberg & Lawlis, 1984). Cultivating more positive images of combating the illness process will at least improve coping with the illness and may positively improve long-term survival and wellness (Achterberg, 1985).

Hypnosis

Hypnosis involves the use of words and techniques to induce in the patient an altered state of consciousness (trance), in which the patient is more susceptible to therapeutic suggestions and more capable of behavior change and life transformation (Yapko, 2003). The therapeutic relationship, trust, and rapport are critical to the success of hypnosis treatment. The therapist uses a variety of strategies, including relaxation techniques, imagery, and direct instructions to induce a trance state (induction phase), and then uses further strategies, such as counting downward or dissociative techniques to further deepen the trance state and increase the patient's readiness for change (deepening stage). During hypnosis, attention is narrowed or focused on the voice and words spoken by the professional. Once the patient is in an adequate hypnotic or trance state, the work of the therapist moves to developing and presenting therapeutic suggestions relevant to the person's needs and goals (suggestion phase). Therapeutic suggestions are the core feature of the "work" of hypnosis (Young, 2005). After hypnosis, the person may or may not consciously recall the suggestions but regardless will begin to implement them to initiate changes in behavior.

Conclusion

Finally, the pathway to health must be personalized. For example, the internal message that has been warped over time can be modified by biofeedback, relaxation therapies, and hypnosis. Specific maladaptive behaviors that have become part of the person's repertoire can be modified by behavior therapy. If the person's primary problem is maladaptive thinking, negative attitudes, and a pessimistic view of life, then CBT will be included in the overall multimodal intervention. If the person has developed a hypersensitivity to stressful situations, then dialectical behavior therapy should be implemented. Finally, if the person suffers from poverty of spirit, then spiritual development and counseling should be included in the overall treatment.

We recommend that the detailed assessment process be the guide for the interventions that are chosen and that all clients begin with the Level One interventions. Recall that these self-care behaviors can reestablish the normal body-mind rhythms and encourage the person to begin with simple change strategies that have a high probability of success. Skipping the Level One interventions and beginning with the Level Two or Three interventions do not establish the platform for change. Those with clinical mood or anxiety disorders may already be consulting a mental health provider so may already be engaged in Level Three interventions. Nonetheless, we recommend that the early processes of behavioral change, which emphasize the basic care of the self, be integrated into the therapeutic context.

References

Achterberg, J. (1985). *Imagery in healing*. Boston: Shambala.
Achterberg, J., & Lawlis, F. (1984). *Imagery and disease: Image Ca, Image Sp, Image Db: A diagnostic tool for behavioral medicine*. Champagn, IL: Institute for Personality and Ability Testing.
Alberti, R., & Emmons, M. (2008). *Your perfect right*. Atascadero, CA: Impact Publishers.
American Psychiatric Association. (2000). *Diagnostic and statistical manual of mental disorders (4th ed., text rev.)*. Washington, DC: American Psychiatric Association.
Baer, R. (2003). Mindfulness training as a clinical intervention: A conceptual and empirical review. *Clinical Psychology: Science and Practice, 10*, 125–143.
Beck, A. T. (1967). *Depression: Causes and treatment*. Philadelphia: University of Pennsylvania Press.
Brody, A. L., Saxena, S., Stoessel, P., Gillies, L. A., Fairbanks, L. A., Alborzian, S., et al. (2001). Regional brain metabolic changes in patients with major depression treated with either Paroxetine or interpersonal therapy: Preliminary findings. *Archives of General Psychiatry, 58*(7), 631–640.
Buscemi, N., Vandermeer, B., Friesen, C., Bialy, L., Tubman, M., Ospina, M., et al. (2005). Manifestations and management of chronic insomnia in adults. *Evidence Report/Technology Assessment (Summary), 125*, 1–10.
Campbell, D. (1997). *The Mozart effect: Tapping the power of music to heal the body, strengthen the mind, and unlock the creative spirit*. New York: Avon Books.
Dalgard, O. S., Bjork, S., & Tambs, K. (1995). Social support, negative life events and mental health. *The British Journal of Psychiatry, 166*, 29–34.
Davis, M., Eshelman, E. R., & McKay, M. (2008a). Breathing. In M. Davis, E. R. Eshelman, & M. Mc Kay (Eds.), *The relaxation and stress reduction workbook* (pp. 27–40). Oakland, CA: New Harbinger Publications, Inc.
Davis, M., Eshelman, E. R., & McKay, M. (2008b). Progressive relaxation. In M. Davis, R. Eshelman, & M. Mc Kay (Eds.), *The relaxation and stress reduction workbook* (pp. 41–46). Oakland, CA: New Harbinger Publications, Inc.
Dinges, D. F., Pack, F., Williams, K., Gillen, K. A., Powell, J. W., Ott, G. E., et al. (1997). Cumulative sleepiness, mood disturbance, and psychomotor vigilance performance decrements during a week of sleep restricted to 4–5 hours per night. *Sleep, 20*, 267–277.

References

Duclos, S. E., & Laird, J. D. (2001). The deliberate control of emotional experience through control of expressions. *Cognition & Emotion, 15*(1), 27–56.

Eriksen, H. R. A., Olff, M., Murison, R., & Ursine, H. (1999). The time dimension in stress responses: Relevance for survival and health. *Psychiatry Research, 85*, 39–50.

Flack, W. F., Jr., Laird, J. D., & Cavallaro, L. A. (1999). Separate and combined effects of facial expressions and bodily postures on emotional feelings. *European Journal of Social Psychology, 29*(2/3), 203–217.

Fruzzetti, A. E., & Iverson, K. M. (2004). Mindfulness, acceptance, validation and "individual" psychopathology in couples. In S. C. Hayes, V. M. Follette, & M. M. Linehan (Eds.), *Mindfulness and acceptance* (pp. 168–192). New York: The Guilford Press.

Giardino, N. D., Lehrer, P. M., & Feldman, J. M. (2000). The role of oscillations in self-regulation: Their contribution to homeostasis. In D. Kenny, J. G. Carlson, J. F. McGuigan, & J. L. Sheppard (Eds.), *Stress and health: Research and clinical application* (pp. 27–51). Amsterdam, Netherlands: Harwood Academic Publishers.

Goleman, D. (2006). *Social intelligence*. New York: Random House.

Gordon, J. S. (2008). *Unstuck: Your guide to the seven-stage journey out of depression*. New York: The Penguin Press.

Hamilton, N. A., Catley, D., & Karlson, C. (2007). Sleep and the affective response to stress and pain. *Health Psychology, 26*, 288–295.

Hayes, S. C., & Pierson, H. (2005). Acceptance and commitment therapy. In A. Freeman, S. H. Felgoise, A. M. Nezu, C. M. Nezu, & M. A. Reinecke (Eds.), *Encyclopedia of cognitive behavioral therapy, Part I* (pp. 1–4). New York: Springer.

Hayes, S. C., Strosahl, K. D., & Wilson, K. G. (2003). *Acceptance and commitment therapy: An experiential approach to behavior change*. New York: Guilford.

Holmes, J. (1994). Brief dynamic psychotherapy. *Advances in Psychiatric Treatment, 1*, 9–15.

Hughes, J. W., Tomlinson, A., Blumenthal, J. A., Davidson, J., Sketch, M. H., & Watkins, L. L. (2004). Social support and religiosity as coping strategies for anxiety in hospitalized cardiac patients. *Annals of Behavioral Medicine, 28*(3), 179–185.

Jevning, R., Anand, R., & Biedebach, M. (1996). Effects on regional cerebral blood flow of transcendental meditation. *Physiology & Behavior, 59*(3), 399–402.

Kandel, E. R. (1998). A new intellectual framework for psychiatry. *The American Journal of Psychiatry, 155*(4), 457–469.

Kabat-Zinn, J. (1994). *Wherever you go, there you are: Mindfulness meditation in everyday life*. New York: Hyperion.

Lau, M. A., Segal, Z. V., & Zaretsky, A. E. (2003). Cognitive-behavioral therapies for the medical clinic. In D. Moss, A. McGrady, T. C. Davies, & I. Wickramasekera (Eds.), *Handbook of mind-body medicine for primary care* (pp. 167–179). Thousand Oaks, CA: Sage.

Lazar, S. W., Kerr, C. E., Wasserman, R. H., Gray, J. R., Greve, D. N., Treadway, M. T., et al. (2005). Meditation experience is associated with increased cortical thickness. *Neuroreport, 16*(17), 1893–1897.

Lehrer, P., & Carrington, P. (2003). Progressive relaxation, autogenic training and meditation. In D. Moss, A. McGrady, T. C. Davies, & I. Wickramasekera (Eds.), *Handbook of mind-body medicine for primary care* (pp. 137–149). Thousand Oaks, CA: Sage.

Leproult, R., Copinschi, G., Buxton, O., & Van Cauter, E. (1997). Sleep loss results in an elevation of cortisol levels the next evening. *Sleep, 20*, 865–870.

Linehan, M. M., Schmidt, H., Dimeff, L. A., Craft, J. C., Kanter, J., & Comtois, K. A. (1999). Dialectical behavior therapy for patients with borderline personality disorder and drug dependence. *The American Journal on Addictions, 8*(4), 279–292.

McCall, T. (2007). *Yoga as medicine: The Yogic prescription for health and healing*. New York: Bantam Books.

McEwen, B. S. (2003). Early life influences on life-long patterns of behavior and health. *Mental Retardation and Developmental Disabilities Research Reviews, 9*, 149–154.

Murphy, S. (2005). Imagery: Inner theater becomes reality. In S. Murphy (Ed.), *The sport psych handbook* (pp. 128–151). Champaign, IL: Human Kinetics.

Neff, K. D., Kirkpatrick, K. L., & Rude, S. S. (2007). Self compassion and adaptive psychological functioning. *Journal of Research in Personality, 41,* 139–154.

Norman, G. J., & Mills, P. J. (2004). Keeping it simple: Encouraging walking as a means of active living. *Annals of Behavioral Medicine, 28*(3), 149–151.

Olstad, R., Sexton, H., & Sogaard, A. J. (2001). The Finnmark Study. A prospective population study of the social support buffer hypothesis, specific stressors and mental distress. *Social Psychiatry and Psychiatric Epidemiology, 36,* 582–589.

Pennebaker, J. W. (1999). Forming a story: The health benefits of narrative. *Journal of Clinical Psychology, 55*(10), 1243–1254.

Sapolsky, R. M. (2003). Stress and plasticity in the limbic system. *Neurochemical Research, 28,* 1735–1742.

Schore, A. N. (2002). Dysregulation of the right brain: A fundamental mechanism of traumatic attachment and the psychopathogenesis of post traumatic stress disorder. *The Australian and New Zealand Journal of Psychiatry, 36,* 9–30.

Schwartz, N. M., & Schwartz, M. S. (2003). Definitions of biofeedback and applied psychophysiology. In M. S. Schwartz & F. Andrasik (Eds.), *Biofeedback: A practitioner's guide* (3rd ed., pp. 27–39). New York: The Guilford Press.

Segal, Z. V., Teasdale, J. D., & Williams, J. M. G. (2004). Mindfulness-based cognitive therapy: Theoretical rationale and empirical status. In S. C. Hayes, V. M. Follette, & M. M. Linehan (Eds.), *Mindfulness and acceptance* (pp. 45–65). New York: The Guilford Press.

Shaffer, F., & Moss, D. (2006). Biofeedback. In C.-S. Yuan & E. J. Bieber (Eds.), *Textbook of complementary and alternative medicine* (2nd ed., pp. 291–312). Abingdon, Oxfordshire, UK: Informa Healthcare.

Sime, W. (2007). Exercise therapy for stress management. In P. M. Lehrer, R. L. Woolfolk, & W. E. Sime (Eds.), *Principles and practice of stress management* (3rd ed., pp. 333–359). New York: Guilford Press.

Surcinelli, P., Rossi, N., Montebarocci, O., & Baldaro, B. (2010). Adult attachment styles and psychological disease: Examining the mediating role of personality traits. *Journal of Psychology, 144*(6), 523–535.

Teasdale, J. D., Segal, Z. V., & Williams, J. M. G. (1995). How does cognitive therapy prevent depressive relapse and why should attentional control (mindfulness) training help? *Behavior Research and Therapy, 33,* 25–39.

Van Dixhoorn, J. (2007). Whole-body breathing. A systems perspective on respiratory retraining. In P. M. Lehrer, R. L. Woolfolk, & W. E. Sime (Eds.), *Principles and practice of stress management* (3rd ed., pp. 291–332). New York: Guilford Press.

Watanabe, E., Fukuda, S., Hara, H., Maeda, Y., Ohira, H., & Shirakawa, T. (2006). Differences in relaxation by means of guided imagery in a healthy community sample. *Alternative Therapies, 12*(2), 60–65.

Widmaier, E. P., Raff, H., & Strang, K. (2004). *Vander, Sherman & Luciano's human physiology* (9th ed.). Boston: McGraw Hill.

Yapko, M. (2003). *Trancework: An introduction to the practice of clinical hypnosis* (3rd ed.). New York: Brunner-Routledge.

Young, J. S. (2005). A wellness perspective on the management of stress. In J. E. Myers & T. J. Sweeney (Eds.), *Counseling for wellness: Theory, research and practice* (pp. 207–215). Alexandria, VA: American Counseling Association.

Yucha, C., & Montgomery, D. (2008). *Evidence-based practice in biofeedback and neurofeedback.* Wheat Ridge, CO: Association for Applied Psychophysiology and Biofeedback.

Zohar, D., Tzischinsky, O., Epstein, R., & Lavie, P. (2005). The effects of sleep loss on medical residents' emotional reactions to work events: A cognitive-energy model. *Sleep, 28,* 47–54.

Part II
Applications to Common Illnesses

Chapter 7
Substance Abuse Disorders

Abstract Substance abuse is a major public health problem, with high prevalence in the US population, and many associated economic costs. The problem of substance abuse is a useful example for better understanding the paradox and the challenge of chronic illness. Substance abuse has significant genetic heritability, along with elements of individual choice and family influence. There are also identifiable pathophysiological changes accompanying substance abuse, the presence of objective diagnostic criteria, and a relapse rate similar to many other chronic diseases. The pathways approach for substance abuse is illustrated by a case narrative involving a 46-year-old alcoholic woman.

Keywords Substance abuse • Alcohol abuse • Drug abuse • Tobacco use

Introduction

This chapter will discuss the Pathways Model as applied to substance abuse, including alcohol abuse, illicit drug use, and tobacco use. Substance abuse is a serious problem in its own right, with significant effects in undermining health. Substance abuse is also a good model for understanding the challenges of chronic illness. We need to shift conceptual paradigms, modify treatment approaches, and adjust personal expectations when we face illnesses that persist over a lifetime.

The Pathways Model understands chronic illnesses as products of multiple causes—heredity, neurochemistry, lifestyle, social stress, and behavior. The individual travels many pathways during the onset of conditions that later become chronic. The individual must discover novel pathways in recovering health, including a new emphasis on self-care and lifestyle change. There is no single treatment and no cure, and recovery is typically lifelong, requiring many supports.

Substance Abuse Prevalence and Costs

Substance abuse is a major public health problem, bringing enormous suffering to individuals and families. Broadly, substance abuse refers to abuse of alcohol, illicit drugs, prescription medication abuse, and cigarette smoking. The World Health Organization (WHO) distinguishes among substance misuse, abuse, and dependence (WHO, n.d.). Misuse of a substance refers to use for a purpose "not consistent with medical or legal guidelines." Misuse may include excessive alcohol or drug use on a single occasion or intermittently, which does not produce serious consequences for the individual or the family. WHO defines abuse in language borrowed from the American Psychiatric Association's *Diagnostic and Statistical Manual, third edition* (American Psychiatric Association, 1987). Substance abuse is defined as a "maladaptive" pattern of use indicated by "continued use despite knowledge of having a persistent or recurrent social, occupational, psychological or physical problem that is caused or exacerbated by the use [or by] recurrent use in situations in which it is physically hazardous" (WHO). Accordingly, persisting in a pattern of use in spite of substantial negative consequences is abuse. Dependence refers to a "state of needing or depending on something or someone for support or to function or survive" (WHO). Substance dependence on alcohol or a drug indicates a personal loss of control over the use and is frequently used interchangeably with addiction.

According to Hasin, Stinson, Ogburn, and Grant (2007), 8.5% of adults in the United States report having experienced alcohol use problems in the past 12 months, and 30.3% report having experienced an alcohol use problem in their lifetime. The mean duration of the substance abuse is nearly 4 years. Holman, English, Milne, and Winter (1996) reported that men who drink 4 drinks per day or more and women who drink 2 drinks per day or more show increased mortality. Alcohol is implicated in causing 22,073 deaths per year, not including suicides and homicides. Deaths from liver disease related to alcohol abuse number 13,050 per year (Heron et al., 2009). 51.9% of Americans or 130.6 million Americans reported being current drinkers in a 2009 survey (SAMHSA, 2010).

The rates of illicit drug use (or "street drug" use) in the United States are high and are increasing. In the 2009 National Survey on Drug Use and Health (NSDUH), an estimated 21.8 million Americans age 12 or older, or 8.7% of the population, used illicit drugs within the past month (SAMHSA, 2010). This included 16.7 million marijuana users, 1.6 million cocaine users, and 1.3 million users of hallucinogens. The same 2009 survey showed that 7.0 million Americans used psychoactive drugs nonmedically. Heron et al. (2009) reported that 38,396 Americans died of drug-induced causes in 2006. This number has increased steadily, at least since 1999.

In 2009, 60.7 million Americans age 12 and older were current users of a tobacco product. This represents 27.7% of the US population. 58.7 million Americans reported cigarette use, 13.3 million smoke cigars, 8.6 million report smokeless tobacco use, and 2.1 million smoke tobacco in a pipe. 15.3% of pregnant women reported cigarette use in the past month. In teen females (ages 15–17), the rate of smoking was actually higher for the pregnant females (20.6%) than for the nonpregnant (13.9%).

The National Institute on Drug Abuse estimates that the annual costs of substance abuse exceed 500 billion dollars. This figure includes direct health-care costs for treating the substance abuse, the community costs of crime by substance abusers, lost work productivity, and the costs of related social problems. The cost was 185 billion dollars for alcohol abuse, 181 billion for illicit drugs, and 168 billion for tobacco (NIDA, 2008).

According to the 2009 NSDUH, in 2009, 23.5 million Americans age 12 years or older needed treatment for an illicit drug or alcohol problem, and only 2.6 received treatment at a specialized treatment facility (SAMHSA, 2010). There is a broad social ambivalence about substance abuse treatment, reflected in comparatively poor reimbursement for substance abuse care. Reimbursements are significantly more restricted than for diagnosed medical problems, such as cancer or cardiovascular disorders. More than 48% of those Americans who received specialized treatment for substance abuse paid from their own savings and earnings. In 2009, 1.1 million Americans perceived a need for substance abuse treatment and received no treatment. Of these, 371,000 "made an effort" to obtain treatment for substance abuse and were unable to obtain treatment (SAMHSA, p. 84).

Paradigms for Substance Abuse Problems

There is a tension within the general population and within the health-care system about how to understand and treat the substance abuser, especially the alcohol and drug abuser. This tension results in a contradictory treatment of the substance abuser, and a relative reluctance to provide and fund intensive and high-quality treatment. There are three prominent models of etiology of substance abuse.

The first model treats substance abuse as a *social problem with moral dimensions*. The substance abuser is regarded as a person who makes a bad or wrong choice, and engages in illegal and antisocial behavior (Morse, 2004). The problem is approached with interdiction and punishment to discourage further immoral behavior. Loue (2003) shows how the paradigm of disease may coexist with a simultaneous trend toward increasingly harsh criminalization. The prime example is the intoxicated individual, who is apprehended while driving. Initially the intervention will combine punishment and psychoeducation: The individual will face a fine and suspension of driving privileges, along with court-ordered attendance at "drunk driver classes." With repeated offenses, the response shifts to a more punitive one over time, with longer license suspensions and incarceration.

The second model treats substance abuse as a *health problem or disease*, and the health-care approach calls for prevention, identification, and treatment (Kritz et al., 2009; McLellan, Lewis, O'Brien, & Kieber, 2000). Effective treatment presumes routine screening of patients at each primary care and specialty medical visit. Ironically, the health-care model for substance abuse is not widely practiced within the health-care system. Some physicians conclude from the high relapse rates in patients undergoing treatment for substance abuse that treatment is useless and neglect to ask even simple substance abuse screening questions. Managed healthcare benefits have also resulted in a watering down of treatment programs, with residential treatment stays shortened, and in many cases "intensive outpatient treatment" substituted for residential care.

The third model is the *addictions model*, and the treatment orientation emphasizes addiction, relapse, and a lifetime recovery process, supported by regular recovery activities (Cook, 1988a, 1988b). The primary frame of reference is the 12-step recovery model of Alcoholics Anonymous, although there is also a growing neurobiological emphasis in addiction-oriented research (Goldstein & Volkow, 2002). There is a growing network of recovery-oriented treatment programs and recovery literature supporting this model. The first step in AA is to accept that "we were powerless over alcohol, that our lives had become unmanageable." This acceptance of powerlessness serves as an antidote to the ubiquitous belief of many substance abusers, that they can just exert will power and quit when they wish.

The addictions model overlaps significantly with the health problem model, emphasizing that alcoholism and substance abuse are an addictive disease, genetically based, with a biological basis for addiction and relapse.

The Health Problem Model for Substance Abuse: An Acute Versus Chronic Disease Model?

Unrealistic expectations lead to discouragement and inaction by health professionals. The relapse rate for individuals completing substance abuse treatment programs is very high. Marlatt (1979) reported that the average time from initial abstinence to relapse for tobacco, alcohol, and the opiates ranged from 4 to 32 days. More recently, NIDA (2009) cited relapse rates at 6-month follow-up to drug abuse treatment ranging from 40 to 60%. Several studies have shown gender differences, with males relapsing consistently at higher rates than women and women on average participating in more treatment sessions per month than men (Fiorentine, Anglin, Gil-Rivas, & Taylor, 1997; Stocker, 1998).

Many physicians do not question patients about substance use during routine medical visits (Fleming & Barry, 1991), because of their beliefs that substance abuse treatment fails anyway. McLellan et al. (2000) challenged this very common attitude in an article that presents a strong case for viewing substance abuse as a chronic condition, showing many of the attributes of other chronic conditions, and requiring a modified set of treatment expectations from professionals. Substance abuse resembles other chronic conditions in many attributes. It has similarities in heritability, pathophysiology, diagnosis, course of the condition, treatment, compliance and adherence problems, and a relapsing and remitting course. Reconceptualizing substance abuse as a chronic condition to be managed transforms the approach for treatment.

The substance abuse research and treatment community supports this shift in paradigms, and many publications within the substance abuse field emphasize that health professionals need to shift their understanding, accept that the average substance

Table 7.1 Genetic heritability: substance abuse and chronic illness (McLellan et al., 2000)

Condition	Heritability
Substance abuse	
Heroin dependency (males)	0.34
Alcohol dependency (males)	0.55
Marijuana dependency (females)	0.52
Cigarette dependency (both genders)	0.61
Chronic illness	
Hypertension	0.25–0.50
Type 2 diabetes	0.80
Type 1 diabetes	0.30–0.55
Adult onset asthma	0.36–0.70

abuser will benefit from interventions, but that interventions will be required on a repeated basis over a lifetime (NIDA, 2009). More recently, O'Connor, Nyquist, and McLellan (2011) have argued for a more central place for addiction medicine in graduate medical education for primary care. This chapter relies extensively on the McLellan et al. (2000) article and later follow-ups by McLellan (2007), which describe a critical shift in medical understanding of substance abuse and addictions.

Chronic Diseases Show a Relatively Strong Genetic Component. The tendency to develop substance dependence is known to run in families, with sons of alcoholics at particular risk for more severe dependence. McLellan et al. point to twin research to support the strong heritability of substance abuse. Current estimates are that the heritability of various addictions range from 0.34 to 0.61. These figures are very similar to the heritability of hypertension (0.25–0.50), type 2 diabetes (0.80), and asthma (0.36–0.70). Table 7.1 shows the comparisons.

Like other illnesses, a single gene is not responsible for vulnerability to substances, but multiple genes affect a person's responses to alcohol and other substances. For example, a variant in the gene that produces the enzyme aldehyde dehydrogenase (ALDH1) causes some individuals to experience unpleasant effects from ingesting alcohol. Persons of Asian descent are more likely to have this variant and are a lower risk for substance abuse (Dick, 2006).

Chronic Diseases Show a Measurable Pathophysiology. In chronic illnesses, researchers identify changes in a variety of physiological systems, showing a systemic dysregulation of the nervous system, the neuroendocrine systems, and neurochemistry. Substance abuse follows this pattern, with indications of disturbance in many physiological systems, beginning with the brain. The ventral tegmental (VT) area of the brain connects the limbic cortex (the emotional brain) through the midbrain to the nucleus accumbens. The ventral tegmental system, in combination with the brain's dopamine system, produces feelings of euphoria during substance abuse.

Neurochemically, alcohol, cocaine, opiates and nicotine impact on the dopamine system, by diverse pathways. Cocaine increases synaptic dopamine and blocks dopamine reuptake into presynaptic neurons. Opiates and alcohol impact on endogenous opioids and γ-aminobutyric acid (GABA) systems. Animals receiving electrical stimulation of dopamine systems rapidly learn to press a lever thousands of times and ignore normal needs for food, water, and rest. Similarly, addictive drugs produce "supranormal" stimulation of the dopamine reward circuitry (McLellan et al., 2000). One of the challenges to individuals attempting to cease drug and alcohol use is that following periods of substance abuse, the dopamine system seems to provide almost no pleasure response without the addictive substance. Many addicts ignore enormous social and relational consequences and persist in their substance use, and report that they only feel positive when using.

In addition, the electrophysiology of the brain may be disturbed in substance abusers. Early research reported a deficiency of alpha, theta, and delta rhythms, and excesses in beta range cortical activity in alcoholics (Pollock et al., 1983). Many alcoholics report that they cannot relax without alcohol, which corresponds to a deficit in slow-wave cortical activity. After alcohol ingestion, alpha range activity increases in magnitude and slows in dominant frequency. This effect is enhanced in men and in those with a family history of alcoholism. Slow "dreamy" brain waves dominate over fast focused activity in EEG during substance use. These electrophysiological findings also serve as the basis for the "Peniston protocol," a treatment approach integrating EEG biofeedback training with substance abuse treatment (Peniston & Kulkosky, 1989; Sokkhadze, Cannon, & Trudeau, 2008). The case study in this chapter will illustrate the use of the Peniston protocol. In summary, the effect of chronic substance abuse is a dysregulation of multiple physiological systems, which is also a marker of other chronic illnesses.

Chronic Diseases Normally Follow a Relapsing and Remitting Course. Individuals with diabetes, hypertension, and asthma show a gradual progression (worsening) of the disease over time, but they also show episodes of worsening condition followed by spontaneous improvements. Substance abuse follows a similar course. The individual may abuse less severely for a time and then may suffer a crisis of intense abuse. Overall, the substance abuse tends to progress, and the individual's overall functioning will deteriorate, with social, occupational, and even spiritual impairments.

McLellan et al. (2000) point out that we do not expect one course of treatment to cure diabetes, hypertension, or heart disease. Rather, one expects these conditions to linger long term, and effective health care focuses on "managing" the disease and improving self-care. The relapse rates for substance abuse (40–60%) are quite comparable to those of several chronic conditions, including diabetes mellitus (30–50%), hypertension (50–70%), and asthma (50–70%) (NIDA, 2009, 11–12) (Table 7.2).

Objective Diagnostic Criteria. One of the markers for an illness is the presence of objective symptoms and reliable biological markers for the condition. While there is no blood test or imaging scan that can reliably identify a substance abuser, there are a number of measurable, objective symptoms and markers. The Diagnostic and Statistical Manual of Mental Disorders provides seven diagnostic criteria for substance dependence, and three of these criteria must be present for the diagnosis of addiction. Tolerance, withdrawal, and the need for larger amounts of the substance

Table 7.2 Comparison of relapse rates for substance abuse and common chronic illnesses (McLellan et al., 2000)

Condition	Relapse rates (%)
Substance abuse	40–60
Diabetes mellitus	30–50
Hypertension	50–70
Asthma	50–70

Table 7.3 Seven criteria for substance dependence (American Psychiatric Association, 2000)

DSM-IV-TR Diagnostic criteria for substance dependence
Tolerance: either (a) a need for markedly increased amounts of substance to achieve intoxication or the desired effect or (b) markedly reduced effect with continued use of the same amount of substance
Withdrawal: either (a) the characteristic withdrawal syndrome for the substance or (b) the same or closely related substance is taken to relieve or avoid withdrawal symptoms
The substance is taken in larger amounts or over longer periods than intended
There is a persistent desire or unsuccessful efforts to cut down or control substance use
A great deal of time is spent in activities necessary to obtain the substance, use the substance, or recover from its effects
Important social, occupational, or recreational activities are given up or reduced because of substance abuse
The substance use is continued despite knowing of having a persistent physical or psychological problem that is likely to have been caused or exacerbated by the substance (e.g., continued drinking despite recognition that an ulcer was made worse by alcohol use)

to produce the same effect are indications that a neurobiological process is present in addictions (Table 7.3).

The Role of Personal Responsibility. Critics of the illness model for substance abuse emphasize that the alcoholic makes a choice to take the first drink. Yet this coexistence of voluntary and involuntary elements marks each of the chronic illnesses. Hypertension has a heritability component, yet each day the individual makes choices in diet and activity that exacerbate the disease. The person with diabetes has a recognized abnormality in glucose metabolism, yet sedentary lifestyle and poor dietary choices promote weight gain and compound the variance in blood sugars. Alcoholics Anonymous emphasizes that the alcoholic is powerless over alcohol and that his/her life has become unmanageable (AA, 2004). Yet AA also provides an elaborate structure and network of self-help to assist each individual in becoming accountable to himself, to a sponsor, and to other alcoholics in the fellowship of AA. Recognizing the disease and its power becomes the vehicle for a new level of personal responsibility. This provides an excellent model for any chronic illness.

The Pathways Model: The Case of Alice

Alice was a 46-year-old career reporter, a mother of three natural children, living with her second husband. She came to me for psychological evaluation in tears and repeatedly covered her face in shame. She had met me once at a career fair, in which she was a shining example for her profession, articulate and proudly describing the joys of journalism to high school students. Alice was arrested 6 days prior to her intake interview, for driving under the influence of alcohol. She acknowledged habitual excessive drinking and progressive loss of control over alcohol in her life, since age 16, when she left home after a conflict with her parents. Her husband and children had teased her about her intoxication at times, but she had masked the severity of the problem until her arrest. Only one coworker, a woman herself in process of recovery from alcohol and cocaine abuse, had recognized the magnitude of her problem and urged Alice to seek help.

Alice initially pleaded with me to compose letters to downplay her alcohol problem and persuade the judge to throw out the legal charges. She pointed out that her arrest was a fluke. She had become afraid of arrest in the past several years and carefully limited her alcohol use to the house. That night, her daughter, a middle school honor student, had suddenly remembered a science assignment and begged her mother to take the car and obtain some poster paper for the project. Alice drove carefully, but a burned out brake light led to her being pulled over. The absence of insurance papers in the car led to more questions, and suddenly the police officer required a breathalyzer. She earned a 0.20 blood level on the breathalyzer, twice the level required for prosecution, and suddenly faced arrest. Nevertheless, Alice acknowledged the real alcohol problem that had escalated in recent months.

Alice reported in her initial interview that all alcohol use had stopped with the arrest. She experienced agitation, shakiness, and nightmares during her withdrawal, but described herself as "through the worst of it." Her physician had offered to hospitalize her for detoxification, and she declined, determined to "do it myself." Yet without alcohol and with the stress of her arrest and the subsequent newspaper report of her arraignment, Alice's anxiety escalated to the point of chronic daily tension and edginess and panic attacks three to five times a week. Looking back, Alice recognized a pattern of severe recurrent anxiety and worry throughout her adult years, worse during times of marital and work stress, but almost never entirely absent. Alcohol moderated the anxiety, and whenever Alice's anxiety and worry increased, her drinking did as well. In her panic attacks, Alice experienced fears of complete exposure of her alcohol problems to her business colleagues and to her mother. She also experienced an unmanageable worry that she was losing her mind and everyone around her would soon know.

Alice also reported disturbed sleep. For the past 6 months, she had been working a second job as a waitress, to manage the mortgage payments, since her husband's overtime pay was slashed. The irregular work hours contributed to a lifelong pattern of very light and erratic sleep, seemingly reactive to nightmares and nighttime ruminations. While discussing her sleep problems, Alice also disclosed use of up to six high-caffeine energy drinks each day, to aid her in remaining awake and alert, in spite of sleep deprivation. The caffeine intake exacerbated the sleep problem, with an edgy irritability persisting into the night, for several hours after her last energy drink.

Level One Interventions. Alice's initial Level One intervention was mindful breathing. Alice had studied yoga for weight loss the previous year and was able to demonstrate effective diaphragmatic breathing in her first session. She was able to experience a calming effect within the first 2 minutes of mindful breathing during her first interview but admitted she had entirely forgotten about her positive experiences with paced, slow diaphragmatic breathing that she had learned during the yoga class.

Alice was also encouraged to reduce the number of energy drinks taken to two daily, with none after 4 PM, and to keep a daily log of caffeine use, anxiety levels, and quality and length of sleep.

Alice began using paced, mindful breathing daily and expressed surprise at the calming effect. She began to use the breathing as a coping strategy each time conflict emerged at home and noticed that both her husband and middle school age daughter also seemed calmer following Alice's use of relaxation. Nonetheless, conflicts continued at home, aggravated by the daughter's embarrassment and anger at her mother's arrest. However, Alice found herself talking more calmly with her daughter about both of their emotions, in a new and unfamiliar way.

Giving up the energy drinks presented a challenge for Alice. She decided to stop rather than reduce caffeine and was surprised at the change. She fell asleep driving in the first week without caffeine and nearly collided with another car. She also dozed off in a news conference at work, eliciting a reprimand from her editor. Episodes of extreme edginess and irritability were frequent. By the end of the week, however, she began to sleep more restfully through the night. In the second week without caffeine, she felt calmer, with increasing energy and less drowsiness.

Level Two Interventions. Given her level of emotional reactivity, Alice's first Level Two intervention was the cultivation of mindfulness—learning to view experience with attention and acceptance, and without judgment. Alice began her study of mindfulness using a CD from Jon Kabat-Zinn (2006) and signed up for an upcoming class on mindfulness through her church. As she cultivated mindfulness, Alice seemed to respond more slowly and thoughtfully, as she consciously sought to observe and not judge events.

Alice reported that her growing practice of mindfulness had a calming effect rippling through her family and workplace. Her daughter still argued frequently, angry about her school friends reading about her mother's arrest. Yet the daughter sought her mother out more, talked more, and began to show affection to her mother. Alice began to see her daughter differently, through the mindful lens, as a young woman struggling with her own emotions and challenges. She was surprised at seeing her daughter this way, as a separate human being in her own right, and also surprised to realize that this perception had never occurred before.

On her own, Alice decided to resume yoga. Use of mindful breathing reminded her how much she had enjoyed yoga. The yoga asanas further moderated her anxiety and jittery feelings. She felt good taking time for herself away from her two jobs and the family. The yoga practices also reinforced her reduced emotional reactivity. The treatment team affirmed her motivation to use yoga but did not record this as part of her official Level Two plan. There was concern that Alice would probably not be able to keep up with yoga given the rest of her program.

The primary therapist referred Alice to Alcoholics Anonymous (AA) and suggested the traditional "90 in 90"—90 meetings in her first 90 days of sobriety. Alice's court caseworker had earlier emphasized AA attendance and Alice was required to turn in a log of meetings attended. Alice resisted AA initially, but began to comply because of the court requirement. She spent the better part of one treatment session lampooning recovery dialog in the AA sessions, and protesting against the declaration of powerlessness in the AA first step. Alice's therapist encouraged her to initially "just be there" in AA sessions, and practice her mindfulness presence.

After her initial reluctance, Alice became gradually more enthused about 12-step work and began to read recovery-oriented literature. She selected a sponsor and asked the sponsor to hold her accountable for abstinence from alcohol. When her spouse became resentful of her time spent away at AA meetings, she "twisted his arm" until he attended Al-Anon with her, the 12-step-based program for partners and family members. He had never admitted to himself that Alice was an alcoholic, and he had coached her initially to comply with treatment on the surface, just enough to obtain a lighter sentence. He became more supportive after seeing several respected families present, listening to their similar experiences with a family member's drinking, and hearing their common challenges around the recovery process.

As expected, Alice found the demands of AA overwhelming and soon dropped her yoga class. But, she made a promise to herself to return to the yoga in the future, once she felt more confident of reaching some kind of maintenance level, at which point two to three AA meetings in a week might suffice.

Level Three Interventions. Alice's Level Three interventions included biofeedback and neurofeedback. Alice began with *heart rate variability (HRV) biofeedback*, using her mindful breathing skills to drive larger heart rate variations. HRV biofeedback was chosen both because of Alice's joy in mastering mindful breathing and as an added tool to assist her with anxiety management.

The biofeedback instruments were used to display for Alice the process of her own breathing, in a line graph display tracking each inhalation and exhalations as a rise and then fall in the line graph. A parallel line graph showed her how her heart rate increased with each inhalation and decreased with each exhalation. The treatment team identified the optimal breath rate, which researcher Paul Lehrer calls the "resonance frequency," at which the largest oscillations in heart rate occur (Lehrer, Vaschillo, & Vaschillo, 2000). In Alice's case, breathing at 6.5 breaths a minute produced the optimal HRV and a deeper subjective sense of relaxation.

She found that the biofeedback HRV practice increased her control over her breathing and enabled her to manage anxiety episodes more effectively. Alice also found herself feeling excited at controlling her physiology, after years of feeling that her body and alcohol use were out of her control. In Alice's case, the HRV biofeedback served as preparation for her second Level Three intervention, *EEG neurofeedback*, following the Peniston protocol for substance abuse treatment neurofeedback is synonymous with EEG biofeedback.

The Peniston Neurofeedback Protocol was inspired by early clinical work at the Menninger Clinic, conducted by biofeedback pioneers Elmer and Alyce Green and Dale Walters. Later Eugene Peniston perfected a specific combination of therapeutic elements in controlled research studies with severe alcoholic combat veterans in a Veterans Administration hospital, many of whom also showed signs of PTSD (Peniston & Kulkosky, 1989). The protocol is based on the research finding, mentioned earlier, that the EEG of alcoholics and substance abusers shows serious abnormalities. A recent article reviewed the research on the Peniston protocol and rated it as "probably efficacious" for substance abuse disorders (Sokkhadze et al., 2008).

The Peniston protocol includes several components. EEG biofeedback instruments are used to train alcoholics to increase alpha and theta range (slow-wave) cortical activity, producing a state of deeply relaxed consciousness. The alpha/theta states are used therapeutically to enable emotional abreaction of past traumatic memories and painful emotional experiences. During the alpha/theta states, patients are also guided to visualize successful abstinence and greater feelings of social ease, without the use of alcohol. The Peniston protocol also includes autogenic training and thermal biofeedback (hand-warming training guided by biofeedback instrumentation) to produce deep autonomic nervous system relaxation.

Alice was initially uneasy about the state of consciousness she experienced with alpha/theta training. She felt "loose" and out of control. However, over the course of several sessions, she reconceptualized it as a new deeper kind of control. She felt excited to really feel herself vividly present as she visualized being at ease at a work party without alcohol and also pictured herself in job interviews, pursuing alternate job positions with greater confidence.

During therapy, Alice also abreacted a number of painful emotional episodes from her childhood years and the difficult years during her first marriage. She was shocked at the intensity of the feelings yet connected the visual images that flooded her with the nightmares that had disturbed her sleep during most of her adult years. She had been abused emotionally and physically as a child and then experienced physical abuse in the first marriage. She had always told herself that these events were "past tense," done, and not affecting her. Yet in the twilight state of consciousness induced by alpha/theta training, she experienced both recognition of the intensity of her past pain and a sense of deeper healing. The nightmares also stopped after 10 weeks of alpha/theta sessions.

Case Summary. In summary, substance abuse is a chronic condition, with biological, familial, and individual components. The natural history of substance abuse is typically characterized by remissions and relapses, and repeated treatment is often needed. The Pathways Model does not erase the power of addiction but provides a useful stepwise organization for interventions.

Alice, whose case was presented above, showed a long-term comorbidity of generalized anxiety disorder with severe alcoholism. In retrospect, there were also indications of posttraumatic stress disorder, with her sleep disturbed by nightmare images of past abuse. Nevertheless, Alice had functioned at a high level in her profession and compartmentalized the alcohol abuse to nighttime drinking. Once faced with the shame of arrest, she mustered the ability to channel her admirable personal determination into the recovery process, integrating a variety of Level One, Level Two, and Level Three changes in her life within a period of 6 months.

Her Level One interventions included mindful breathing and an elimination of the high-caffeine energy drinks she had abused daily. These Level One interventions, along with abstinence from daily alcohol use, served to begin the restoration of normal biological cycles of sleep and wakefulness and to give her an initial tool for self-calming.

Her Level Two interventions were mindfulness training and Alcoholics Anonymous. The mindfulness training augmented her self-calming. She developed an ability to absorb events in a more detached and peaceful fashion, which impacted positively on her relationships at home. The AA attendance was central to her entire recovery process, but she initially resisted it. Over time, the deeper understanding of addiction that came with participation in AA and reading AA educational material guided much of her personal thinking about her life.

Alice's Level Three interventions included biofeedback and neurofeedback. She experienced the HRV biofeedback as a natural extension of her breath practices and of her mindfulness. She expressed a deeper level of calm and self-acceptance with each additional HRV biofeedback session. The alpha/theta states bothered her at first but became a tool for a useful rehearsal in her mind of successful coping without alcohol. Finally, the alpha/theta training also served to help her in healing some of the painful memories that had haunted her dreams.

Alice thrived on this combination of Level One, Two, and Three treatments. She felt alive and excited about her life in a new way. Nevertheless, part of the patient education process included an emphasis on substance abuse education. The real risk of relapse was emphasized, the need for ongoing recovery-oriented support activities and the need for lifelong self-care.

At her final visit, Alice expressed a growing confidence in her sobriety. Alice felt like a new person in many ways. She discontinued her second job early in the treatment process yet found that the family funds could be managed to cover their needs. Her family reported pride in her transformation, and both spouse and the angry daughter expressed gratitude that she had been arrested, triggering the whole process of change. At 5 years, her positive life changes continued.

References

Alcoholics Anonymous. (2004). *Twelve steps and twelve traditions*. New York, NY: Alcoholics Anonymous World Services.

American Psychiatric Association. (1987). *Diagnostic and statistical manual of mental disorders (3rd ed., Revised)*. Washington, DC: American Psychiatric Association.

American Psychiatric Association. (2000). *Diagnostic and statistical manual of mental disorders (4th ed., Text Revision)*. Washington, DC: American Psychiatric Association.

Cook, C. (1988a). The Minnesota Model in the management of drug and alcohol dependency: Miracle, method or myth? Part I. The philosophy and the programme. *British Journal of Addictions, 83*(6), 625–634.

References

Cook, C. (1988b). The Minnesota Model in the management of drug and alcohol dependency: Miracle, method or myth? Part II. Evidence and conclusions. *British Journal of Addictions, 83*(7), 735–748.

Dick, D. M. (2006). Endophenotypes successfully lead to gene identification; results from the collaborative study on the genetics of alcoholism. *Behavioral Genetics, 36*(1), 112–126.

Fiorentine, R., Anglin, M. D., Gil-Rivas, V., & Taylor, E. (1997). Drug treatment: Explaining the gender paradox. *Substance Use and Misuse, 32*(6), 653–678.

Fleming, M. F., Barry, K. L., & MacDonald, R. (1991). The Alcohol Use Disorders Identification Test (AUDIT) in a College Sample. *International Journal of Addictions, 26*, 1173–1185.

Goldstein, R. Z., & Volkow, N. D. (2002). Drug addiction and its underlying neurobiological basis: Neuroimaging evidence for the involvement of the frontal cortex. *The American Journal of Psychiatry, 159*(10), 1642–1652. doi:10.1176/appi.ajp. 159.10.1642.

Hasin, D. S., Stinson, F. S., Ogburn, E., & Grant, B. F. (2007). Prevalence, correlates, disability, and comorbidity of DSM-IV alcohol abuse and dependence in the United States: Results from the National Epidemiologic Survey on Alcohol and Related Conditions. *Archives of General Psychiatry, 64*, 830–842.

Heron, M. P., Hoyert, D. L., Murphy, S. L., Xu, J. Q., Kochanek, K. D., & Tejada-Vera, B. (2009). Deaths: Final data for 2006. *National Vital Statistics Reports, 57*(14), 1–136. Available at http://www.cdc.gov/nchs/data/nvsr/nvsr57/nvsr57_14.pdf.

Holman, C. D., English, D. R., Milne, E., & Winter, M. G. (1996). Meta-analysis of alcohol and all-cause mortality: A validation of NHMRC recommendations. *The Medical Journal of Australia, 164*, 141–145.

Kabat-Zinn, J. (2006). *Mindfulness for beginners: Explore the infinite potential that lies within this very moment.* (CD). Louisville, CO: Sounds True, Inc.

Kritz, S., Chu, M., John-Hull, C., Madray, C., Louie, B., & Brown, L. (2009). Opioid dependence as a chronic disease: The interrelationships between length of stay, methadone dose, and age on treatment outcome at an urban opioid treatment program. *Journal of Addictive Diseases, 28*(1), 53–56.

Lehrer, P. M., Vaschillo, E., & Vaschillo, B. (2000). Resonant frequency biofeedback training to increase cardiac variability. Rationale and manual for training. *Applied Psychophysiology and Biofeedback, 25*(3), 177–191.

Loue, S. (2003). The criminalization of the addictions. *Journal of Legal Medicine, 24*(3), 281. doi:10.1080/01947640390231948.

Marlatt, G. A. (1979). A cognitive-behavioral model of the relapse process. In N. A. Krasnegor (Ed.), *Behavioral analysis and treatment of substance abuse. National Institute on Drug Abuse, research monograph no. 25..* Washington, US: Govt. Printing Office.

McLellan, A. T. (2007). Reducing heavy drinking: A public health strategy and a treatment goal? *Journal of Substance Abuse Treatment, 33*(1), 81–83.

McLellan, A. T., Lewis, D. C., O'Brien, C. P., & Kieber, H. D. (2000). Drug dependency: A chronic medical illness. *Journal of the American Medical Association, 284*(13), 1689–1695.

Morse, S. J. (2004). Medicine and morals, craving and compulsion. *Substance Use & Misuse, 39*(3), 437–460. doi:10.1081/JA-120029985.

O'Connor, P. G., Nyquist, J. G., & McLellan, A. T. (2011). Integrating addiction medicine into graduate medical education in primary care: The time has come. *Annals of Internal Medicine, 154*(1), 56–59.

Peniston, E. G., & Kulkosky, P. J. (1989). Alpha-theta brainwave training and beta endorphin levels in alcoholics. *Alcoholism: Clinical and Experimental Results, 13*(2), 271–279.

Pollock, V. E., Volavka, J., Goodwin, D. W., Mednick, S. A., Gabrielli, W. F., Knop, J., et al. (1983). The EEG after alcohol in men at risk for alcoholism. *Archives of General Psychiatry, 40*, 857–864.

Sokkhadze, E. M., Cannon, R. L., & Trudeau, D. (2008). EEG biofeedback as a treatment for substance use disorders: Review, rating of efficacy and recommendations for further research. *Applied Psychophysiology and Biofeedback, 33*(1), 1–28.

Stocker, S. (1998). Men and women in drug abuse treatment relapse at different rates and for different reasons. *NIDA Notes, 13*(4), 1–4. Available at http://www.aegisuniversity.com/Nida%20Notes%20-%20Drug%20Abuse%20Treatment/Men%20and%20Women%20in%20Drug%20Abuse%20Treatment%20Relapse%20at%20Different%20Rates%20and%20for%20Different%20Reasons.pdf.

Substance Abuse and Mental Health Services Administration (SAMHSA). (2010). *Results from the 2009 National Survey on Drug Use and Health: Volume I. Summary of National Findings (Office of Applied Studies, NSDUH Series H-38A, HHS Publication No. SMA 10-4586Findings)*. Rockville, MD. Available at http://www.oas.samhsa.gov/NSDUH/2k9NSDUH/2k9ResultsP.pdf.

U.S. Department of Health and Human Services, National Institutes of Health, National Institute on Drug Abuse. (2008). *Understanding drug abuse and addiction*. Retrieved January 5, 2013, from http://drugabuse.gov/PDF/InfoFacts/Understanding08.pdf.

U.S. Department of Health and Human Services, National Institutes of Health, National Institute on Drug Abuse. (2009). *Principles of drug addiction treatment: A research-based guide* (2nd ed.). (NIH Publication No. 09–4180). Retrieved January 5, 2013, from http://www.nida.nih.gov/PDF/PODAT/PODAT.pdf.

World Health Organization. (no date). *Lexicon of alcohol and drug terms published by the World Health Organization*. Website of the World Health Organization. Available at http://www.who.int/substance_abuse/terminology/who_lexicon/en/.

Chapter 8
Depression

Abstract Depression is a serious disorder, affecting 12 % of adult males and 25 % of adult females in the United States, and approximately 121 million people worldwide. Depression frequently progresses to a chronic condition, often producing disability. The social, economic, and medical costs are substantial. Depression has a strong heritability, based on a polygenic transmission. Environmental factors contribute substantially to the onset, maintenance, and chronicity of depression, in the form of depressed parents, social learning, stressful life events, separation and loss, and psychological trauma. Pathways approaches to healing depression draw on nutrition, exercise, social support, imagery, psychotherapy, and a variety of mind-body and complementary therapies.

Keywords Depression • Anxiety • Mood • Prevalence • Neurobiological mechanisms • Integrative treatment

Introduction

Clinical depression is a disabling problem affecting mood, physical health, and thinking, characterized by sad mood, loss of motivation or interest, fatigue, absence of joy, irritability, hopelessness, and a number of physical and behavioral symptoms. Clinical depression goes beyond everyday sadness or discouragement. It is more severe, pervasive, and longer lasting and undermines social relationships, occupational functioning, and ability to manage everyday life. Current psychiatric diagnostic nomenclature distinguishes major depression, dysthymic disorder, bipolar disorder, adjustment reactions with depressive mood to common stressors, and depression, not otherwise specified (APA, 2000).

Clinical Depression: Incidence and Costs

One recent report estimates that depression affects 25% of women and 12% of men in the United States in their lifetime and is frequently a chronic disorder (Gelenberg, 2010). The more episodes an individual experiences, the higher the risk for future depressive episodes, worsening the course of the disorder with each episode.

Major population studies support these estimates of incidence and chronicity. According to the National Institute of Mental Health Epidemiological Catchment Area (ECA) study, conducted between 1980 and 1985, the 1-year prevalence of mood disorders in the United States was 9.5%, and the lifetime prevalence was reported as 20.8% (Robins & Regier, 1991). The National Comorbidity Survey (NCS), conducted between 1990 and 1992, produced a slightly higher estimate for 1-year prevalence of 11.1% for all mood disorders (Kessler et al., 1994).

Looking at specific depressive disorders, 6.7% of the US adult population suffers a major depressive episode in any 1-year period and 16.5% in their lifetime (Kessler, Chiu, Demler, & Walters, 2005; Kessler, Berglund, Demler, Jin, & Walters, 2005). For dysthymic disorder, a chronic low level of depression, with many cognitive and emotional symptoms, 1.5% of the adult population suffers dysthymia each year, and 2.5% of the adult population suffers this disorder in their lifetimes (Kessler, Chiu, Demler, & Walters, 2005).

Both the ECA and NCS studies were exhaustive population studies, the ECA study covering 18.571 households and 2,290 institutional residents, 18 years or older, and the NCS study 8,098 adolescents and adults. Estimates for persons with depression, based on the NCS study, show that about 51.7% of persons with depression receive health-care services for their depression, and only 38% of persons receiving care are getting adequate treatment (Wang et al., 2005). Thus approximately 70% of depressed persons continue to suffer, lacking adequate professional help for their disorder.

The surveys also showed that particular groups are more vulnerable to depression. For example, women are 50% more likely to experience a mood disorder in their lifetime than men; non-Hispanic blacks are 40% less likely, and Hispanics 20% less likely than non-Hispanic whites to suffer a mood disorder in their lifetime (Robins & Regier, 1991). Focusing specifically on major depression, women are 70% more likely than men to suffer a depressive episode in their lifetime, and individuals 30–44 years old are 120% more likely than persons over 60 to suffer a depressive episode (Kessler, Berglund, Demler, Jin, & Walters, 2005; NIMH, 2011).

Depression is not merely a disorder of the affluent West. Currently, between 2 and 15% of the world population suffers with clinical depression (Moussavvi et al., 2007). The World Health Organization estimates that depression affects 121 million persons worldwide (WHO, 2012). Globally, less than 25% of persons with depression have access to effective treatment (WHO).

Human, economic, and medical costs of depression are vast, both in the United States and globally, although surveys produce widely varying estimates of the actual costs. The National Alliance on Mental Illness (NAMI, 2011) reports that 15% of depressed persons in the United States take their own life, resulting in 30,000 deaths per year. As one of the leading causes of disability, depression robs individuals, families, and industry of personal productivity. Depression is a leading cause for absenteeism from the workplace and low productivity on the job (PWMH, 2012). NAMI reports that workplace costs (direct and indirect) in the United States exceed $34 billion per year (2011). Medical costs include both the direct cost of treating depression and those of increased utilization of medical care for other illnesses. Depressed patients ask for medical care more frequently, often presenting physical symptoms to primary care or specialty clinics. A study by Henk, Katzelnick, Kobak, Gresit, and Jefferson (1996) examined 50,000 patients within a health maintenance organization, identified a subgroup of high utilizers, and found that those high utilizers with depression had an average of $1,498 more medical costs in 1 year than nondepressed patients. This figure represents increased use of general medical services, as well as the direct costs of treating depression.

Mechanisms and Models for Depression

Genetics

Depression is a disorder that is clearly affected by multiple pathways. A meta-analysis of twin studies estimated the heritability of major depression to be 37% (Sullivan, Neale, & Kendler, 2000). Efforts to isolate specific genes contributing to this heritability have as yet been inconclusive. Gene studies to date suggest that depression is polygenic in nature, that is, that multiple genes interact, each exerting relatively small effects on the vulnerability to depression (Demirkan et al., 2011). Genes involved in neurotransmitter circuits and in reactivity to stress are implicated (Levinson, 2006; Lopez-Leon et al., 2008). The evidence also suggests that there is a shared genetic basis for depression and anxiety.

Genetics define the first pathway predisposing an individual to clinical depression.

Neurochemical and Neuroscience Models of Depression

Much of the pharmacologic approach to depression emerged from the monoamine theory, which states that a deficiency in the neurotransmitter chemical serotonin is one of the biological bases for depression. The selective serotonergic reuptake inhibitor (SSRI) class of medications enhances the availability of serotonin in the synapse and has been widely accepted as a first-line treatment for depression. Other research targeted deficiencies in dopamine and norepinephrine or combined deficiencies of two neurotransmitters. Additional neurochemical systems have also been investigated for their role in the etiology of depression, including cholinergic, glutamatergic, GABAegic, glucocorticoid, and peptidergic systems (Drevets, Price, & Furey, 2008).

The advent of neuroimaging has also made it possible to investigate abnormalities in brain structure and function, producing "neurocircuitry models" for depression. Neural networks including the medial prefrontal cortex, the medial and caudolateral orbital cortex, the amygdala, the hippocampus, and ventromedial areas of the basal ganglia appear to be involved in the regulation of normal mood, and deficiencies in these circuits are implicated in the etiology of depression. Drevets et al. (2008) and Price and Drevets (2012) discussed current neurocircuitry models in greater detail and proposed that dysfunction "in and between the medial prefrontal cortex and related limbic structures" can account for the various emotional, cognitive, neurochemical, autonomic, and other manifestations of depression.

Neurochemistry and neurocircuitry describe the neurophysiological processes accompanying depression. The original pathways leading to depression may be genetic or psychosocial or an interaction of the two; neurophysiological dysregulation contributes to the chronicity of depression and its resistance to treatment.

Environmental Factors

Environmental factors contribute significantly to depression. Silberg, Maes, and Eaves (2010) emphasized that the depressed parent contributes to the child's genetic risk for depression, but the presence of a depressed parent, with her/his mood, modeling, and overt behavior, in the home contributes further to the child's vulnerability to depression.

As discussed in Chap. 3, Psychosocial Pathways to Illness and Health, separation and loss, emotional trauma, and stressful life events all can serve as significant triggers for illness, including depression and anxiety. A recent study in the Netherlands of adults with depression or anxiety found that 18.4% reported a stressful life event in childhood and 57.8% reported childhood trauma. Those with childhood emotional neglect or psychological abuse were more likely to suffer chronic depression and/or anxiety (Hovens et al., 2012). Grieving individuals are also at increased risk for clinical depression and anxiety. Boelen and van den Bout (2005) studied 1,321 bereaved individuals and confirmed their heightened risk for three distinct clusters of emotional symptoms: complicated grief, clinical depression, and anxiety disorders.

Separation and loss, stressful life events, and trauma are all pathways to depression. In some cases, early losses or trauma predisposes the individual to later life depression. In other cases, the loss or traumatic event is the immediate trigger setting the depressive episode into play.

Comorbidity with Other Disorders

Depression is frequently found in individuals also bearing other diagnoses, including anxiety, substance abuse, and chronic medical illness. According to the National Comorbidity Study Replication, 59% of persons with major depression also have been diagnosed in their lifetime with an anxiety disorder. Depression also is frequently comorbid with a variety of medical illnesses, especially chronic conditions (Katon & Ciechanowski, 2002). The likelihood of comorbidities also increases with successive episodes of depression. A recent Spanish study of patients in primary care showed that 71.1% of first-episode depressed patients reported the presence of at least one medical condition and 88.6% of patients with recurrent episodes reported one or more medical condition (Gili et al., 2011). Using cardiac disease as an example, the World Mental Health Survey found a twofold increased risk for depression in patients with heart disease, compared to patients without heart disease (Ormel et al., 2007). Rudisch and Nemeroff (2003) found prevalence rates for depression in patients with coronary artery disease ranging between 17 and 27%.

A serious vicious circle is evident between depression and illness. Premorbid depression, with its associated cognitions and behaviors, increases the patient's vulnerability for illness. Living with illness is stressful and discouraging and frequently triggers depressive episodes. Depression also reduces patient compliance with medical care and self-management practices, such as in diabetes, thus worsening the course of illness (Di Matteo, Lepper, & Croghan, 2000). When chronically ill patients are also depressed, their quality of life is lowered and mortality and morbidity increase, compared to nondepressed individuals with the same illness (Baumeister, Hutter, Bengel, & Härter, 2011; Herrmann-Lingen & Buss, 2006). For example, depression clearly lowers heart rate variability and increases morbidity and mortality in patients following myocardial infarction (Barth, Schumacher, & Herrmann-Lingen, 2004; Carney et al., 2001).

Comorbidities are important to consider in developing treatment plans for a patient. Assisting a depressed patient to better manage stress or moderate anxiety frequently reduces the severity of depressed mood. Depressed patients also suffering an anxiety disorder are more likely to attempt suicide (Bronisch & Wittchen, 1994). Depression in combination with a chronic physical illness also elevates suicidality and lowers health-related quality of life (Katon & Ciechanowski, 2002; Moussavvi et al., 2007).

Moussavvi et al. (2007) reviewed World Health Surveys in 60 nations and reported that while 3.2% of respondents suffered from depression alone, between 9.3 and 23% of respondents with one or more chronic physical illness also reported depression. Consistently across the 60 countries, those depressed individuals with one or more chronic illness had the worst health scores of any group. Their conclusion was that depression produces the greatest decrement in health, compared with other chronic diseases. This is consistent and lends support to the 1996 projection that depression will be the second highest source of disease burden, globally, by the year 2020, second only to ischemic heart disease (Murry & Lopez, 1996).

Comorbidities are pathways to depression. Anxiety, substance abuse, and chronic illness frequently accompany depression. The presence of depression renders the individual more vulnerable to medical problems becoming chronic and undermines the individual's ability to comply with medical care and carry out effective illness self-management. In turn, the presence of the anxiety, substance abuse, or chronic medical condition may trigger depression or exacerbate its intensity. Treating the depression improves the prognosis of the comorbid illness and vice versa.

Interventions

Medication

The NICE guidelines for the treatment of depression recommend pharmacological and/or psychological interventions (Churchill et al., 2010; NICE, 2009). The first line of treatment for the average depressed patient in primary care is antidepressant medication (NICE, 2009). In addition, the number of depressed outpatients receiving medication alone has increased between 1998 and 2007, from 44.1 to 57.4% (Olfson & Marcus, 2010). Direct advertising of medications to the consumer has increased the frequency of patients requesting specific medications, and medical education favors pharmaceutical intervention. The physician today has a large number of medications to consider, including several categories based on the drug's actions.

The most widely used category of antidepressant currently is the selective serotonin reuptake inhibitors (SSRIs), including fluoxetine (Prozac), sertraline (Zoloft), citalopram (Celexa), paroxetine (Paxil), escitalopram (Lexapro), and vilazodone (Viibryd), which serve to enhance the availability of serotonin in the synapse (NIMH, 2012). These agents have a lower side effect profile than the tricyclics and MAOIs but can still cause drowsiness, dry mouth, weight gain, impotence, and other bothersome side effects. They are unlikely to be lethal in overdose.

Also widely used are several categories of medication targeting combinations of neurotransmitters: norepinephrine-dopamine reuptake inhibitors such as bupropion (Wellbutrin), and serotonin-norepinephrine reuptake inhibitors such as desvenlafaxine (Pristiq) and duloxetine (Cymbalta). One additional category of medications, norepinephrine reuptake inhibitors such as atomoxetine (Strattera), is more often utilized for attention disorders than for clinical depression.

An older class of antidepressants still in widespread use is the tricyclic antidepressants, such as amitriptyline (Elavil). These medications enhance the availability of synaptic norepinephrine and serotonin, but in usual doses produce many adverse effects, such as increased heart rate, dry mouth, constipation, impotence, and other unpleasant effects. They are also frequently lethal in overdoses. Today, they are most often used at lower doses in patients with chronic pain or insomnia to moderate pain, enhance sleep, and lift mood with fewer significant side effects.

The monoamine oxidase inhibitors (MAOIs) such as phenelzine (Nardil) block the action of enzyme monoamine oxidase, which breaks down several neurotransmitters. They are effective in improving mood but are rarely used due to potentially fatal interactions with foods containing tyramine. However, a newer generation MAOI, moclobemide (Manerix), is being increasingly prescribed, because it has the mood lifting effectiveness of the older MAOIs without the dangerous interactions with food.

Treatment with a single medication is frequently not sufficient to remediate depression (Moller et al., 2012). Psychiatric physicians are more likely than primary care physicians to utilize combinations of two or more antidepressant medications or add additional categories of medications such as anxiolytics, neuroleptics, or mood stabilizers, to augment the effects of the antidepressant medicine. However, the risk of adverse effects increases exponentially with polypharmacy.

Medications seem to offer quick and effective relief from a troubling problem. However, in spite of the availability of newer medications, patients continue to suffer adverse effects, and many medications lose efficacy over time. Patients grow frustrated with side effects and with the need to make repeated changes in medication or dosage. Frequently, patients with a positive improvement in mood and minimal adverse effects will still discontinue early, because of inadequate education about the medication, discomfort with taking medication, or the cost of medication. Eaddy and Regan (2003) analyzed data on 740,000 patients prescribed with SSRIs and reported that 50% of the patients failed to adhere to the medication regimen for 60 days and only 28% were compliant at 6 months.

Antidepressant medication is a widely followed pathway to recovery. Adverse effects and persistence of depression in spite of medication call for the individual to utilize other pathways as well.

Psychotherapy

Survey research has shown that patients prefer psychological intervention over antidepressant medication (Riedel-Heller, Matschinger, & Angermeyer, 2005). Yet, many physicians express reluctance to refer for psychotherapy because of patient resistance, poor insurance reimbursement for the costs of psychotherapy, and psychotherapists' neglect of communication with the referring physician. When researchers examined physician's failure to provide recommended combination treatments for depression, physician's attributed over 75% of the barriers to patient-centered factors such as patient resistance and noncompliance (Nutting et al., 2002). The likelihood of a successful referral and physician satisfaction with referral increase when the psychotherapist is on site within primary care, in integrated care practices (Gallo et al., 2004). Adding case management services also reduces dropouts from psychotherapy, even in high-risk populations (Miranda, Azocar, Organista, Munoz, & Lieberman, 1996).

Several forms of psychotherapy are widely utilized for depression, including cognitive behavioral therapy, interpersonal psychotherapy, brief dynamic psychotherapy, and, increasingly the so-called new wave therapies—mindfulness-based psychotherapy and acceptance and commitment therapy (Hofmann & Asmundson, 2008). These psychotherapy approaches have been discussed in Chapter Six on Pathways Interventions.

Research on psychotherapy shows consistent empirical support for psychotherapy for depression. Large effect sizes have been shown for cognitive behavioral therapy (Weerasekera, 2010) and interpersonal psychotherapy (DeMello, de Jesus, Bacaltchuk, Verdeli, & Neugebauer, 2005; Weerasekera, 2010), and moderate to large effect sizes for brief dynamic psychotherapy (Driessen et al., 2010; Weerasekera, 2010). Generally, psychotherapy has performed as well as medication in research studies. Once treatment ends, psychotherapy effects are more enduring than medication effects, thus reducing the risk of relapse (Hollon et al., 2005; Hougaard & Jorgensen, 2007). In severe or complex cases, especially, a combination of psychotherapy and medication produces better results than those that are achieved with either treatment alone (Hollon et al., 2005; Hougaard & Jorgensen, 2007).

Cognitive behavioral therapy and interpersonal psychotherapy have been most widely investigated, but efforts to identify a specific type of psychotherapy as most effective have produced mixed results. Chambless and Ollendick (2001) reviewed all available well constructed studies of clinical efficacy and clinical effectiveness. Clinical efficacy refers to the ability of a therapy to perform well under the controlled conditions of a research study. Clinical effectiveness refers to the ability of a therapy to perform well under the real-world conditions of a typical clinic. Efficacy studies include more homogeneous samples, excluding any patients with multiple diagnoses. Effectiveness studies must include a wider range of diverse patients, some with comorbidities, others with intolerance to certain medicines.

For children and adolescents, cognitive behavioral therapy was more effective than supportive therapy or nondirective therapy in reducing the symptoms of depression, including major depression (Chambless & Ollendick, 2001). In several efficacy studies with adults, psychotherapy was shown to be effective in treating depression, but no significant differences were found among cognitive behavioral therapy, interpersonal therapy, and brief dynamic psychotherapy (Elkin et al., 1989; Thompson, Gallagher, & Steinmetz Breckenridge, 1987). Studies of clinical effectiveness showed higher drop out rates than efficacy studies and, in some cases, included significantly more treatment sessions. Nevertheless, these studies also showed that psychotherapy (primarily CBT in these studies) produced significant reductions in depressive symptoms (Chambless & Ollendick, 2001).

Critics of the effort to identify specific forms of psychotherapy that have the greatest clinical efficacy or clinical effectiveness point out that there are other variables that predict therapeutic effect. For example, although CBT has been shown repeatedly to have strong efficacy and clinical effectiveness for depression, CBT also has the highest drop out rate in many studies, and problem solving psychotherapy has the lowest drop out rate (Cuijpers, van Straten, Andersson, & van Oppen, 2008). Patients who drop out do not benefit from treatment.

Elliott, Bohart, Watson, and Greenberg (2011) have argued that therapists showing more empathy have produced better treatment outcomes, regardless of the specific form of psychotherapy. Churchill et al. (2010) have recommended research on integrative forms of psychotherapy, drawing on several forms of therapeutic intervention, according to patient needs. In clinical practice, a high percentage of psychotherapists utilize an eclectic or integrative form of psychotherapy and not one specific approach.

Psychotherapy is a powerful pathway to health for depressed patients. A number of forms of psychotherapy have been shown to be as effective as medication for mild to moderate depression. For severe depression, the combination of psychotherapy plus medication produces more improvement, and the improvement is more long-lasting than either treatment alone. The therapist's empathy is a critical factor in improving mood, regardless of therapeutic model. Integrative therapy drawing on interventions from several treatment approaches allows for individualizing the treatment for the individual patient.

Exercise

Exercise has long been a common sense strategy for coping with depressed mood. Several studies have investigated the relationship between the intensity, frequency, and duration of exercise and mood. A review by Teychenne, Ball, and Salmon (2008) showed that physical activity, in both short and long durations, was associated with improved mood. Physical activity of more vigorous intensity was associated with greater reductions in depression than less vigorous activity. Nevertheless, activity of any intensity produced improvements in mood (Teychenne et al.). In other words, exercise need not be strenuous to affect mood. A recent study of over 40,000 Norwegians examined the relationship between physically active leisure time and depression and anxiety (Harvey, Hotopf, Overland, & Mykletun, 2010). The results showed that persons engaging in regular leisure-time activity, of any intensity, were less likely to report symptoms of depression. The study concluded that higher levels of social support and social engagement could explain some of the effects of exercise on mood, but direct biological effects on mood were also probable. Conversely, Teychenne, Ball, and Salmon (2010) conducted a separate review of studies of sedentary behavior and concluded that sedentary behavior was consistently associated with an increased risk for depression.

A recent Cochrane Collaborative review examined 144 clinical trials on the use of exercise as a *treatment* for depression and found only 28 of the studies were methodologically adequate for inclusion in the meta-analysis (Mead et al., 2010). The studies included a variety of forms of exercise, including walking, treadmill walking, running, bicycling, aerobic training, aerobic dance, resistance training, and Qigong. The final review showed that exercise has a large clinical effect on depressed mood, with reductions in symptom severity. The effects were comparable to cognitive therapy and antidepressant medication. The authors called for several improvements in research and concluded that even the studies included in their analysis showed flaws limiting the conclusions.

Physical exercise, movement, and increased leisure activity in a variety of forms are effective pathways for moderating depression and improving mood. Conversely, sedentary behavior is a pathway toward depression and other illnesses. The Pathways Model calls for beginning with simple movement (Level One) and progressing to more vigorous aerobic exercise (Level Two).

Nutrition

Many depressed individuals and their families are frustrated with adverse effects of medication and seek nutritional interventions as an alternative. As is the case with exercise, nutritional change, herbal medicine, and nutritional supplements have long been suggested for individuals with depression, but the quality of research has been uneven, and findings often inconsistent. The following discussion highlights some of the better documented strategies for applying dietary change, herbal medicine, and nutritional supplements for depression.

When integrated into a program of comprehensive lifestyle change, dietary changes can alleviate illness and improve wellness. Dean Ornish has established a solid evidence base for his comprehensive program for lifestyle change in cardiac rehabilitation (Ornish, 1996; Ornish et al., 1998; Silberman et al., 2010). The Ornish program includes a whole foods, plant-based (vegetarian) diet, smoking cessation, physical exercise, stress management, yoga, and meditation. In a series of clinical trials, culminating in multicenter studies, Ornish and colleagues showed that many measurable aspects of cardiac illness—including triglyceride levels, cholesterol levels, blood pressure, and atherosclerosis—could be reversed by this comprehensive program in lifestyle change.

More recently, the Ornish program was applied in an investigation of a depressed group within a larger cardiac illness population (Pischke, Frenda, Ornish, & Weidner, 2010). The study followed 997 depressed men and women enrolled in the "high-risk" arm of the Multisite Cardiac Lifestyle Intervention Program. On enrolling, the depressed patients exhibited more adverse medical status, consumed more dietary fat, and practiced less stress management than nondepressed patients. Treated with a program targeting diet, exercise, and stress management, 248 of the depressed patients became euthymic.

Several herbal medicines may provide some therapeutic benefit for persons with depression. The research to date is strongest on St. John's wort. Extracts of St. John's Wort (*Hypericum perforatum*) have been found effective in over 40 clinical trials for mild to moderate depression, with results comparable to tricyclic and SSRI medications, and fewer adverse effects (Ernst, Pittler, Wider, & Boddy, 2006; Kasper, Caraci, Forti, Drago, & Aguglia, 2010). St. John's Wort has a serotonergic mechanism of action, and caution should be used in combining it with SSRI medications. There is also an emerging body of research supporting other herbal preparations, including sage (*Salvia officinalis* or *Salvia sclarea*), saffron petal (*Crocus sativus*), and lavender (*Lavandula*) for depression (Dwyer, Whitten, & Hawrelak, 2011; Natural Standards, 2012; Seol et al., 2010).

A number of other nutritional supplements and other natural preparations are also potentially helpful for depression. Research has shown some efficacy for the hormone dehydroepiandrosterone (DHEA) in reducing depression. One study specifically found DHEA to be effective in treating depression with midlife onset (Schmidt et al., 2005). DHEA is a precursor to male and female sex hormones and should be taken under medical supervision because of its potential serious interactions with several medications. It should not be combined with antidepressant medication (Natural Standards, 2012).

Folate (vitamin B9) has been recommended for depressed patients (Alpert & Fava, 1997). Fifteen percent to 38% of adults diagnosed with depressive disorders have been shown to be deficient in folate. There is also evidence for low folate levels contributing to poor response to antidepressant medications, specifically SSRIs (Alpert & Fava, 1997). The benefits of folate for depression may be limited to those persons who are deficient in folate, and research is not strong enough to suggest replacing conventional medication with folate (Natural Standards, 2012).

Functional medicine is a relatively newer field within alternative medicine utilizing a more strategic approach to nutritional interventions for health and healing. Functional medicine is based on a systemic biological approach (Jones, 2006; Schimmel & Penzer, 1997). The functional medicine practitioner utilizes diagnostic laboratory testing to identify specific deficiencies, or problems in absorption, and designs interventions to address these problems rather than simply prescribing the same herbs or nutritional supplements for all persons with the same diagnosis.

Healthy eating, nutritional supplements, and herbal preparations are widely used pathways to healing. Functional medicine offers the potential for more strategic and targeted uses of herbs and nutritional supplements.

Mind-Body Therapies

Many mind-body therapies have been utilized for depression, and at least anecdotal reports have claimed clinical efficacy for many mind-body interventions in reducing symptoms of depression.

Mindfulness Training. Mindfulness is a form of mental awareness derived from Buddhist meditation practices. Used as a life skill, mindfulness involves "paying attention in a particular way: on purpose, in the present moment, and non-judgmentally" (Kabat-Zinn, 1994, p. 4). Mindfulness training has been found in several studies to have significantly moderated depression symptoms (Teasdale, 1997). In addition, it has been applied successfully for the treatment of "treatment-resistant depression" (Eisendrath, Chartier, & McLane, 2011) and in recurrent major depressive disorder (Teasdale et al., 2000; Piet & Hougaard, 2011).

Hypnosis for Depression. For many years, hypnosis training included an admonition that hypnosis might exacerbate depressed mood and hypnosis was contraindicated for depression (Yapko, 1992). Michael Yapko (1992, 1997) challenged these widely accepted tenets and developed an approach for the hypnotically assisted treatment for depression. Recently, an entire issue of the *International Journal of Clinical and Experimental Hypnosis* was dedicated to evidence-based research documenting the clinical effectiveness of hypnosis for the treatment of depression (Alladin, 2010; Yapko, 2010).

Hypnotic therapy for depression utilizes a variety of hypnotic techniques (Alladin & Alibhai, 2007; Yapko, 2010). Yapko emphasized the phenomenological similarity of depression and hypnosis: Both involve a narrowed focus; are powerfully influenced by our relationships with others; involve cognitive expectancies, negative or positive; and involve "believed-in imagination" (Yapko, 2010). Hypnosis can be used strategically, utilizing each of these similarities for therapeutic effects. Hypnosis can refocus the patient, guiding the narrowed focus of the depressed individual to a focus on past moments of joy and hope. The positive hypnotic relationship can be a tool in overcoming the negative relationship experiences often highlighted in depression. The hypnotic state can redirect expectancies in positive directions. Hypnosis can also suggest a deep absorption in a believed-in positive imaginal experience. Finally, Yapko also emphasized that the hypnotic treatment of many of the conditions comorbid with depression, whether anxiety, substance abuse, or medical conditions, also regularly moderated the depression.

Biofeedback Interventions for Depression. Early biofeedback texts cautioned that severe depression could be a contraindication for the use of biofeedback. Over time, it became apparent that biofeedback-assisted relaxation therapy offered relief for the depressed individual who is overwhelmed by life stress and anxiety. A 2008 review of the outcomes research on depression rated a variety of biofeedback approaches as *possibly efficacious* for depressive disorders (Yucha & Montgomery, 2008). Today, biofeedback and relaxation-oriented interventions are widely used to reduce anxiety, moderate physiological tensions, and induce greater feelings of personal agency and empowerment (Gilbert & Moss, 2003; Moss, 1998).

In addition, two newer biofeedback protocols offer specific interventions to moderate depressive symptoms, serving to supplement psychotherapeutic and complementary approaches. Karavidas et al. (2007) conducted a pilot study utilizing heart rate variability biofeedback with 11 individuals with major depression. The participants showed significant improvement in depressive symptoms on the Beck Depression Inventory and Hamilton Depression Scale. Larger controlled studies are needed to confirm the efficacy of HRV biofeedback for depression.

Peter Rosenfeld developed a treatment protocol using EEG biofeedback for depressed patients. He drew on the neuroscience research of Richard Davidson (1995), showing a frontal asymmetry in hemispheric activation in depressed individuals. Persons with greater right frontal activation showed a disposition toward an avoidant and depressive reaction when stressful events occurred, and those with greater left frontal activation tended to react with an approach/problem solving reaction under stress, with more positive mood. In a series of small studies of EEG training to modify brain asymmetry, even patients with severe treatment-resistant depression showed improved mood after the intervention (Baehr, Rosenfeld, & Baehr, 1997; Rosenfeld, 2000). Baehr and Rosenfeld (2003) report training over 50 depressed patients, using over 30 sessions of EEG neurofeedback training, to modify the frontal asymmetry pattern and improve mood. Larger-scale independent studies are needed, to validate their findings.

Other Mind-Body Approaches. Many other mind-body approaches have been utilized clinically with depressed patients, including music therapy (Erkkila et al., 2011), dance therapy (Akandere & Demir, 2011; Koch, Morlinghaus, & Fuchs, 2007), expressive arts therapy (Rogers, 2011), guided imagery (Apostolo & Kolcaba, 2009; Brewin et al., 2009), and a variety of forms of meditation. Gordon (2008) popularized a comprehensive application of mind-body interventions—including breath training, imagery, nutrition, movement, and verbal expression—for clinical depression. Mind-body therapies are attractive to consumers, because they produce less adverse effects. Their therapeutic effects drawn on the body's own healing resources and seek to reregulate disturbed neurophysiological systems. Patient education is important, however, because patients oriented to medical interventions expect an immediate effect and often become frustrated early in the treatment process.

Medications often have noticeable beneficial effects on day one or, in the case of antidepressants, within 3–4 weeks, without effort on the patient's part. Mind-body healing techniques are behavioral skills that require practice and repetition before they acquire effectiveness. Just as one would not expect to play the piano skillfully on day one, it is not practical to expect the effects of meditation or relaxation in the first week. On the other hand, medications often lose their effectiveness over time, and higher doses or changes in medications become necessary. Mind-body techniques, however, gain effectiveness with practice and lead to more effective lifelong self-regulation. The longer an individual practices yoga or engages in progressive muscle relaxation, the more extensive and powerful the effects. A practical and very simple conclusion follows: For immediate, short-term benefit, turn to medication and physical medicine. For long-term benefit, with minimal adverse effects, turn to mind-body healing techniques.

Mind-body practices offer natural pathways for healing depression. They can augment mainstream treatments and, in some cases, replace them. The depressed human being benefits from discovering that he or she can make a change and it makes a difference in his or her body.

Integrative Treatment Combining Multiple Interventions

Taking heart disease as an example, an exhaustive review by the Cochrane Collaboration examined both psychological and pharmacological interventions for patients with coronary artery disease and comorbid depression. The review produced discouraging results, showing that both psychological interventions and pharmacological interventions produced positive but small effects on depression outcomes. The pharmacological results were marred by significant adverse reactions to medication, and there was no evidence that psychological interventions reduced mortality, reduced the risk for further cardiac events, or improved the physical dimension of health-related quality of life. The authors called for additional better designed studies but also concluded that single interventions are insufficient for patients with depression and CAD and that multimodal and collaborative interventions are necessary (Baumeister, Hutter, & Bengal, 2011). The National Institute for Clinical Excellence guidelines for adults suffering depression in combination with a physical illness call for psychological interventions as first-line interventions because of the adverse effects of antidepressants and the resulting "poor risk-benefit ratio" (Baumeister, Hutter, & Bengal; NICE, 2009).

Reviews of outcome studies on patients with depression in the absence of medical illness lead to similar conclusions. Even the best studies on antidepressant medications and on cognitive behavioral therapy interventions show three things. Significant numbers of patients do not complete the treatment regimen. High percentages of patients do not improve. And many improved patients, labeled as treatment successes, report reduced levels of depression but persistence of many depressive symptoms and continued diminishment of quality of life. The concept of multimodal interventions, of packaging several interventions, appears to be one reasonable response to these challenges.

The Pathways Model organizes multiple interventions into a three-level system and presents a useful framework for integrative treatment in the care of a depressed human being. Many mildly and moderately depressed individuals may direct their own recovery with Level One and Level Two interventions, while most severely depressed individuals will benefit from the entire spectrum of Levels One, Two, and Three.

Pathways Interventions: The Case of Abigail

This case study was chosen to show the applicability of the Pathways Model for challenging and difficult patients and not just the moderate cases. The patient in this case study initially seemed a good candidate for involuntary hospital-based care but responded positively when invited to participate in her own recovery.

Initial Visit and Assessment

Contact with Abigail began with a telephone call from her primary care physician, who asked: "Will a member of your staff accompany me on a home visit to evaluate a severely depressed 39 year old mom?" Home visits are no longer common in primary care or in clinical and health psychology. In this case, however, the physician was persuaded by the family to accommodate this patient, and he recruited the psychotherapist. Abigail was a 39-year-old divorced mother of a 6-year-old daughter, Mandy. Abigail's older sister Ruthi asked the physician to intervene because of concern for her niece's welfare. Previously employed as an accountant, Abigail had not worked since her daughter's birth.

Upon arriving at the house at 2:30 PM, the physician and therapist found Abigail sitting in her pajamas in the living room, rocking in a chair, with the curtains drawn. She was well oriented but downcast, with minimal eye contact, staring at the floor through much of the interview. Abigail admitted eating no lunch but had planned to prepare a meal for her daughter Mandy.

Abigail had been in good health, with one episode of depression prior to her pregnancy. That first incident came on when her older sister (Ruthi) left home for college when Abigail was 12. Abigail's premorbid temperament and manner were described as acerbic, cynical, and bitter, but without melancholia. The onset of depression was evident 2 days following the daughter Mandy's birth.

Abigail's mother was a teacher, who suffered a postpartum depression following Abigail's birth. The mother became reclusive, bonded poorly with Abigail, and left most of the infant and child care to Ruthi, her firstborn. The mother committed suicide by medication overdose on Abigail's fourth birthday. Subsequently, the father began to drink excessively and, on several occasions during childhood, awoke Abigail in the night to scream about her causing the mother's death.

Ruthi was a nurturing sister and caregiver, and Abigail recalled childhood as painful but mostly happy. The depression triggered by Ruthi's departure for college was severe but resolved within 3 months. Abigail herself was an excellent student and earned a master's degree in accounting. She was successful in accounting work and developed a reputation for attention to detail. During Abigail's last year of college, her father moved geographically, remarried, and broke off contact with both daughters.

Abigail married after graduate school, and her relationship with her husband Edward seemed positive until the onset of her depression. The husband divorced her 8 months following their daughter's birth and accepted a job out of state. Edward provided child support and sent birthday cards, but had not visited Mandy or Abigail in 2 years. He was contacted by Ruthi but declined to become involved in addressing the current problems.

Abigail reported sadness and tearfulness initially after the birth and intense fears of being a terrible mother. She became compulsively attentive to the baby at first, bathing her several times a day, sleeping on the floor next to the crib, and changing her diapers and clothing constantly. Over time, she reported decrements in appetite and energy, weight loss, absence of joy even in caring for Mandy, and sleep disturbance with delayed onset and early morning awakening. Times of uncontrolled crying occurred frequently.

Initially, Abigail requested and received antidepressant medication but experienced sedation from the medicine and refused further medication. By the time her spouse Edward left, she was sitting and staring much of each day, eating sporadically, and declining any activity outside the home. Her sister Ruthi began to help Abigail with child care and shopping for the family.

Abigail's depression moderated several times, to a degree that she began to discuss job seeking. But each time, unexpected financial problems, or arguments with a relative or neighbor, provoked relapses in depressed mood. When Mandy began first grade, Abigail abruptly slid back into inactivity and severe depression.

Abigail's symptoms supported the diagnosis of a major depressive disorder, recurrent and severe. She completed a Beck Depression Inventory in her first clinic visit and earned a score of 42, placing her in the extreme depression range. She also completed a Beck Anxiety Self-Rating Scale and earned a score of 41 or severe. A secondary diagnosis of post-traumatic stress disorder was added, and an obsessional cognitive style noted. She admitted frequent flashbacks and nightmares of scenes from her traumatic childhood. In spite of depression, she exhibited a vigilant overly alert perceptual style and frequent startle reactions. She reported near-constant anxiety and obsessional ruminations about replaying her mothers' life.

Pathways Assessment: Relevant Pathways. Abigail's family history suggested a genetic disposition to depression, with a history of three generations of depressed women. She reported disturbed early bonding due to the loss of her mother. She acknowledged traumatic experiences with a depressed and intoxicated father. Her obsessional cognitive style was a strength in her profession but also contributed to Abigail replaying negative self-messages. Her postpartum depression onset suggested an initial hormonal disturbance as a trigger for the depression, while her lack of movement and activity was a likely contributor to the maintenance of her depression.

Additional pathways contributors to the chronicity and severity of her depression included disturbed sleep with delayed onset and early morning awakening; constant anxiety, with breath holding, sighing, and episodes of hyperventilation, lack of social supports, loneliness, and isolation; an absence of any rewarding activities or relationships; and ineffective interpersonal skills, with alternating passivity and irritability. It is important to notice that many of these factors—such as sleep disturbance—can be at the same time symptoms of depression and factors contributing to continuity of severe depression over time.

Pathways Assessment: Readiness for Change. Abigail admitted a deep sense of hopelessness and pessimism. She doubted that any medical treatment would help her and questioned how any action on her own part could make a difference. Following Prochaska's readiness for change model, Abigail seemed to be stuck at the "pre-contemplation stage." She displayed a pervasive lack of any awareness that life can be improved by a change in her behavior (Prochaska & Velicer, 1997).

Pathways Interventions

The treatment team of physician and psychologist was worried, about the virtual neglect of the child and Abigail's suicide risk. In a second visit, the psychologist and physician jointly conducted a suicide risk assessment. On the Beck Depression Inventory, Abigail had responded to the suicide question with the response: "I have thoughts of killing myself, but would not carry them out." On questioning, Abigail acknowledged thoughts of death one or two times each week but explained that she was determined to remain alive to provide care for her daughter and see her grow to adulthood. She did not wish to cause her daughter Mandy the kind of emotional pain that her own mother's suicide had triggered in Abigail. She denied any specific plan for taking her life and denied engaging in any mental or behavioral preparations for suicidal action.

In this second visit, with Abigail and her sister Ruthi, a narrow set of options were defined and presented to Abigail. She was asked to choose between (1) involuntary hospitalization and transfer of custody for Mandy and (2) a twice-weekly outpatient treatment program with her full cooperation, including medication for depression. Abigail wished to avoid hospitalization and loss of custody at all costs and signed a written treatment contract.

Level One: Medication. Abigail feared medication side effects and knew that her mother had died with an overdose of antidepressants. Nevertheless, her physician persuaded her to accept a prescription for Lexapro, an SSRI with a relatively low side effects profile and lower lethality for overdose. Abigail felt a lift in energy in the third week on Lexapro. Her physician gradually increased the dosage to 60 mg, due to the powerful obsessional ruminations. Abigail admitted that it seemed easier to set her worries and troubling thoughts aside, since she had begun the medication.

Level One: *Movement*. Initially, psychotherapy consisted of supportive psychotherapy, building trust, and monitoring of Level One Interventions—what Abigail called baby steps. Abigail agreed to increase movement—walking to her rural mailbox and back twice daily, then after a week walking to her sister's home less than a city block away, and then walking daily to a nearby park with Mandy. Abigail was surprised that she started to enjoy the walks, especially the beauty of the nearby park. She also admitted enjoying more contact with her sister.

Level One: *Soothing*. Abigail was encouraged to continue rocking whenever anxious, and this was labeled as a "self-soothing coping skill." She had been ashamed of "rocking like a mental patient," and this cognitive reframing brought a smile to her face. She also was encouraged to hum and pray when anxious and found herself humming songs that her sister had sung to her in childhood. The praying led to recalling bedtime prayers from childhood.

Prolonging Level One. Abigail was kept in Level One interventions longer than usual because the Level One activities seemed to be reducing her anxiety, and she continued to be pessimistic about skill building and self-regulation.

Level One: *Sleep*. Abigail was educated about sleep hygiene and asked to study her sleep environment and habits. She identified that her bedroom had a number of reminders of her failed marriage, including her ex-husband's clothing and several photos. Her sister helped her remove reminders of the past and helped her to repaint the walls in a soothing lavender color. Abigail began to play soft music in the bedroom, to shut out neighborhood noise.

Level One: *Breathing*. Initially, Abigail was taught a very simple mindful breathing routine as an aid to sleep onset. The routine emphasized breathing from the abdomen, pursing the lips on the exhalation, and taking large relaxed, effortless breaths, at a rate about six per minute. The breathing helped Abigail in shortening sleep onset time and reducing her feelings of being "wired" and edgy. She was encouraged to practice her mindful breathing throughout the day, especially whenever she was tense or worried.

Level Two: *Yoga*. Abigail had pursued yoga in college and had very positive feelings about Eastern practices and fitness. She signed up for a twice-weekly beginning-level Hatha yoga class at a nearby yoga studio. Her sister attended with her, which Abigail welcomed. Abigail found the postures and the yogic breathing soothing and felt more comfortable in her body after 3 weeks of yoga classes and home practice.

Level Two: *Emotional Journaling*. The Pennebaker expressive writing format was reviewed with Abigail, and she showed interest in expressing herself on paper. She was given a copy of the Pennebaker (2004) *Writing to Heal* guide for journaling. She was invited to write once daily for about 20 minutes, following the Pennebaker guidelines. Abigail began to write frantically, journaling twice daily for about 40 minutes a session, until her writing triggered an intense episode of sobbing and shaking. After reporting this reaction to the therapy team, she was advised to take a several days break from journaling and began again, with the guidance to journal no more than once a day, for 15–20 minutes, and to stop whenever the process became too painful. She cried often during her journaling but began to feel a lifting of the heavy subjective weight around her mother's death.

Level Two: A Support Group. Abigail enjoyed several encounters with other mothers in the nearby park, and one invited her to attend a mothers' support group, at a nearby church. Abigail checked out the group through this new friend and was assured that there was no proselytizing or heavy religious messages. For the first time, she began venting to her treatment team about an oppressive religious dogmatism in her childhood home and church. She began attending the support group and found more common ground emotionally than she expected. She was relieved to learn that many of her reactions to daughter Mandy were common and "normal" reactions shared by other women. She also began to visit other mothers and arrange play dates through them for Mandy. She asked her treatment team to give her "Level Two credits" for the support group.

Level Three: Heart Rate Variability Biofeedback. Abigail observed biofeedback equipment in clinic offices and asked whether biofeedback could help her relax. She had calmed significantly, primarily through her mindful breathing, yoga, and expressive writing, yet still found her upper body muscles tight, her hands and arms jittery, and her mind racing. Much of her anxiety seemed post-traumatic. She admitted listening for footsteps in the night and tensing as she recalled her father's accusing voice.

Abigail's therapist discussed respiratory biofeedback and heart rate variability (HRV) training as useful tools decreasing anxiety and tension. The therapist gave her an article by Maria Karavidas on the usefulness of HRV training for major depression (Karavidas et al., 2007). Depression lowers the variability of the heart; HRV training restores normal variability and lifts mood.

Abigail began with respiratory biofeedback training, learning to pace her breathing more evenly and with less effort. Next her therapist assessed Abigail's *resonance frequency*, the breathing rate that produced for Abigail the highest magnitude in heart rate oscillations (Lehrer, Vaschillo, & Vaschillo, 2000). Abbey began to train at this optimal breathing frequency, 5.5 breaths per minute. Breathing at this rate gradually increased the amplitude of her heart rate oscillations, from an initial 8 beats to a sustained mean of 24 beats.

Abigail felt she had "mastered" the heart rate variability skills in about 4 sessions, assisted by her previous experience with yoga and mindful breathing. Her therapist strongly encouraged her to continue with the training, and by 12 sessions, Abigail reported much more impressive results. Abigail was convinced she could calm herself now, in the face of any stressful situation. She reported that she could feel her mood lighten each time she practiced at her resonance frequency at home.

Level Three: Hypnosis and Hypnotherapy. After Abigail's sixth session of HRV biofeedback, her therapist invited her to accept some sessions of hypnosis and hypnotically enhanced psychotherapy. Initially, Abigail's therapist used trance-induction to enhance her depth of relaxation, and she found herself relaxed to a deeper level than ever before.

Abigail's therapist next invited her into a series of age regressions, dwelling on the happy and playful moments in Abigail's childhood days with Ruthi. Following Yapco's principle that both depression and hypnosis share the quality of a heightened focus, Abigail's focus was guided to peak moments in the sunnier periods of her childhood years. As hypothesized, the healthiest core of Abigail's psyche seemed to anchor around Ruthi's devotion to "Abbey." Abigail left the therapy session several times humming or softly singing songs from her summer vacations with Ruthi, and the two sisters reconnected with several cousins who had been playmates in childhood. The age regressions also triggered painful awareness of losses related to the mother's death but also a growing awareness that her childhood had been a mixture of joys and tears.

Abigail exhibited several abreactions of emotion and spontaneous upsurges of childhood memories during and after her HRV and hypnosis sessions. The abreactions were alternately joyful and sad, but the intensity of the sad and traumatic episodes began to wear on Abigail. She expressed that she had not realized that the treatment process could be so exhausting and painful. Abigail learned to utilize self-hypnosis between sessions, returning to a safe place via imagery and watching her painful memories through a tinted window. Both the dissociative suggestions and the relaxation served to desensitize her from the traumatic emotions accompanying the memories. Gradually, her memories became more factual and less painful.

Other treatment options for post-traumatic stress disorder were discussed, but the hypnotic trance-work seemed to desensitize her trauma adequately, and her mood improved perceptibly.

Abigail Today

This particular case study is still in process. Three years have passed since Abigail's physician called and initiated the interventions. Abigail now is employed in a half-time book-keeping job, with less responsibility and less stress than her original job. She sees her sister and several new friends regularly and enjoys Mandy's soccer games and dance recitals. Abigail's Beck Depression Inventory and Beck Anxiety scores have moderated dramatically since her initial evaluation:

Beck Depression Inventory at 3 years—14 (mild)
Beck Anxiety Self-Rating Scale at 3 years—9 (mild)

She reports sleeping 7–8 hours most nights, and jokes that her appetite is now a little too good. Abigail now prefers her childhood nickname of Abbey. She began to date, but the beginnings of closeness frightened her, and she retreated from these relationships. She still occasionally awakens with a nightmare of her father's screaming episodes. She wrote to her father, thinking to resolve the trauma by a face-to-face meeting, but the letter came back unopened, stamped "Refused."

Abigail continues to use mindful breathing, yoga, journaling, and friendships as her everyday coping strategies. She has a breath "pacer" on her iPhone™ and practices breathing at her resonance frequency several times a week. She continues, at her own request, to utilize intermittent hypnosis and psychotherapy sessions to place frustrations into perspective and refresh her relaxation and self-hypnosis skills.

References

Akandere, M., & Demir, M. (2011). The effect of dance over depression. *Collegium Antropologicum, 35*(3), 651–656.

Alladin, A. (2010). Evidence-based hypnotherapy for depression. *International Journal of Clinical and Experimental Hypnosis, 58*(2), 165–185. doi:10.1080/00207140903523194.

Alladin, A., & Alibhai, A. (2007). Cognitive hypnotherapy for depression: An empirical investigation. *International Journal of Clinical and Experimental Hypnosis, 55*(2), 147–166.

Alpert, J. E., & Fava, M. (1997). Nutrition and depression: The role of folate. *Nutrition Reviews, 55*(5), 145–149. doi:10.1111/j.1753-4887.1997.tb06468.x.

American Psychiatric Association. (2000). *Diagnostic and statistical manual of mental disorders (4th ed., text revision)*. Washington, DC: American Psychiatric Association.

Apostolo, J. L., & Kolcaba, K. (2009). The effects of guided imagery on comfort, depression, anxiety, and stress of psychiatric inpatients with depressive disorders. *Archives of Psychiatric Nursing, 23*(6), 403–411.

Baehr, E., & Rosenfeld, J. P. (2003). Mood disorders. In D. Moss, A. McGrady, T. Davies, & I. Wickramasekera (Eds.), *Handbook of mind-body medicine in primary care* (pp. 377–392). Thousand Oaks, CA: Sage Publications.

Baehr, E., Rosenfeld, J. P., & Baehr, R. (1997). The clinical use of an alpha asymmetry protocol in the neurofeedback treatment of depression: Two case studies. *Journal of Neurotherapy, 2*(3), 10–23.

Barth, J., Schumacher, M., & Herrmann-Lingen, C. (2004). Depression as a risk factor for mortality in patients with coronary heart disease: A meta-analysis. *Psychosomatic Medicine, 66*, 802–813.

Baumeister, H., Hutter, N., & Bengal, J. (2011). Psychological and pharmacological interventions for depression in patients with coronary artery disease (Review). *The Cochrane Library, 9*, 1–75.

Baumeister, H., Hutter, N., Bengel, J., & Härter, M. (2011). Quality of life in medically ill persons with comorbid mental disorders: A systematic review and meta-analysis. *Psychotherapy and Psychosomatics, 80*, 275–286.

Boelen, P. A., & van den Bout, J. (2005). Complicated grief, depression, and anxiety as distinct post loss syndromes. *The American Journal of Psychiatry, 162*(11), 2175–2177.

Brewin, C. R., Wheatley, J., Patel, T., Fearon, P., Hackmann, A., Wells, A., et al. (2009). Imagery rescripting as a brief stand-alone treatment for depressed patients with intrusive memories. *Behavior Research and Therapy, 47*(7), 569–576.

Bronisch, T., & Wittchen, H.-U. (1994). Suicidal ideation and suicide attempts: Comorbidity with depression, anxiety disorders, and substance abuse disorder. *European Archives of Psychiatry and Clinical Neuroscience, 244*(2), 93–98. doi:10.1007/BF02193525.

Carney, R. M., Blumenthal, J. A., Stein, P. K., Watkins, L., Catellier, D., Berkman, L. F., et al. (2001). Depression, heart rate variability, and acute myocardial infarction. *Circulation, 104*(17), 2024–2028.

Chambless, D. R., & Ollendick, T. H. (2001). Empirically supported psychological interventions: Controversies and evidence. *Annual Review of Psychology, 52*, 685–716.

Churchill, R., Davies, P., Caldwell, D., Moore, T. H. M., Jones, H., Lewis, G., et al. (2010). Interpersonal, cognitive analytic and other integrative therapies versus treatment as usual for depression (Protocol). *The Cochrane Library, 9*, 1–18.

Cuijpers, P., van Straten, A., Andersson, G., & van Oppen, P. (2008). Psychotherapy for depression in adults: A meta-analysis of comparative outcome studies. *Journal of Clinical and Consulting Psychology, 76*(6), 909–922.

Davidson, R. J. (1995). Cerebral asymmetry, emotional and affective style. In R. J. Davidson & K. Hugdahl (Eds.), *Brain asymmetry* (pp. 362–387). Cambridge, MA: MIT Press.

DeMello, M. F., de Jesus, M. J., Bacaltchuk, J., Verdeli, H., & Neugebauer, R. (2005). A systematic review of research findings on the efficacy of interpersonal therapy for depressive disorders. *European Archives of Psychiatry and Clinical Neuroscience, 255*(2), 75–81.

Demirkan, A., Penninx, B. W. J. H., Hek, K., Wray, N. R., Amin, N., Aulchenko, Y. S., et al. (2011). Genetic risk profiles for depression and anxiety in adult and elderly cohorts. *Molecular Psychiatry, 16*, 773–783.

Di Matteo, M. R., Lepper, H. S., & Croghan, T. W. (2000). Depression is a risk factor for noncompliance with medical treatment. *Archives of Internal Medicine, 160*, 2101–2107.

Drevets, W. C., Price, J. L., & Furey, M. L. (2008). Brain structural and functional abnormalities in mood disorders: Implications for neurocircuitry models of depression. *Brain Structure & Function, 213*(1–2), 93–118.

Driessen, E., Cuijpers, P., DeMat, S. C. M., Abbass, A. A., de JOnghe, F., & Dekker, J. J. M. (2010). The efficacy of short term psychodynamic psychotherapy for depression: A meta-analysis. *Clinical Psychology Review, 30*(1), 25–36.

Dwyer, A. V., Whitten, D. L., & Hawrelak, J. A. (2011). Herbal medicines, other than St. John's Wort, in the treatment of depression: A systematic review. *Alternative Medicine Review, 16*(1), 40–49.

Eaddy, M., & Regan, T. (2003, October). *Real world six-month immediate-release SSRIs nonadherence*. Program and abstracts of the Disease Management Association of America 5th Annual Disease Management Leadership Forum. Chicago, Illinois.

Eisendrath, S., Chartier, M., & McLane, M. (2011). Adapting mindfulness-based cognitive therapy for treatment-resistant depression: A clinical case study. *Cognitive and Behavioral Practice, 18*(3), 362–370.

Elkin, I., Shea, T., Watkins, J. T., Imber, S. D., Sotsky, S. M., Collins, J. F., et al. (1989). National Institute of Mental Health Treatment of Depression Collaborative Research Program: General effectiveness of treatments. *Archives of General Psychiatry, 46*, 971–982.

Elliott, R., Bohart, A. C., Watson, J. C., & Greenberg, L. S. (2011). Empathy. In J. C. Norcross (Ed.), *Psychotherapy relationships that work* (2nd ed.). New York: Oxford University Press.

Erkkila, J., Punkanen, M., Fachner, J., Ala-Ruona, E., Pöntiö, I., Tervaniemi, M., et al. (2011). Individual music therapy for depression: Randomized controlled trial. *The British Journal of Psychiatry, 199*(2), 132–139.

Ernst, E., Pittler, M. H., Wider, B., & Boddy, K. (2006). *The desktop guide to complementary and alternative medicine* (2nd ed.). Edinburgh: Mosby/Elsevier.

Gallo, J. J., Zubritsky, C., Maxwell, J., Nazar, M., Bogner, H. R., Quijano, L. M., et al. (2004). Primary care clinicians evaluate integrated care and referral models of behavioral health care for older adults: Results from a multisite effectiveness trial (PRISM-E). *Annals of Family Medicine, 2*(4), 305–309. doi:10.1370/afm.116.

Gelenberg, A. J. (2010). The prevalence and impact of depression. *The Journal of Clinical Psychiatry, 71*(3), e06. doi:10.4088/JCP.8001tx17c.

Gilbert, C., & Moss, D. (2003). Basic tools: Biofeedback and biological monitoring. In D. Moss, A. McGrady, T. Davies, & I. Wickramaskera (Eds.), *Handbook of mind-body medicine in primary care: Behavioral and physiological tools* (pp. 109–122). Thousand Oaks, CA: Sage.

Gili, M., Garcia-Toro, M., Vives, M., Armengol, S., Garcia-Campayo, J., Soriano, J. B., et al. (2011). Medical comorbidity in recurrent versus first-episode depressive patients. *Acta Psychiatrica Scandinavica, 123*(3), 220–227. doi:10.1111/j.1600-0447.2010.01646.x.

Gordon, J. (2008). *Unstuck: Your guide to the seven stage journey out of depression*. New York, NY: Penguin.

Harvey, S. B., Hotopf, M., Overland, S., & Mykletun, A. (2010). Physical activity and common mental disorders. *The British Journal of Psychiatry, 197*, 357–364. doi:10.1192/bjp.bp. 109.075176.

Henk, H. J., Katzelnick, D. J., Kobak, K. A., Gresit, J. H., & Jefferson, J. W. (1996). Medical costs attributed to depression among patients with a history of high medical expenses in a health maintenance organization. *Archives of General Psychiatry, 53*(10), 899–904.

Herrmann-Lingen, C., & Buss, U. (2006). Anxiety and depression in patients with coronary heart disease. In J. Jordan, B. Bardé, & A. M. Zeiher (Eds.), *Contributions toward evidence-based psychocardiology: A systematic review of the literature* (pp. 125–157). Washington, DC: American Psychological Association.

Hofmann, S. G., & Asmundson, G. J. G. (2008). Acceptance and mindfulness-based therapy: New wave or old hat. *Clinical Psychology Review, 28*(1), 1–16.

Hollon, S. D., Jarrett, R. B., Nierenberg, A. A., Thase, M. E., Trivedi, M., & Rush, J. (2005). Psychotherapy and medication in the treatment of adult and geriatric depression: Which monotherapy or combined treatment. *The Journal of Clinical Psychiatry, 66*(4), 455–468.

Hougaard, E., & Jorgensen, M. B. (2007). Psychological treatment of depression [article in Danish]. *Ugeskrift for Laeger, 169*(16), 1444–1447.

Hovens, J. G., Giltay, E. J., Wiersma, J. E., Spinhoven, P., Penninx, B. W., & Zitman, F. G. (2012). Impact of childhood life events and trauma on the course of depressive and anxiety disorders. *Acta Psychiatrica Scandinavica, 126*(3), 198–2007. doi:10.1111/j.1600-0447.2011.01828.x.

Jones, D. S. (Ed.). (2006). *Textbook of functional medicine*. Gig Harbor, WA: Institute of Functional Medicine.

Kabat-Zinn, J. (1994). *Wherever you go, there you are*. New York: Hyperion.

Karavidas, M., Lehrer, P., Vaschillo, E., Vaschillo, B., Marin, H., Buyske, S., et al. (2007). Preliminary results of an open label study of heart rate variability biofeedback for the treatment of major depression. *Applied Psychophysiology and Biofeedback, 32*(1), 19–30.

Kasper, S., Caraci, F., Forti, B., Drago, F., & Aguglia, E. (2010). Efficacy and tolerability of Hypericum extract for the treatment of mild to moderate depression. *European Neuropsychopharmacology, 20*(11), 747–765.

Katon, W., & Ciechanowski, P. (2002). Impact of major depression on chronic medical illness. *Psychosomatic Research, 53*, 859–863.

Kessler, R. C., Chiu, W. T., Demler, O., & Walters, E. E. (2005). Prevalence, severity, and comorbidity of twelve-month DSM-IV disorders in the National Co-morbidity Survey Replication (NCS-R). *Archives of General Psychiatry, 62*(6), 617–627.

Kessler, R. C., Berglund, P. A., Demler, O., Jin, R., & Walters, E. E. (2005). Lifetime prevalence and age-of-onset distributions of DSM-IV disorders in the National Co-morbidity Survey Replication (NCS-R). *Archives of General Psychiatry, 62*(6), 593–602.

Kessler, R. C., McGonagle, K. A., Zhao, S., Nelson, C. B., Hughes, M., Eshleman, S., et al. (1994). Lifetime and 12-month prevalence of DSM-III-R psychiatric disorders in the United States: Results from the National Comorbidity Survey. *Archives of General Psychiatry, 51*, 8–19.

Koch, S. C., Morlinghaus, K., & Fuchs, T. (2007). The joy dance: Specific effects of a single dance intervention on psychiatric patients with depression. *The Arts in Psychotherapy, 34*(4), 340–349.

Lehrer, P. M., Vaschillo, E., & Vaschillo, B. (2000). Resonant frequency biofeedback training to increase cardiac variability. Rationale and manual for training. *Applied Psychophysiology and Biofeedback, 25*(3), 177–191.

Levinson, D. F. (2006). The genetics of depression: A review. *Biological Psychiatry, 60*, 84–92.

Lopez-Leon, S., Janssens, A. C., Gonzalez-Zuloeta Ladd, A. M., Del-Favero, J., Claes, S. J., Oostra, B. A., et al. (2008). Meta-analyses of genetic studies on major depressive disorder. *Molecular Psychiatry, 13*, 772–785.

Mead, G. E., Morley, W., Campbell, I. P., Greig, C. A., McMurdo, M., & Lawlor, D. A. (2010). Exercise for depression (Review). *The Cochrane Library, 1*, 1–61.

Miranda, J., Azocar, F., Organista, K. C., Munoz, R. F., & Lieberman, A. (1996). Recruiting and retaining low-income Latinos in psychotherapy research. *Journal of Consulting and Clinical Psychology, 64*(5), 868–874.

Moller, H. J., Bitter, I., Bobes, J., Fountoulakis, K., Hoschl, C., & Kasper, S. (2012). Position statement of the European Psychiatric Association (EPA) on the value of antidepressants in the treatment of unipolar depression. *European Psychiatry, 27*, 114–128.

Moss, D. (1998). Biofeedback, mind-body medicine, and the higher limits of human nature. In D. Moss (Ed.), *Humanistic and transpersonal psychology: An historical and biographical sourcebook* (pp. 145–161). Westport, Connecticut: Greenwood Press.

Moussavvi, S., Chatterji, S., Verdes, E., Tandon, A., Patel, V., & Ustun, B. (2007). Depression, chronic diseases, and decrements in health: Results from the World Health Surveys. *The Lancet, 370*, 851–858.

Murry, C. J. L., & Lopez, A. D. (Eds.). (1996). *The global burden of disease: A comprehensive assessment of mortality and disability from diseases, injuries, and risk factors in 1990 and projected to 2020*. Cambridge, MA: Harvard University Press.

National Alliance on Mental Illness (NAMI). (2011). *The impact and cost of mental illness: The case of depression*. National Institute on Mental Illness website. http://www.nami.org/Template.

References

cfm?Section=Policymakers_Toolkit&Template=/ContentManagement/ContentDisplay.cfm&ContentID=19043.

National Institute for Health and Clinical Excellence (NICE). (2009). *Depression: The treatment and management of depression in adults (update)*. Clinical guideline 90 2009. Retrieved July 26, 2011, from http://guidance.nice.org.uk/CG90.

National Institute of Mental Health (NIMH). (2011). *Health topics*. Statistics. National Institute of Mental Health website. http://www.nimh.nih.gov/statistics/index.shtml.

National Institute of Mental Health (NIMH). (2012). *What medications are used to treat depression?* National Institute of Mental Health. http://www.nimh.nih.gov/health/publications/mental-health-medications/what-medications-are-used-to-treat-depression.shtml.

Natural Standards. (2012). *Depression*. Natural Standards bottom line monograph. http://www.naturalstandrad.com.

Nutting, P. A., Rost, K. M., Dickinson, M., Werner, J. J., Dickinson, P., Smith, J. L., et al. (2002). Barriers to initiating depression treatment in primary care practice. *Journal of General Internal Medicine, 17*, 103–111.

Olfson, M., & Marcus, S. C. (2010). National trends in outpatient psychotherapy. *The American Journal of Psychiatry, 167*, 1456–1463.

Ormel, J., Von Korff, M., Burger, H., Scott, K., Demyttenaere, K., Huang, Y. Q., et al. (2007). Mental disorders among persons with heart disease. Results from World Mental Health surveys. *General Hospital Psychiatry, 29*, 325–334.

Ornish, D. (1996). *Dr. Dean Ornish's program for reversing heart disease*. New York, NY: Ivy Books/Ballantine Books.

Ornish, D., Scherwitz, L., Billings, J., Brown, S. E., Gould, K. L., Merritt, T. A., et al. (1998). Intensive lifestyle changes for reversal of coronary heart disease Five-year follow-up of the Lifestyle Heart Trial. *Journal of the American Medical Association, 280*, 2001–2007.

Partnership for Workplace Mental Health (PWMH). (2012). *Depression cost calculator*. Partnership for Workplace Mental Health, American Psychiatric Foundation website. http://www.workplacementalhealth.org/Business-Case/Depression-Calculator.aspx.

Pennebaker, J. W. (2004). *Writing to heal: A guided journal for recovering from trauma and emotional upheaval*. Oakland, CA: New Harbinger Press.

Piet, J., & Hougaard, E. (2011). The effect of mindfulness-based cognitive therapy for prevention of relapse in recurrent major depressive disorder: A systematic review and meta-analysis. *Clinical Psychology Review, 31*(6), 1032–1040.

Pischke, C. R., Frenda, S., Ornish, D., & Weidner, G. (2010). Lifestyle changes are related to reductions in depression in persons with elevated coronary risk factors. *Psychological Health, 25*(9), 1077–1100.

Price, J. L., & Drevets, W. C. (2012). Neural circuits underlying the pathophysiology of mood disorders. *Trends in Cognitive Sciences, 16*(1), 61–71.

Prochaska, J. O., & Velicer, W. F. (1997). The transtheoretical model of health behavior change. *American Journal of Health Promotion, 12*, 38–48.

Riedel-Heller, S. G., Matschinger, H., & Angermeyer, M. C. (2005). Mental disorders—who and what might help? Help-seeking and treatment preferences of the lay public. *Social Psychiatry and Psychiatric Epidemiology, 40*(2), 167–174.

Robins, L., & Regier, D. (Eds.). (1991). *Psychiatric disorders in America: The epidemiologic catchment area study*. New York, NY: Free Press.

Rogers, N. (2011). *The creative connection for groups: Person centered expressive arts for healing and social change*. Palo Alto, CA: Science and Behavior Books.

Rosenfeld, J. P. (2000). An EEG biofeedback protocol for affective disorders. *Clinical Electroencephalography, 31*(1), 7–12.

Rudisch, B., & Nemeroff, C. B. (2003). Epidemiology of comorbid coronary artery disease and depression. *Biological Psychiatry, 54*, 227–240.

Schimmel, H., & Penzer, V. (1997). *Functional medicine: The origins and treatment of disease* (2nd ed.). Heidelberg, Germany: Karl F. Haug.

Schmidt, P. J., Daly, R. C., Bloch, M., Smith, M. J., Danaceau, M. A., St. Clair, L. S., et al. (2005). Dehydroepiandrosterone monotherapy in midlife-onset major and minor depression. *Archives of General Psychiatry, 62*, 154–162.

Seol, G. H., Shim, H. S., Kim, P. J., Moon, H. K., Lee, K. H., Shim, I., et al. (2010). Antidepressant-like effect of Salvia sclarea is explained by modulation of dopamine activities in rats. *Ethnopharmacology, 130*(1), 187–190.

Silberg, J. L., Maes, H., & Eaves, L. J. (2010). Genetic and environmental influences on the transmission of parental depression to children's depression and conduct disturbance: An extended Children-of-Twins study. *Journal of Child Psychology and Psychiatry, 51*(6), 734–744. doi:10.1111/j.1469-7610.2010.02205.x.

Silberman, A., Banthia, R., Estay, I. S., Kemp, C., Studley, J., Hareras, D., et al. (2010). The effectiveness and efficacy of an intensive cardiac rehabilitation program in 24 sites. *American Journal of Health Promotion, 24*(4), 260–266.

Sullivan, P. F., Neale, M. C., & Kendler, K. S. (2000). Genetic epidemiology of major depression: Review and meta-analysis. *The American Journal of Psychiatry, 157*, 1552–1562.

Teasdale, J. D. (1997). The relationship between cognition and emotion. The mind-in-place in mood disorders. In D. M. Clark & C. G. Fairbarn (Eds.), *Science and practice of cognitive behavioral therapy* (pp. 67–93). Oxford, England: Oxford University Press.

Teasdale, J. D., Segal, Z. V., Williams, J. M. G., Ridgeway, V. A., Soulsby, J. M., & Lau, M. A. (2000). Prevention of relapse recurrence in major depression by mindfulness based cognitive therapy. *Journal of Consulting and Clinical Psychology, 68*(4), 615–623.

Teychenne, M., Ball, K., & Salmon, J. (2008). Physical activity and likelihood of depression in adults: A review. *Preventive Medicine, 46*, 397–411.

Teychenne, M., Ball, K., & Salmon, J. (2010). Sedentary behavior and depression among adults: A review. *International Journal of Behavioral Medicine, 17*(4), 246–254.

Thompson, L. W., Gallagher, E., & Steinmetz Breckenridge, J. (1987). Comparative effectiveness of psychotherapies for depressed elders. *Journal of Consulting and Clinical Psychology, 55*, 385–390.

Wang, P. S., Lane, M., Olfson, M., Pincus, H. A., Wells, K. B., & Kessler, R. C. (2005). Twelve month use of mental health services in the United States. *Archives of General Psychiatry, 62*(6), 629–640.

Weerasekera, P. (2010). Psychotherapy for the practicing psychiatrist: Promoting evidence-based practice. *Focus, 8*, 3–18.

World Health Organization. (2012). *Depression*. World Health Organization website. http://www.who.int/mental_health/management/depression/definition/en/.

Yapko, M. (1992). *Hypnosis and the treatment of depressions: Strategies for change*. New York: Brunner/Mazel.

Yapko, M. (1997). *Breaking the patterns of depression*. New York: Random House/Doubleday.

Yapko, M. D. (2010). Hypnosis in the treatment of depression: An overdue approach for encouraging skillful mood management. *International Journal of Clinical and Experimental Hypnosis, 58*(2), 137–146.

Yucha, C., & Montgomery, D. (2008). *Evidence-based practice of biofeedback and neurofeedback*. Wheat Ridge, CO: Association for Applied Psychophysiology and Biofeedback.

Chapter 9
Anxiety

Abstract Anxiety disorders manifest themselves as uncomfortable emotions, over-arousal of biological systems and changes in self-care behaviors. Interventions must address each of these categories of anxiety responses to help patients return to health. This chapter describes two clinical cases to demonstrate the use of the Pathways Model in anxiety disorders.

Keywords Anxiety disorders • Physiological mechanisms • Breath training • Relaxation • Biofeedback • Cognitive behavioral therapy

Introduction

Anxiety disorders are the most common of the mental health disorders. The anxiety disorders have an estimated lifetime prevalence of about 28 % and an earlier median age of onset (11 years) than the mood disorders or substance abuse disorders (Kessler, Berglund, Demler, Jin, & Walters, 2005). International prevalence studies suggest that symptoms of anxiety are reported in every country studied and in most locales comorbidity with substance abuse is also high. For individuals with more than one anxiety disorder, functional impairment is magnified (Kroenke, Spitzer, Williams, Monahan, & Lowe, 2007).

Within the anxiety disorders classification, phobias and generalized anxiety disorder symptoms are frequently described by patients, while panic disorder and PTSD are less common. Adjustment disorder with anxiety or with mixed anxiety and depression probably has a higher prevalence than any of the anxiety disorders. But in many cases, problems coping with a specific stressor often resolve on their own or with peer support, so this disorder is less frequently brought for clinical attention and diagnosed. Similarly, impulse control disorder, in its own category, may be related to anxiety. Hasty, poorly considered decisions are often made in response to a stressful situation. Anxious persons often do not have the clarity of thought or coping techniques to make a good decision, so they undertake thoughtless action in order to end the uncomfortable feelings and indecisiveness. Other behaviors, also driven by anxiety, are seemingly so automatic that the person cannot identify feelings or thought process until after the actions are complete.

Brief Descriptions of the Anxiety Disorders

Generalized anxiety disorder is characterized by chronic worry, tension, and anxiety that have been ongoing for at least 6 months. Continued overarousal is exhausting, so the person feels fatigued much of the time and has trouble calming down enough to fall sleep. Any disruption in circadian rhythm imposed by work or travel will accentuate the insomnia. The diagnostic criterion for panic disorder is repeated panic attacks. The attack is experienced as a rapid increase in anxiety that typically peaks within 10 min and then de-escalates. The anxiety manifests itself as rapid heartbeat, quick breaths, and a sense of impeding catastrophe. Situations most likely to produce panic-type symptoms are those that are novel, perceived as out of one's control, and potentially harmful. Acute stress disorder and posttraumatic stress disorder (PTSD) are responses to severe stressors in the short time frame (acute) or over months or years (PTSD) (APA, 2000). Persons exposed to trauma remain hyper-activated; they reexperience the trauma when awake or during dream sleep and they seek to avoid reminders of the trauma. There are other anxiety provoking memories that do not qualify as trauma, but seem to have almost as serious an effect as situations that are strictly defined as traumatic, such as acute embarrassment or public criticism. The effects of perceived trauma continue to affect the exposed individuals many years after the original event occurred (Schore, 2002). For example, abuse histories in women are associated with prolonged dysregulation of stress response systems lasting decades. Women studied by Girdler, Leserman, Bunevicius, Klatkin, Pedersen, and Light (2007) did not have current medical or psychiatric illness, yet had higher prevalence of premenstrual dysphoric disorder (PMDD), more marked BP, and vascular resistance responses to stress. Phobias of objects, situations, or social engagement are characterized by anxiety when confronted with the object or situation. Although the triggering factor is sometimes not remembered, the phobic reaction continues.

Anxious emotions and worried thoughts are mirrored in physiological activity (Mussgay & Ruddel, 2004). As described in detail in an earlier chapter, the sympathetic nervous system and the endocrine hormones—cortisol and catecholamines—are the prime responders to real or recreated stressful events (Bremner, Krystal, Southwick, & Charney, 1996). What is unique to the anxiety disorders is that the physiological manifestations of the emotion are themselves sources of anxiety. The cycle tends to repeat, emotion → physiology → emotion and so on. Understanding this positive feedback system is critical for the education of patients and the design of effective mind–body interventions.

Psychological and Physiological Characteristics of Anxiety

Fear is healthy and necessary for survival in the animal kingdom. Almost every animal and the highest order animal, the human has programmed fear responses hardwired in the brain. People are more likely to fear things that have the potential to cause harm. Fears are partially inherited and partially learned through social learning (observation) and conditioning (Tompkins & Martinez, 2010). Many fears are adaptive so that people can protect themselves from negative events or people that have harmed them in the past. Repetitive thinking and recreating in imagery negative events that occurred in the past are associated with neuroendocrine responses, particularly cortisol in the case of social stressors that elicit fear (Lovallo & Thomas, 2000).

Not only are traumatic events recreated in the mind but rumination about moderately negative events also mobilizes the neuroendocrine system (salivary cortisol), particularly in socially embarrassing situations. Cortisol increases when a "transgressor" has produced fear (McCullough, Orsulak, Brandon, & Akers, 2007). Fear may mediate the rumination/cortisol link. Catecholamines are elevated in persons with PTSD (Young & Breslau, 2004). In evaluating a person with an anxiety disorder, the fear factor should be explored for its potential to continue to recreate painful images and the associated physiological responses.

In addition, research shows that abnormal respiration frequently accompanies the anxiety disorders (Wilhelm, Gevirtz, & Roth, 2001). Rapid breathing, shallow breathing, breath holding, and other forms of maladaptive respiration can be measured by biofeedback instrumentation, and these breath patterns contribute to the anxiety (Timmons & Ley, 1994). Irregular or rapid breathing produces a depletion of carbon dioxide in the airways and bloodstream, called hypocapnia, causing a number of the symptoms commonly associated with anxiety, including chest pain, shortness of breath, dizziness, confusion, irregular heartbeat, and tingling in the fingers and hands. Patients' worries about these respiration-related symptoms then exacerbate the physiological dysregulation, in a vicious cycle of physiological arousal and cognitive alarm. Assisting patients to restore smooth, regular-paced breathing is a useful tool in managing individual anxiety episodes, and frequently assists in the process of recovery.

The Case of Suzette

Some clients do not endorse terms like anxious or worried, nor do they identify their life events as negative. Their problems are better described as "over-activation" or "over-arousal." To illustrate this, the case of Suzette will be described. Suzette was a 41-year-old woman who described herself as energetic, busy, and enthusiastic, while also admitting to sometimes feeling overwhelmed and overcommitted with responsibilities. After Suzette stated: "My life is wonderful" for the second time, the therapist responded: "Why are you here?"

During the initial evaluation, Suzette revealed that she was the mother of twins, had one other child, worked full time, and did a lot of volunteer work involving her children. Her husband also worked full time and because of a long commute, got home after the children had eaten dinner. Suzette was referred to our care because of fluctuating heart rate, occasional periods of elevated blood pressure, chest pain, and nausea. Medical evaluation by a cardiologist did not reveal coronary artery disease or sustained hypertension, and the symptoms were considered to be stress related. Suzette reluctantly agreed to the referral to the Behavioral Medicine Clinic. Suzette grew up in a quiet household, the only child of parents who were older than those of most of her friends. She was often lonely and bored. Her parents denied her contact with friends and did not encourage her to engage in school clubs or athletics. She married Russ, whom she met in college when she was 24. Suzette described her relationship with Russ as "great," and believed that she was a good mother and was performing well at work. She hoped that she would not be asked to give up any of her activities.

Some people are energized beyond the system's tolerance level. Genetic predisposition to react forms the foundation. Hyper-excitability of the brain and over-stimulation by both negative and positive events creates anxiety. Multiple activities represent sources of energy that transfer to the person and increase responsiveness. In the world of performance, it is well known that the environment, other people, noise, lights, and music can be used as ways to activate and prepare for optimal performance. Outside of situations where the person consciously wishes to energize, because they are fatigued or emotionally flat, there is usually little awareness of this process. The person with anxiety disorders only realizes that they are uncomfortable and have symptoms, which they do not understand.

Close examination of the work of McEwen (2004) allows an explanation for the deleterious effects of over-activation. Allostatic load is increased by repeated stimuli and little time for recovery, regardless of the positive or negative valence of these events (McEwen & Lasley, 2003). The stress responses systems, including increased cortisol and adrenergic sympathetic activity, react whether the event is positive or negative, as long as the event requires adaptation or coping with change. The stress responses are conditioned or learned by the nervous system. This same system reacts mindlessly in the present as it reacted so many times in the past. Vestigial response patterns remain, just as the appendix is a vestigial organ that serves little purpose now. Memory fragments mixed with unconscious drivers of behavior can produce actions that the patient finds hard to explain.

Intervention Plan

Education and Level One Intervention

The intervention plan for Suzette began with providing information about the biological responses to stress, using the work of McEwen (2004) to assist patient education. For Suzette, we explained her reactions to positive and negative events in terms of the cumulative life events model (Holmes & Rahe, 1967). We did not directly confront her beliefs that her life is "wonderful," and focused the dialogue for the most part on bodily responses, which was actually where her symptoms resided. The Level One interventions most appropriate for Suzette were breathing and soothing. The practitioner introduced a slow, mindful breathing technique and recommended daily practice. The constant over-activation was addressed by self-soothing exercises, such as rocking or praying. Since Suzette was involved with her church and reported having a regular time for prayer, the calming effects of prayer were emphasized. Tied to the soothing effects of these activities, Suzette was presented with information about environmental energy and advised not to draw energy from other people, noise, or light. She was encouraged to keep music soft, sit in dim light, maintain temperature in the cool range, and avoid overheating. She was also encouraged to stay away from large groups of people and fast conversation. Through Suzette's volunteer work at her children's school, she had observed the effects of preperformance anxiety resulting in near panic and impaired performance. The childrens' anxiety manifested itself as forgetting lines or singing incorrect musical notes.

Level Two Interventions

Relaxation was necessary to calm Suzette's overactive system. Progressive relaxation seemed optimal to begin stress management (Level Two), since Suzette was used to action and might have found it difficult to sit still. Daily practice of progressive relaxation was recommended, but this was met with resistance. So, a brief, modified tense-relax exercise was offered and Suzette accepted this instruction. She began to practice during her lunch break at work and again when she got home from work. After training in active relaxation, Suzette accepted instruction in passive relaxation with thermal biofeedback (Level Three). She was surprised that she could control her hand temperature.

Level Three Interventions

This evidence became a spring board for a second Level Three intervention, cognitive behavioral therapy (CBT). Suzette began to realize that she had tried to "be all things to all people." She learned that work performance did not always have to be perfect and did not always require her entire attention. Her children actually felt proud when she gave them responsibility for packing their own lunches and making sure that gym clothes were in their book bags. Suzette developed several cue words that she used to calm down when she noticed that she was excited and began to experience chest pain. For example, Suzette realized that she was talking very quickly at a party where there were a lot of people there and the music was loud. She sought a quieter area of the room and talked to one or two people, instead of staying with the loudest group—to whom she was drawn.

Change was slow, partially because Suzette refused to come to therapy more than once a month. At the beginning of each session, she told the therapist that the *next* session would be her last. However, the improvement, particularly in chest pain proved to Suzette that she and the therapist were on the right track. One year later, Suzette reported no chest pain, no nausea and her blood pressure had stabilized. Rapid talking and quick breathing were useful signals. Her awareness level was acute so she monitored breathing during the day, and slowed down when she felt short of breath. Treatment was terminated.

Case Summary

In summary, Suzette presented with a pattern of chronic physiological over-activation, accompanied by irregular heart rate, elevated blood pressure, chest pain, and insomnia. She responded positively to Level One interventions of education about stress, mindful breathing, self-soothing, and lifestyle modifications involving reduced exposure to overstimulation, Level Two activity involving a modified relaxation exercise, and Level Three interventions including passive relaxation with thermal biofeedback and CBT. After 1 year of reluctantly engaging in behavioral health counseling, Suzette had significantly modified her lifestyle, regularly applied slow, mindful breathing, and reported a cessation of her physiological symptoms.

The Case of Bernie

Bernie was a 50-year-old pediatrician who requested treatment for "stress management." He reported blurred vision, some problems with memory, and severe neck pain. During the evaluation, Bernie described his very busy practice and his community. He wanted to be a doctor since he was in high school and enjoyed the challenges of caring for sick children. But he said that during the past few years "medicine has changed" "parents have changed," and "kids have changed." Bernie recruited two new pediatricians into the practice because he wanted to get more involved in the local physicians' organization. He was elected by his peers to the vice president's position and this would lead to the presidency in a few years. During his term, he became increasingly disillusioned with his colleagues. Instances of pettiness, cruel criticism of other doctors were frequent. Few were willing to work together. There were disagreements about direction and about the methods for achieving the few common goals. Bernie felt a sense of sadness and anxiety as he spent more time in administrative work and less time in his practice. His visual problems were a source of great worry, since there was a history of glaucoma on his father's side. Further, the almost constant neck pain made Bernie question how much longer he could stand and bend over to examine a baby. Sometimes the pain was so severe that it affected his thinking and memory. It took him a little longer to recall the dosage of a common medication. At the evaluation session, he spoke of his early days of practice almost with reverence; he recalled the wonder at seeing the growth of his infant patients to childhood and teenage years. However, increasing insurance-driven pressures for shorter visits and larger weekly billings seemed to have turned a natural optimist into someone with a pessimistic viewpoint about himself, his practice, and the future of medicine.

An optimistic viewpoint is "a significant predictor of positive physical health outcomes." The review by Rasmussen and Scheier (2009) highlights the effects of optimism on illness and health. Although the pathways that mediate this effect are not known, the mental state of optimism can be cultivated in patients with several techniques. In an anxious, worried person, like Bernie, pessimism had become his usual mental state; he increasingly felt that something awful was going to happen to him.

Research by Kendler, Hettema, Butera, Gardner, and Prescott (2003) sought to identify the specific factors underlying the life events that were associated with major depression, anxiety or mixed anxiety and depression. Generalized anxiety disorder is predictable by feelings of loss, danger, or threat. There is some overlap between GAD and mixed anxiety and depression which is also predicted by life events involving loss, but in addition, feelings of entrapment and humiliation were found to be important. Entrapment refers to the belief that an already stressful situation will worsen; the person is stuck in a situation and past attempts to improve the situation have gone wrong.

In our evaluation of Bernie, we concluded that he had primary generalized anxiety disorder and secondary dysthymia. Bernie had already had an in-depth assessment by his ophthalmologist and his neurologist. Fortunately, the ophthalmologist reported that his eyes were normal. The neurologist found no nerve damage, but severe muscle spasms and age appropriate arthritis. Memory testing found no impairment. Despite these generally positive results and reassurance from his own physicians, Bernie's thoughts of losing his sight, no longer being able to bend over a sick child, or failing to remember what drug to prescribe remained Bernie's worst fears.

Research on stress identifies the likely mechanisms driving Bernie's symptoms. The hippocampus and amygdala play major roles in learning and memory. The hippocampus organizes episodic and declarative memories, such as names of places, people and things, and context (the time and place of events). This structure also acts to shut off the stress response. The amygdala functions in procedural memory including learned skills or sequences of events. It is also involved in long-term memory, emotional associations, and anticipation of stressful events (McEwen & Lasley, 2003). Long-term potentiation (LTP) derives from short high frequency stimulation of neurons, which later increases the potency of these particular neuronal signals (Purves et al., 1997). LTP has been documented in the hippocampus, the amygdala, the neocortex, and cerebellum. Stress affects memory, particularly for detail, since the stress response system is designed for responses to easily visible stressors. The stress hormones, particularly glucocorticoids, affect real-time processing of information and memories of emotional events (Birnbaum et al., 2004; Bremner et al., 2004).

The sense of control over one's own body is particularly important in persons with anxiety. Rapid heart rate, blurred vision, and pain without physical cause convey a message of loss of control (Tompkins & Martinez, 2010). Bernie had trained himself to disregard some useful bodily signals (rapid breathing, fatigue) while overfocusing on others (blurred vision, pain). If the patient perceives risk or threat as high and personal or other resources as low, the stress experience intensifies. Bernie believed that many aspects of his life were becoming more difficult to control, including his body, his medical practice, and his colleagues.

Interventions: Level One

The Level One intervention recommended for Bernie was the "relaxing sigh" followed by slow-paced breathing (Davis, Eshelman, & McKay, 2008). Baseline breath rate was 16 per minute and Bernie was instructed to pace his breath first to 12, then 10, and then 6 breaths per minute. This simple technique began to help Bernie relax, but he needed to begin the exercise with a sigh. Mindful breathing directed his attention inward in a positive way, instead of attending only to pain, discomfort, or problems (Grossman, Niemann, Schmidt, & Walach, 2004). Most importantly, he felt that he gained control over one physiological response. Evidence supports the belief that neuroendocrine responses to stress can be reduced by perceived acquired control over a potential threat, by familiarity with the stressor, and by social support (Abelson, Liberzon, Young, & Khan, 2005).

In-depth discussions regarding the effects of anxiety on vision reviewed for Bernie that both the sympathetic and the parasympathetic nervous systems innervate the eye. The former dilates the pupil and aids in focusing on objects at a distance; the latter does the opposite (Widmaier, Raff, & Strang, 2004). Of course, Bernie knew the nerve pathways to the eye, but had never realized that stress might be affecting his ability to see clearly. It was likely that the acute stress response was dilating the pupil and interfering with focus on close objects such as the fine print of drug package inserts. After a week of daily practicing, he was instructed to do relaxed breathing and then attempt to read the package insert under low stress conditions.

The second Level One intervention was movement. Bernie had become quite sedentary in the past few years. Long hours at the office and the daily experiences of pain resulted in mental fatigue and physical tiredness. Therefore, he was instructed to take a few minutes several times a day to move his body, either to swing his arms (without causing further pain) or to walk a short distance.

Interventions: Level Two

The Level Two interventions were passive relaxation using autogenic phrases and emotional journaling. Autogenic exercises focused on sensations of heaviness in the muscles and warming the hands. Simple relaxation phrases directed first towards the lower body, then the central, and finally the upper body and head are repeated (Davis et al., 2008). At first, it was important to support each intervention with research findings to increase the credibility of the treatment. Later, Bernie became more trusting and either looked up the references on his own or no longer asked for them. Establishing a regular routine was critical to Bernie's success. People with anxiety are comforted by sameness and dependability of routines and familiar places. Bernie was told to maintain his immediate environment as constant as he could, for example, he should take the same route to work each day. He should instruct his office manager to keep the arrangement of the charts as it was and not change. The two new pediatricians had requested to remodel their offices and the reception area; Bernie agreed to the office remodeling, but postponed it for 3 months. The anxious person does not cope well with even small changes so the delay was welcome (Knez, 2005). It was important that Bernie felt comfortable in his surroundings again and began to experience that the daily stressors were things that he had coped with previously with little difficulty.

Written expression has positive effects on health and sense of well-being (Pennebaker & Seagal, 1999). Writing about traumatic experiences is associated with positive health benefits through an integration or summarization of events that allows the person a new perspective. In addition, expectancies of the beneficial effects of writing about stressful experiences play an important role (Langen & Schuler, 2007). Although Bernie's experiences during the past few years would not be classified by most clinicians as traumatic, he tended to ruminate about decisions that he had made and replay contentious conversations with his colleagues. Bernie had read about the benefits of journaling and asked for instructions, which were provided. Daily writing about negative experiences provided a greater sense of clarity about his recent choices regarding where he devoted time and energy.

Interventions: Level Three

Bernie's Level Three interventions were CBT and SEMG biofeedback. Relaxation supplemented with biofeedback was very difficult for Bernie. His automatic bracing response maintained high levels of neck and shoulder tension. Initially, awareness of pain increased when Bernie began to relax his muscles, but with encouragement he was able to tolerate the short-lived increase without protective bracing. His tension levels decreased significantly with biofeedback and daily practice of breathing and passive relaxation. CBT focused on countering negative thoughts about his practice, medicine in general, and his colleagues. Although some of his concerns were, in fact, real and accurate, Bernie had added layers of catastrophic thinking to the realistic concerns. Bernie's journaling was used to support the CBT. Bernie brought his writings to our sessions and this material was then used for a detailed analysis of negative thoughts and beliefs. During the 6 months of therapy, Bernie came to realize that his real love was taking care of sick children. When his neck pain decreased, he started enjoying his clinic days again. He recovered the joys of caring for infants and children, who became well under his care. He decided that he would complete his term as vice president but not continue on as president in the physician's association.

Case Summary

In summary, Bernie presented with symptoms of Generalized Anxiety Disorder, and dysthymia, blurred vision, short-term memory deficits, and neck pain. Work stress and a growing pessimism about his medical practice and his profession, along with fears about his deteriorating condition, made his life a burden. Bernie responded positively to a Level One intervention combining the "relaxing sigh" and paced, mindful breathing. His Level Two interventions included Autogenic Training and emotional journaling. His Level Three treatment included CBT and SEMG biofeedback. During 6 months of therapy, Bernie successfully reduced the muscle tension in his neck and shoulders, and experienced relief from the frightening neck pain. He also experienced a lessening pessimism and a recovery of the joy in his pediatric practice.

References

Abelson, J. L., Liberzon, I., Young, E. A., & Khan, S. (2005). Cognitive modulation of the endocrine stress response to a pharmacological challenge in normal and panic disorder subjects. *Archives of General Psychiatry, 62*, 668–675.
American Psychiatric Association. (2000). *Diagnostic and statistical manual of mental disorders* (4th ed.). Washington, DC: American Psychiatric Association.
Birnbaum, S. G., Yaun, P. X., Wang, M., Vijayraghavan, S., Bloom, A. K., Davis, D. J., et al. (2004). Protein kinase over activity impairs prefrontal cortical regulation of working memory. *Science, 306*, 882–884.
Bremner, D., Krystal, J. H., Southwick, S. M., & Charney, D. S. (1996). Noradrenergic mechanisms in stress and anxiety. *Synapse, 23*(1), 39–51.
Bremner, J. D., Vythilingam, M., Vermetten, E., Anderson, G., Newcomer, J. W., & Charney, D. S. (2004). Effects of glucocorticoids on declarative memory function in major depression. *Biological Psychiatry, 55*, 811–815.
Davis, E., Eshelman, E. R., & McKay, M. (2008). *The relaxation & stress reduction workbook* (6th ed.). Oakland: New Harbinger.
Girdler, S. S., Leserman, J., Bunevicius, R., Klatzkin, R., Pedersen, C. A., & Light, K. C. (2007). Persistent alterations in biological profiles in women with abuse histories: Influence of premenstrual dysphoric disorder. *Health Psychology, 26*(2), 201–213.
Grossman, P., Niemann, L., Schmidt, S., & Walach, H. (2004). Mindfulness based stress-reduction and health benefits: A meta-analysis. *Journal of Psychosomatic Research, 57*(1), 35–43.
Holmes, T., & Rahe, R. H. (1967). The social readjustment rating scale. *Journal of Psychosomatic Research, 11*(2), 213–218.
Kendler, K. S., Hettema, J. M., Butera, F., Gardner, C. O., & Prescott, C. A. (2003). Life event dimensions of loss, humiliation, entrapment, and danger in the prediction of onsets of major depression and generalized anxiety. *Archives of General Psychiatry, 60*, 789–796.

References

Kessler, R. C. F., Berglund, P., Demler, O., Jin, R., & Walters, E. E. (2005). Lifetime prevalence and age-of-onset distributions of DSM-IV disorders in the national comorbidity survey replication. *Archives of General Psychiatry, 62*, 593–602.

Knez, I. (2005). Attachment and identity as related to a place and its perceived climate. *Journal of Environmental Psychology, 25*(2), 207–218.

Kroenke, K., Spitzer, R. L., Williams, J. B. W., Monahan, P. O., & Lowe, B. (2007). Anxiety disorders in primary care: Prevalence, impairment, comorbidity, and detection. *Annals of Internal Medicine, 146*, 317–325.

Langen, T. A., & Schuler, J. (2007). Effects of written emotional expression: The role of positive expectancies. *Health Psychology, 26*(2), 174–182.

Lovallo, W. R., & Thomas, T. R. (2000). Stress hormones in psychophysiological research: Emotional, behavioral, and cognitive implications. In J. T. Cacioppo, L. G. Tassinary, & G. Berntson (Eds.), *Handbook of psychophysiology* (pp. 342–367). New York: Cambridge University Press.

McCullough, M. E., Orsulak, P., Brandon, A., & Akers, L. (2007). Rumination, fear, and cortisol: An in vivo study of interpersonal transgressions. *Health Psychology, 26*(1), 126–132.

McEwen, B. S. (2004). *The end of stress as we know it*. Washington, DC: The Dana.

McEwen, B., & Lasley, E. N. (2003). Allostatic load: When protection gives way to damage. *Advances, 19*(1), 28–33.

Mussgay, L., & Ruddel, H. (2004). Autonomic dysfunctions in patients with anxiety throughout therapy. *Journal of Psychophysiology, 18*(1), 27–37.

Pennebaker, J. W., & Seagal, J. D. (1999). Forming a story: The health benefits of narrative. *Journal of Clinical Psychology, 55*, 1243–1254.

Purves, D., Augustine, G. J., Fitzpatrick, D., Katz, L. C., LaMantia, A. S., & McNamara, J. O. (1997). *Neuroscience* (pp. 440–446). Sunderland: Sinauer Associates.

Rasmussen, H. N., & Scheier, M. F. (2009). Optimism and physical health: A meta-analytic review. *Annals of Behavioral Medicine, 37*, 239–256.

Schore, A. N. (2002). Dysregulation of the right brain: A fundamental mechanism of traumatic attachment and the psychopathogenesis of post traumatic stress disorder. *The Australian and New Zealand Journal of Psychiatry, 36*, 9–30.

Timmons, B., & Ley, R. (1994). *Behavioral and psychological approaches to breathing disorders*. NY: Plenum.

Tompkins, M. A., & Martinez, K. A. (2010). *A Teen's guide to managing anxiety and panic*. Washington, DC: Magination Press.

Widmaier, E. P., Raff, H., & Strang, K. (2004). *Vander, Sherman & Luciano's human physiology* (9th ed.). Boston: McGraw Hill.

Wilhelm, F. H., Gevirtz, R., & Roth, W. T. (2001). Respiratory dysregulation in anxiety, functional cardiac, and pain disorders: Assessment, phenomenology, and treatment. *Behavior Modification, 25*(4), 513–545. doi:10.1177/0145445501254003.

Young, E. A., & Breslau, N. (2004). Cortisol and catecholamines in posttraumatic stress disorder. *Archives of General Psychiatry, 61*, 394–401.

Chapter 10
Diabetes and Obesity

Abstract Type 2 diabetes mellitus and obesity are two interrelated disorders that share etiological factors, including heredity, maladaptive behaviors, and distress. The prevalence of both disorders has increased over the past decade, particularly in ethnic minority groups. Understanding the role of choice-driven behaviors in the course of diabetes forms the basis for the Pathways interventions described in this chapter. The case narrative introduced here exemplifies the effects of stress and negative mood states on weight and glycemic stability and the reinstitution of positive mood and improved physiological control after intervention.

Keywords Diabetes mellitus • Obesity • Metabolic syndrome • Self-management

Definitions and Standard Management

Type 2 diabetes mellitus (DM) is defined as hyperglycemia (elevated blood glucose), coupled with cellular insulin resistance. The person with DM may produce sufficient or excessive quantities of insulin; however, adequate glucose does not enter the cells because the cell membranes have developed resistance. Average blood glucose is indicated by a blood test called glycosylated hemoglobin (HbA1c), which represents the values of blood glucose averaged over an approximately 3-month period; normal values are 6% or less (American Diabetes Association, 2009). Prior to the last decade, the onset of type 2 DM was associated with middle or late adulthood, but the increases in obesity in the U.S. young adult population have been paralleled by significant increases in new cases of type 2 DM, particularly in ethnic minorities (Center for Disease Control and Prevention, 2008; Ogden et al., 2006). The condition of prediabetes or glucose intolerance is now identified as a critical period during which the onset of diabetes can be slowed or prevented. Diet, exercise, problem-solving nutritional challenges, and sometimes medical management are recommended for prediabetes (Hankonen, Absetz, Haukkala, & Uutela, 2009; Knowler et al., 2002). It is important to intervene early, as soon as HbA1c levels begin to rise, since HbA1c is predictive, not only of future diabetes but also of increased risk for cardiovascular disease (Tsenkova, Love, Singer, & Ryff, 2008).

Type 2 DM is one of the group of disorders of metabolism that also includes essential hypertension, hyperlipidemia, and obesity. The overlapping genetic and maladaptive behavioral etiologies (inactivity, overeating, and stress) of these disorders led to the definition of the "metabolic syndrome." In this chapter, diabetes and obesity will be addressed, while hypertension and heart disease will be the focus of Chap. 11. It was decided to separate the components of the metabolic syndrome for several reasons. The prevalence of obesity, the most important precursor to diabetes, has been increasing over the past decades, whereas that of heart disease is actually lessening. Secondly, the authors believed that hypertension (elevated blood pressure) and heart disease were best coupled with another cardiovascular disorder, neurocardiogenic syncope (characterized by low blood pressure).

Traditional management of type 2 DM consists of education, oral hypoglycemic agents, diet, and exercise. The ADA recommends an educational program for all patients with diabetes that focuses on understanding the disease and self-management. Medication regimens are adjusted depending on HbA1c values and patients' daily monitoring of blood glucose. Over time, many patients with type 2 diabetes require daily injections of insulin (American Diabetes Association, 2005). Regular physical activity has been demonstrated to produce positive effects beyond weight loss alone, called "residual effects" that are considered as protective against elevated blood glucose and DM (Carnethon & Craft, 2008). Psychological/behavioral interventions have also been implemented for people with type 2 DM to produce better glycemic control, not necessarily to discontinue medical management. The major effective modalities are stress management, including relaxation and biofeedback, and psychotherapy (McGrady & Bailey, 2003; McGrady, 2010).

Psychophysiological Etiology

Multiple factors are associated with the onset of diabetes, including genetic predisposition, stress, insufficient sleep, altered mood, inactivity, and obesity. Stress is often associated with maladaptive eating habits, which predispose to excessive body weight and high blood glucose (Kyrou, Chrousos, & Tsignos, 2006). Chronic stress produces a load on the adaptation system such that the demands for psychological coping become more and more difficult to meet. With repetitive stress, both the physiological and psychological coping systems may not recover in between the stressful episodes. With very strong but intermittent stressful situations, the body and mind again may fail to adjust and instead generate chronic maladaptive responses (McEwen, 2004). Therefore, stress produces not only daily activation of the flight/fight/freeze responses, but also emotional distress, negative thinking, and sometimes, spiritual distress (McGrady, Bourey, & Bailey, 2003).

Negative emotions such as anxiety or depression contribute to the etiology of DM and subsequently, depressed mood and anxious thoughts magnify elevations in blood glucose. For example, depression affects physiological regulation of glucose levels in the blood and tissues, and undermines self-care behaviors (Anderson, Freedland, Clouse, & Lustman, 2001; Fisher, Thorpe, DeVellis, & DeVellis, 2007; Li, Ford, Strine, & Mordad, 2008). The depressed person will not be as active in personal self-management as the person without this negative mood state. Depression leads people to choose more of the comfort foods, to exercise less frequently, and to limit social interactions, all of which are in turn related to obesity and poor glycemic control (Simon et al., 2008). Negative mood seemingly interferes with diabetic patients' ability to benefit from psychophysiological interventions, perhaps due to low compliance (McGinnis, McGrady, Cox, & Grower-Dowling, 2005).

Persons who are anxious and chronically worried about their condition or about life stress are less likely to take the time to prepare adequate meals and to get regular exercise. Anger and hostility represent other negative mood states that impact individuals' self-care in addition to their personal relationships with others (Delahanty et al., 2007). Shared physiological pathways exist between mood and regulation of blood glucose. For example, depressed patients who demonstrated elevated salivary cortisol levels (indicating a type of depression and the presence of chronic stress) also had central obesity, a major predictor of elevated blood glucose (Weber-Hamann et al., 2002).

Obesity, simple to define but difficult to control, results from a discrepancy between energy taken in (food) and energy expenditure (activity and metabolism). In adults, body weight is maintained relatively constant based on communication among peripheral energy stores (fat cells), the gastrointestinal system, and several brain centers that regulate appetite. Signals are received by the hypothalamus, interpreted by higher brain centers to either increase or decrease food intake in order to maintain balance between consumption and the energy needs (Widmaier, Raff, & Strang, 2004).

The major long-term regulatory factor for maintenance of body weight is leptin, which is released by fat cells and travels through the blood stream to the group of neurons which comprise the feeding center in the hypothalamus (Froy, 2009). Leptin combines with receptors in the hypothalamus and produces a signal to decrease appetite and thereby decrease food intake. Other hormones like cortisol, neuropeptide Y, and ghrelin are appetite stimulants. Some of the stimulants are produced in the stomach or small intestine and some in other tissues. The normal feedback system consists of appetite suppression and appetite stimulating substances (Kyrou et al., 2006). Exercise is another powerful contributor to energy usage, appetite, and body weight.

When the leptin system is dysregulated, cell membranes may develop a resistance to leptin similarly to the impedance mentioned earlier of the tissues to insulin (Wang et al., 2001). So, overfeeding or eating too much perpetuates the difficult entry of glucose into the cells, thus, raising the amount of glucose in the blood. The normal signal to decrease feeding is either not received or misinterpreted, and eating continues despite high levels of leptin. The obese person consumes food for comfort and as an emotional placebo not purely for metabolic or energy needs. In central obesity, there is evidence for dysregulation of the hypothalamic pituitary adrenal axis and high cortisol levels (Björntorp, 1992).

In addition, negative emotional states are related to waist-hip ratio which indicates the amount of fat in the abdominal region (Ahlberg et al., 2002). Fat cells (adipocytes) secrete not only leptin, but also proinflammatory molecules such as IL6 and TNF alpha. So, stress not only promotes beta adrenergic activity and inhibits parasympathetic activity, but also induces the release of cytokines from adipocytes, strongly suggesting a clear link among stress, obesity, and inflammatory processes. These relationships are explained in more detail in Chap. 4. Brown fat found in very small amounts in adult humans in the neck and thorax areas has a high metabolic rate; the amount is inversely correlated with body mass index, suggesting a role in adult metabolism (Cypess et al., 2009). In summary, persons with fat concentrated in the abdominal regions demonstrate high plasma cortisol levels, impaired leptin sensitivity, low serotonin, increased free fatty acids, and indicators of chronic, low-level inflammation. Associations exist among stress-induced activity of the autonomic nervous system, emotional distress, and manifestations of metabolic dysregulation.

Socioeconomic status (SES) has been correlated with excessive daily challenges and with physical and psychological distress (Prescott, Godtfredsen, Osler, Schnohr, & Barefoot, 2007). In a lengthy (12 years) exploration of the relationship between SES and the metabolic syndrome, low SES increased the risk for the metabolic syndrome. For example, people of relatively low SES are confronted with more situations requiring adaptation, and use more psychological reserves than people of higher SES. Simply stated, those with more education, better jobs, and higher income are able to draw on and replenish interpersonal, professional, and tangible resources when necessary (Matthews, Gallo, Raikkonen, & Kuller, 2008). Work stress, since it is usually chronic, is another key risk factor for the development of diabetes. Even workplace stress of moderate severity, if it is frequent, is associated with increased blood glucose over time (Chandola, Brunner, & Marmot, 2009). The term "coping" is often used to describe how people handle stressful situations, but coping can be adaptive or maladaptive, leading to resolution of the problem or to harboring negative thoughts and a chronic overarousal. Higher scores (indicating better ability to manage stressful situations) on problem-based coping inventories and positive affect have been correlated with lower values of HbA1c (Tsenkova et al., 2008).

Sleep deprivation has recently been suggested as a harbinger of DM, largely based on the evidence of the effects of poor sleep on regulation of blood glucose (Knutsen & van Cauter, 2008). Lack of sleep or disruptive sleep hinders the regulation of food intake and maintenance of normal body weight (Van Cauter et al., 2004). Leptin, the substance that decreases appetite, is released in smaller amounts in sleep-deprived humans. During slow wave, deep sleep, the stress hormone cortisol is inhibited and growth hormone release increases (Latta et al., 2004; Patel, 2009; Spiegel, Tasali, Leproult, & Van Cauter, 2004). In summary, not only are there normal variations in appetite and metabolism during waking hours, but also during night time sleep. Based on research on shift workers and other people with disrupted sleep the circadian clock may have an essential role in regulating metabolism and energy balance; this clock is linked with lipogenic and adipogenic pathways (Froy, 2009).

In summary, DM is a lifelong illness which requires the use of coping skills and self-management decisions on a daily basis. Interrelationships among behavior, daily stress, mood, and quality of life occur in diabetes perhaps more so than in any other chronic illness (Fisher et al., 2007). Behavioral, psychological, and physiological systems interact on a minute-by-minute basis to maintain glycemic control. Insufficient sleep, unhealthy food choices, and lack of resilience increase risk for the serious complications of this disease.

The Case of Rosa

Rosa was a 35-year-old woman of Italian descent, who was diagnosed with type 2 DM 5 years ago, and treated with an oral hypoglycemic agent. There was a history of diabetes on her father's side. Rosa was approximately 30–35 lbs. overweight; her HbA1c levels were elevated (8.0%) and she struggled with glycemic control. Rosa had been told by her physician that if her blood glucose levels continued to increase then she would be advised to begin insulin to avoid complications, such as neuropathy. The possibility of developing complications and having to take insulin was very frightening to Rosa, and she said that she would do anything to prevent daily injections.

Rosa and her husband Tony had three children, two boys aged 15 and 13 and a 9-year-old girl. Rosa worked part time in a medical office, and on most days she had to complete multiple tasks that required different skill sets, all under time deadlines. When she got home from work she prepared meals for the family. Evenings were usually spent in cleaning and supervising kids' homework during the school year. Meal choices were frequently based on convenience, but were not healthy for a person with diabetes. The family dinner time often consisted of arguments about the kids' behaviors or disagreements about allocation of money. Although Rosa could identify daily stressors, she was not aware of the effects of stress on blood glucose.

Rosa's major sources of stress were her part-time job, her weight, and her 15-year-old son Frankie, who began to get into trouble when he entered ninth grade. As the school work became harder, Frankie struggled and did not put sufficient time into studying; his grades were slipping. Frankie also became belligerent towards his teachers and both Rosa and Tony. Rosa felt helpless about parenting Frankie and anxious that the younger children would model Frankie and start getting into trouble also.

The assessment process for Rosa consisted of 2 weeks of monitoring blood glucose and negative emotional states. She questioned why a psychologist would request blood glucose data, but nonetheless she agreed to do it. Rosa's readiness to change was determined to be at the preparation level (Prochaska et al., 1994). Although her initial motivation was based on fear, the therapist thought that fear would be sufficient to get her through the first few weeks of treatment. Motivational interviewing (Rollnick, Miller, & Butler, 2008; West, DiLillo, Bursac, Gore, & Greene, 2007) was implemented to develop a more mature level of motivation. It was determined that Rosa had mild levels of depression and moderate levels of anxiety, sufficient for a diagnosis of adjustment disorder with depressed and anxious mood.

Level One Interventions. The Level One interventions recommended for Rosa were soothe and feed. Rosa had taken a yoga class a couple of years ago and was still familiar with the breathing techniques. When asked to demonstrate those techniques, she was able to do it without any difficulty. She was advised to resume the daily use of mindful breathing and to institute a period of time every day to spend by herself. Initially, there was a great deal of resistance to this recommendation. Rosa had some feelings of guilt about her time away from home, including work hours and an additional half hour commute each way. However, she agreed that she would try to take 15 min to herself before leaving for work, since there was no one else home at that time.

The next Level One intervention was to apply the mindfulness principle to eating (Albers, 2008). Since her experience of preparing dinner and eating food was quite negative, she did not see how she could slow down this process but agreed to try. After 2 weeks, Rosa returned and reported that she had resumed the breathing exercise and had taken some time for herself only once or twice a week. She was unable to slow down the food preparation or dinner. It was then suggested that Rosa remain at the dinner table after the rest of the family had finished their meals and this suggestion was accepted. During this time, she did allow herself to enjoy the end of the meal. This simple change allowed Rosa some additional time to herself. However, Rosa's mood remained depressed, her anxiety about Frankie ever present, and her blood sugar continued to fluctuate. She continued to mention her fear of having to take insulin.

Level Two Interventions. The Level Two interventions that were recommended were progressive relaxation and exercise. Rosa had already been cleared for an exercise program by her physician and so it was not necessary to begin with simple movement; however, time was certainly an issue in this regard. The therapist guided Rosa in progressive relaxation and instructed her to practice it daily for 15 min. However, Rosa refused the exercise recommendation because of time constraints.

After 2 weeks, Rosa returned in a highly distressed state. Frankie had been picked up riding in a car with an open container of alcohol. Rosa wanted to obtain a lawyer, but Tony was so furious that he was stating that Frankie should go to court alone and take his punishment. Rosa had not begun the progressive relaxation and was focusing all of her attention on her son's difficulties. The result of this session was to reemphasize the basics: to return to the Level One intervention platform and to encourage Rosa to maintain her self-soothing ritual and her personal time at the end of dinner. She questioned whether she should discontinue treatment until "this mess is cleared up."

The principles of motivational interviewing were of great importance and were utilized in this session. Rosa finally agreed that her anxiety was doing nothing to help Frankie, whereas a calmer mental state allowed her to better focus on problem solving. She committed to continue therapy and to take 15 min to relax before work, specifically mindful breathing and progressive relaxation. Interestingly, Tony began to sit at the table with her after dinner. Although Tony wanted to use this time to argue about Frankie, Rosa was firm that this time was devoted to enjoying the end of the meal. However, Rosa asked Tony to stay in the kitchen and help her clean up and then both parents discussed the decisions to be made regarding Frankie. With the preceding 15 min of mindful eating, the family hot topics were easier to discuss.

Level Three Interventions. The Level Three interventions recommended for Rosa consisted of mindfulness meditation, biofeedback, and acceptance and commitment therapy (ACT) (Gregg, Callaghan, Hayes, & Glenn-Lawson, 2007; Hayes, Luoma, Bond, Masuda, & Lillis, 2006; McGinnis et al., 2005). Rosa was advised to use the yoga physical postures that she had learned previously, since she could not commit to other physical exercise, and she agreed to reinstitute yoga practice with a DVD that she had at home (Innes, Bourguignon, & Taylor, 2005). Mindfulness meditation was recommended so that Rosa would be able to focus on the moment, being aware of her feelings and addressing negative thoughts as necessary. Rosa realized that during the course of the work day there were multiple occasions where she could take a few seconds to appreciate completion of a task. Certainly, when Rosa entered therapy, she was unaware of anything positive in her work life, her personal life, or with her family. Everything felt overwhelming and out of control. Daily practice of mindfulness allowed Rosa to slow time down and to find minutes of enjoyment during the course of a normal day. Biofeedback, specifically surface electromyography (SEMG) and temperature biofeedback, was incorporated to give Rosa a sense of control over her physiological responses to stress. She began to see that this sense of control could be applied to her blood glucose, her weight, and her mood.

Rosa eventually asked for an adjustment in her work schedule. Instead of coming in at noon and working until 5 with no breaks, Rosa requested to arrive at the office at 11:00 so that she could take two half-hour breaks during the course of the afternoon. Her employer denied this request. However, compromise was reached in that she would arrive at 11:00, be allowed to take a half-hour break and leave at 4:30. This small change allowed Rosa to have a quiet lunch and relaxation period between 2:00 and 2:30. Getting home a half hour early allowed Rosa more opportunity to prepare healthier meals.

Approximately 6 months into treatment, additional problems with Frankie caused Rosa to have a setback in personal stress management, which was reflected in increased blood glucose. She became overwhelmed again by Frankie's problems. A crisis therapy appointment resulted in the revelation that Rosa identified with Frankie. In her own teenage years, Rosa had contentious times with her parents. Rosa's parents wanted her to go to college, partially because they had never had the opportunity, but she had already met Tony and had no interest in further education. Now Frankie's problems reminded her of these difficult times; she blamed herself, saying: "like mother, like son." Rosa thought that Frankie's actions were her responsibility just as she had blamed her own mother for many years after she left her parents' home. Painfully, Rosa realized that she could not control her son's behavior and therefore, her own past problems in school were her own responsibility and not her parents, based on the choices that she had made.

Rosa's mother was still alive and healthy at the age of 65 although her dad was deceased; so Rosa decided that her mother had a right to know of the problems with her grandson. Interestingly, when Rosa arrived at her mother's home, the smell of cooking onions and garlic in olive oil brought back a flash of memory of family dinners with her parents and siblings. The memory was so vivid that she stopped in the doorway for a minute, transported back, not to the hard times, but to the happy occasions that she had shared with her immediate and her extended large Italian family.

When Rosa explained Frankie's problems to her mother, it resulted in the first honest and open conversation that Rosa had with her mother in many years. Past difficulties between mother and daughter were explored, and Rosa relayed to her mother her newly discovered sense of responsibility for her own actions so many years ago. After the mother-daughter conversation, Rosa decided that she would resume cooking some of the ethnic dishes that she had enjoyed in the past. Mom supplied several spices from her cupboard and shared three or four recipes, which Rosa made over a period of several weeks. Cooking these dishes in Rosa's own kitchen repeatedly triggered only the pleasant memories of childhood.

Eventually, Rosa and Tony agreed on a strategy to deal with Frankie. They communicated to Frankie that mom or dad refused to be blamed for his problems and that he was making conscious decisions about his own life that would have consequences later. They would pay the attorney fees this time and would support Frankie's attendance at his own therapy sessions, but Frankie needed to take responsibility for his own actions, because he was creating his own future; Rosa was not creating it for him.

Rosa's therapy continued for 18 months, at the end of which she had lost 25 lbs and her most recent hemoglobin A1c was 6.5%, a major decrease, although still above normal. Her mood was significantly improved and she felt more positive about the future than she had in a long time. Frankie continued to have his struggles, but Rosa felt confident that she was doing the best that she could. Most of the time the kids still left the table as soon as they were finished, but Rosa and Tony continued to spend additional time after dinner, enjoying a cup of tea together. Sometimes, one of the kids sat with Rosa and Tony, adhering to the mindful eating rule. Rosa committed to continuing the relaxation meditation and positive coping strategies.

Weight loss is notoriously difficult to achieve and to maintain over time. Research confirms the difficulty in losing weight in women experiencing chronic stress and the challenges in keeping stressed obese women in programs designed for weight loss (Kim, Bursac, DiLillo, White, & West, 2009). For Rosa, mindfulness decreased the impact of stress-related eating and her preference for higher fat and sweet tasting foods lessened, facilitating better choices. Healthy eating is not simple, but actually results form a complex series of actions, beginning with shopping lists, consideration of cost, transportation to stores, variety of foods available, and knowledge of food storage and food preparation (Hankonen et al., 2009). Rosa's interest in cooking Italian ethnic foods was helpful in meal planning and providing balanced nutritious food for herself and her family. One of the signal events in therapy was Rosa's visit with her mother and the effects of the smells of her mother's cooking as a memory trigger. For many years particular odors have been known to reproduce entire memories of the past in vivid detail (Proust quoted in Vial, 2009).

The choice of interventions for Rosa considered her lack of skills to manage her diabetes, her need for relief of emotional distress, particularly the burden of guilt for her own and her son's behaviors. As Rosa's treatment progressed, her distress gradually reduced, and her sense of mastery over her diabetes improved. Her past positive experience with yoga provided an initial entry point, which was mindful breathing (Innes et al., 2005). As Rosa acquired skills to help manage her physiological responses to stress, she felt empowered and her blood glucose levels decreased. McGinnis et al. (2005) suggested that biofeedback and relaxation could benefit people with DM, but depressed mood may derail efforts to teach patients to manage their blood glucose. In certain situations, group-based counseling consisting of cognitive restructuring and stress management can be utilized to address the multifaceted problems faced by people with DM. Common challenges include not only the actual number indicating blood glucose, but also the fear of complications, feeling of helplessness, and exaggerated physiological responses to stress (Karlsen, Idsoe, Dirdal, Hanestad, & Bru, 2004). Group sessions mobilize social support as participants share stories of challenges faced and their solutions. Yi, Vitaliano, Smith, Yi, and Weinger (2008) found that stress was less potent in elevating HbA1c in patients who had higher levels of resilience and more positive coping, defined as self-esteem, self-efficacy, self-mastery, and optimism. Resilience buffered the negative effects of stress on blood glucose.

Case Summary

Interventions for Rosa were chosen based on assessment of her needs, her capabilities, and evidence-based behavioral medicine. ACT consisting of mindfulness, values-based action, and acceptance was particularly effective with Rosa. She restored the mindful breathing that she had previously learned in yoga class, gradually instituted mindful eating and was eventually able to accept her diabetes. Self-management improved dramatically. SEMG and thermal biofeedback with relaxation therapy provided Rosa with a renewed sense of control of her physiological responses to stress and opened the possibility that she could also attain glycemic control. Although weight loss was the by-product of these changes and was not addressed directly, Rosa's confidence increased as her weight decreased. Feedback from her physician was very positive regarding her lowered HbA1c levels. She remained on the oral hypoglycemic agent, but the threats of complications and need for insulin were eliminated.

References

Ahlberg, A., Ljung, T., Rosmond, R., McEwen, B., Holm, G., Akesson, H. O., et al. (2002). Depression and anxiety symptoms in relation to anthropometry and metabolism in men. *Psychiatry Research, 112*, 101–110.
Albers, S. (2008). *Eat, drink and be mindful*. Oakland, CA: New Harbinger Publications.
American Diabetes Association. (2005). *Standards for diabetes education 2005*. www.diabetes.org

American Diabetes Association. (2009). Diagnosis and classification of diabetes mellitus. *Diabetes Care, 32*(S1), S62–S67.
Anderson, R. J., Freedland, K. H., Clouse, R. E., & Lustman, P. J. (2001). The prevalence of comorbid depression in adults with diabetes. *Diabetes Care, 24,* 1069–1078.
Björntorp, P. (1992). Regional fat distribution-implications for type II diabetes. *International Journal of Obesity, 16,* S19–S27.
Carnethon, M. R., & Craft, L. L. (2008). Autonomic regulation of the association between exercise and diabetes. *Exercise and Sport Sciences Reviews, 36*(91), 12–18.
Center for Disease Control and Prevention. (2008). *National diabetes fact sheet: General information and national estimates on diabetes in the United States, 2007.* Atlanta, GA; U.S. Department of Health and Human Services, Centers for Disease Control and Prevention, 2008. Retrieved 2007, from, http://www.cdc.gov/diabetes/pubs/pdf.ndfs
Chandola, T., Brunner, E., & Marmot, M. (2009). Chronic stress at work and the metabolic syndrome: Prospective study. *British Medical Journal, 332,* 521–525.
Cypess, A. M., Lehman, S., Williams, G., Tai, I., Rodman, D., Goldfine, A. B., et al. (2009). Identification and importance of brown adipose tissue in adult humans. *The New England Journal of Medicine, 360*(15), 1509–1517.
Delahanty, L. M., Grant, R. W., Wittenberg, E., Bosch, J. L., Wexler, D. J., Cagliero, E., et al. (2007). Association of diabetes-related emotional distress with diabetes treatment in primary care patients with type 2 diabetes. *Diabetic Medicine, 24,* 48–54.
Fisher, E. B., Thorpe, C. T., DeVellis, B. M., & DeVellis, R. F. (2007). Healthy coping, negative emotions, and diabetes management: A systematic review and appraisal. *The Diabetes Educator, 33*(6), 1080–1103.
Froy, O. (2009). Metabolism and circadian rhythms: Implications for obesity. *Endocrinology Review, 31*(1), 1–24.
Gregg, J. A., Callaghan, G. M., Hayes, S. C., & Glenn-Lawson, J. L. (2007). Improving diabetes self-management through acceptance, mindfulness, and values: A randomized controlled trial. *Journal of Consulting and Clinical Psychology, 75*(2), 336–343.
Hankonen, N., Absetz, P., Haukkala, A., & Uutela, A. (2009). Socioeconomic status and psychosocial mechanisms of lifestyle change in a type 2 diabetes prevention trial. *Annals of Behavioral Medicine, 38,* 160–165.
Hayes, S. C., Luoma, J., Bond, F., Masuda, A., & Lillis, J. (2006). Acceptance and commitment therapy: Model, processes, and outcomes. *Behaviour Research and Therapy, 44,* 1–25.
Innes, K. E., Bourguignon, C., & Taylor, A. G. (2005). Risk indices associated with the insulin resistance syndrome, cardiovascular disease, and possible protection with yoga: A systematic review. *The Journal of the American Board of Family Practice, 18,* 491–519.
Karlsen, B., Idsoe, T., Dirdal, I., Hanestad, B. R., & Bru, E. (2004). Effects of a group-based counselling programme on diabetes-related stress, coping, psychological well-being and metabolic control in adults with type 1 or type 2 diabetes. *Patient Education and Counseling, 53,* 299–308.
Kim, K. H., Bursac, Z., DiLillo, V., White, D. B., & West, D. S. (2009). Stress, race, and body weight. *Health Psychology, 28*(1), 131–135.
Knowler, W. C., Barrett-Connor, E., Fowler, S. E., Hamman, R. F., Lachin, J. M., Walker, E. A., et al. (2002). Reduction in the incidence of type 2diabetes with lifestyle intervention or metformin. *The New England Journal of Medicine, 346*(6), 393–403.
Knutsen, K. L., & van Cauter, E. (2008). Associations between sleep loss and increased risk of obesity and diabetes. *Annals of the New York Academy of Sciences, 1129,* 287–304.
Kyrou, J., Chrousos, G. P., & Tsignos, C. (2006). Stress, visceral obesity, and metabolic complications. In G. P. Chrousos & C. Tsigos (Eds.), *Stress, obesity, and metabolic syndrome* (pp. 77–110). New York: Blackwell Publishing.
Latta, F., Nedeltcheva, A., Spiegel, K., Leproult, R., Vandenbril, C., Weiss, R., et al. (2004). Reciprocal interactions between the GH axis and sleep. *Growth Hormone & IGF Research,* Suppl A, S10–7.
Li, C., Ford, E. S., Strine, T. W., & Mordad, A. H. (2008). Prevalence of depression among U.S. adults with diabetes. *Diabetes Care, 31*(1), 105–107.

References

Matthews, K. A., Gallo, L., Raikkonen, K., & Kuller, L. H. (2008). Association between socioeconomic status and metabolic syndrome in women: Testing the reserve capacity model. *Health Psychology, 27*, 576–583.

McEwen, B. (2004). *The end of stress as we know it.*. Washington, DC: The Dana Press.

McGinnis, R. A., McGrady, A., Cox, S., & Grower-Dowling, K. (2005). Biofeedback-assisted relaxation in type 2 diabetes. *Diabetes Care, 28*(9), 2143–2149.

McGrady, A., & Bailey, B. (2003). Diabetes mellitus. In M. S. Schwartz & F. Andrasik (Eds.), *Biofeedback: A practitioner's guide* (pp. 727–749). New York: Guilford Press.

McGrady, A., Bourey, R., & Bailey, B. (2003). The metabolic syndrome: Obesity, type 2 diabetes, hypertension, and hyperlipidemia. In D. Moss, A. McGrady, T. Davies, & I. Wickramasekera (Eds.), *Handbook of mind-body medicine for primary care* (pp. 275–297). Thousand Oaks, CA: Sage.

McGrady, A. (2010). The effects of biofeedback in diabetes and essential hypertension. *Cleveland Clinic Journal of Medicine 77*(3), S68–S71.

Ogden, C. L., Carroll, M. D., Curtin, L. R., McDowell, M. A., Tabak, C. J., & Flegal, K. M. (2006). Prevalence of overweight and obesity in the United States, 1999–2004. *Journal of the American Medical Association, 295*, 1549–1555.

Patel, S. R. (2009). Reduced sleep as an obesity risk factor. *Obesity Reviews, 2*(10), 61–68.

Prescott, E., Godtfredsen, N., Osler, M., Schnohr, P., & Barefoot, J. (2007). Social gradient in the metabolic syndrome not explained by psychosocial and behavioural factors: Evidence from the Copenhagen city heart study. *European Journal of Cardiovascular Prevention and Rehabilitation, 14*, 405–412.

Prochaska, J. O., Velicer, W. F., Rossi, J. S., Goldstein, M. G., Marcus, B. H., & Rakowski, W. (1994). Stages of change and decisional balance for twelve problem behaviors. *Health Psychology, 12*, 39–46.

Rollnick, S., Miller, W. R., & Butler, C. C. (2008). *Motivational interviewing in health care*. NewYork: Guilford Press.

Simon, G. E., Ludman, E. J., Linde, J. A., Operskalski, B. H., Ichikawa, L., Rohde, P., et al. (2008). Association between obesity and depression in the middle-aged women. *General Hospital Psychiatry, 30*, 32–39.

Spiegel, K., Tasali, E., Leproult, R., & Van Cauter, E. (2004). Metabolic consequences of sleep and sleep loss. *Sleep Medicine, 89*, 2119–2126.

Tsenkova, V. K., Love, G. D., Singer, B. H., & Ryff, C. D. (2008). Coping and positive affect predict longitudinal change in glycosylated hemoglobin. *Health Psychology, 27*(3), S163–S171.

Van Cauter, E., Spiegel, K., Tasali, E., & Leproult, R. (2004). Metabolic consequences of sleep and sleep loss. *Sleep Medicine, 9*(1), S23–S28.

Vial, F. (2009). *The unconscious in philosophy and French and European literature: Nineteenth and early twentieth century*. New York, NY: Rodopi.

Wang, J., Obici, S., Morgan, K., Barzilai, N., Feng, Z., & Rossetti, L. (2001). Overfeeding rapidly induces leptin and insulin resistance. *Diabetes, 50*, 2786–2788.

Weber-Hamann, B., Hentschel, F., Kniest, A., Deuschle, M., Colla, M., Lederbogen, F., et al. (2002). Hypercortisolemic depression is associated with increased intra-abdominal fat. *Psychosomatic Medicine, 64*, 274–277.

West, D. S., DiLillo, V., Bursac, Z., Gore, S. A., & Greene, P. G. (2007). Motivational interviewing improves weight loss in women with type 2 diabetes. *Diabetes Care, 30*, 1081–1087.

Widmaier, E. P., Raff, H., & Strang, K. (2004). *Vander Sherman & Luciano's human physiology* (9th ed.). Boston: McGraw Hill.

Yi, J. P., Vitaliano, P. P., Smith, R. E., Yi, J. C., & Weinger, K. (2008). The role of resilience on psychological adjustment and physical health in patients with diabetes. *British Journal of Health Psychology, 13*(2), 311–325.

Chapter 11
Hypertension and Neurocardiogenic Syncope

Abstract Blood pressure is regulated by neural and endocrine systems to maintain sufficient perfusion of tissues during rest and activity. Sustained elevated blood pressure increases risk for heart disease and stroke. In contrast, periods of low perfusion or hypotension are associated with dizziness and syncope, which are risk factors for sudden death. Many psychosocial factors affect blood pressure and its regulation. In this chapter, the Pathways Model is applied to cases of essential hypertension and neurocardiogenic syncope to illustrate the multilevel treatment approach to these psychophysiological disorders.

Keywords Hypertension • Syncope • Depression • Anxiety

Introduction

The terms "psychocardiology" and "behavioral cardiology" have been in use for almost two decades and suggest that psychological and emotional states affect functioning of the cardiovascular system. Perusal of the most respected cardiology scientific journals highlights the relevance of behavioral and emotional factors to practitioners who care for patients with heart disease, stroke, chronic heart failure, and the autonomic disorders (Das & O-Keefe, 2006; Rozanski, Blumenthal, Davidson, Saah, & Kubzansky, 2005). In clinical practice, stress is frequently mentioned in the context of a medical evaluation for irregularities in blood pressure, whether the pressure is too high or too low. Assessment of the risk for cardiac events, such as heart attack, stroke, or loss of consciousness from syncope acknowledges the relevance of psychological factors and maladaptive behaviors (Bigger & Glassman, 2010).

Regulation of Blood Pressure

Blood pressure (BP) values are expressed as systolic/diastolic in millimeters of mercury (mmHg). Systolic BP (SBP) is defined as the maximum pressure that occurs during ejection of blood from the heart, and diastolic BP (DBP) is the minimum pressure that occurs during cardiac relaxation. Mean arterial pressure (MAP) is the average pressure driving blood through all organs except the lungs to ensure adequate perfusion of tissues. MAP is the product of cardiac output (heart rate in beats per minute × stroke volume output (the amount of blood ejected per heart beat)) and the total peripheral resistance (TPR) (Ganong, 2005). Heart rate is influenced by multiple factors including physical movement, breathing, emotional state, and neural activity. Variations in heart rate are normally correlated with breathing in a complex pattern termed respiratory sinus arrhythmia (RSA), where greater heart rate variability (HRV) is a sign of cardiac health (Force, 1996).

TPR is the impediment or resistance to the flow of blood in the arteries, arterioles, and to a lesser extent, the veins. Sympathetic and parasympathetic autonomic neural activity, circulating substances in the blood, and local conditions in the tissues all influence TPR. For example, under stressful conditions, sympathetic nervous system activity increases causing the arterioles to constrict, presenting a larger resistance to the flow of blood. In concert with increased heart rate, a larger TPR raises BP. Rapid responses to stress or physical activity are organized by the nervous system, while long-term changes require renal and endocrine involvement (Widmaier, Raff, Hershel, & Strang, 2006). BP varies throughout the waking hours of the day, depending on physical activity, emotion, and environment. During sleep, persons with normal BP exhibit a drop in both SBP and DBP of about 10%, called "dipping." Family history of hypertension, African American ethnicity, male gender, and negative emotions have been correlated with non-dipping, which results in higher risk for cardiovascular disease (Kario, Schwartz, Davidson, & Pickering, 2001; Linden, Klassen, & Phillips, 2008).

Essential Hypertension

Essential or primary hypertension is defined as chronically elevated BP of unknown origin and is the most common type. The Seventh Report of the Joint National Committee (2003) defined a new category called "prehypertension" formerly "high normal" which denotes SBP between 120 and 139 or DBP between 80 and 89 mmHg. The two stages of hypertension are based on higher levels of SBP and DBP in addition to other risk factors such as age, obesity, presence of type 2 diabetes, hyperlipidemia, and lifestyle factors such as alcohol, high sodium diet, and inactivity. Central to the development of essential hypertension is autonomic imbalance, that is, sympathetic overactivity and underactivity of the parasympathetic system (Brook & Julius, 2000; Sakakibara & Hayano, 1996; Sakakibara, Takeuchi, & Hayano, 1994).

Psychosocial Factors Influencing Blood Pressure

Demographic factors, such as age, gender, and ethnicity strongly affect BP. In general, BP increases with age, but men have higher BP than women only until their mid-sixties (Luke, 1996; Reckelhoff, 2001). Adult African Americans are much more likely to have elevated BP than Caucasians throughout the life span (Winkleby, Kraemer, Ahn, & Warady, 1998; Wright et al., 2008). Understanding the rate of change in BP over time is challenging because adjunctive factors influence the trajectory. Stressful conditions during childhood and low levels of parental education quicken the rate of change (Lehman, Kiefe, Taylor, & Seeman, 2009). In a 15-year longitudinal study, time urgency, competitiveness, and exaggerated achievement orientation were associated with greater than the normal age related increases in BP (Whooley, de Jonge, Vittinghoff, Otte, & Moos, 2008; Yan et al., 2003). Social support is widely believed to buffer the effects of stress on many physiological systems (Schwerdtfer & Friedrich-Mai, 2009). For example, marital status, specifically, being married, influences HRV in a positive way, independently of age (Randall, Bhattacharyya, & Steptoe, 2009). However, offers of support and personal closeness with others have different effects depending on the person's tendency towards hostility. In the high hostile personality type, support does not decrease BP, presumably because negative interactions interfere with the benefits of socialization (Holt-Lunstad, Smith, & Uchino, 2008; Vella, Kamarck, & Shiffman, 2008).

An extensive literature supports the importance of psychological factors such as depression, anger, and anxiety as influences on BP and risk for heart disease (Dimsdale, 2008; Kaplan & Nunes, 2003; Kop, Kuhl, Barasch, Jenny, & Gottlieb, 2010; Kubansky, Davidson, & Rozanski, 2005; Park & Pepine, 2010). Low HRV, an indicator of poor cardiac health, is commonly found in patients with depression who have coronary disease or a recent history of acute myocardial infarction (Carney, Freedland, & Veith, 2005). Even in medically healthy adults, stressful situations produced aberrant autonomic responses to stress in those with higher scores on the Beck Depression Inventory (Hughes & Stoney, 2000). Impaired recovery after stressful situations in depressed individuals is also relevant to risk for heart disease (Salomon, Clift, Karlsdottir, & Rottenberg, 2009). In actuality, depression is an independent and significant risk factor for the development of heart disease and stroke (Surtees et al., 2008), and the relationship appears to be bidirectional (Khawaja, Westermeyer, Gajwani, & Feinstein, 2009).

Behavior is commonly affected by negative emotional states, for example, persons who are depressed will not be as active in their own self-care as those without this negative mood state (Bonnet, Irving, Terra, & Berthez, 2005). Depression impedes individuals from adhering to their medical regimen and cardiac rehabilitation because their attitude is one of defeat (McGrady, McGinnis, Badenhop, Bentle, & Rajput, 2009). Even normal daily tasks seem to require abnormal amounts of energy; additional responsibilities easily overwhelm the depressed person. A sense of mastery or self-efficacy in simple self-care tasks or more challenging activities seems to be influential in maintaining heart health (Barkar, Ali, & Whooley, 2007; Sarkar et al., 2007; Surtees et al., 2010).

Anxious thoughts, worry, and feelings of anxiety are associated with increased stress hormone levels and autonomic dysfunction, manifested as increased heart rate, increased BP, and greater TPR. Repeated, frequent stressful experiences frequently produce chronic dysregulation of the autonomic nervous system (ANS), including decreased sensitivity of the (baro)receptors that monitor pressure and low HRV. Over time, risk for sustained hypertension and heart disease increases (Kubansky et al., 2005; Vijayvergiya, 2008). Other physiological mechanisms currently proposed to explain the effects of generalized anxiety or repeated panic attacks on hypertension or heart disease are subacute chronic inflammation (Sher, 2001) and serotonin deficiency (Davies, Hood, Christmas, & Nutt, 2008). Psychological state not only affects daytime BP but hostility, for example, also interferes with nighttime BP dipping (Mezick et al., 2010).

Case of Marquise

Marquise was a 46-year-old African American male, with a 15-year history of essential hypertension. His medication regimen was based on standard medical therapeutic recommendations (calcium channel blocker and diuretic) (Chobanian et al., 2003). He was married to Chantal, a lawyer, and they had two teenage children. Marquise worked full-time as a certified public accountant and was proud of his reputation for accuracy, but his clients were sometimes put off by his curt manner and impatience. Marquise had little time for outside activities or exercise particularly during tax season. He came home from work very tired in the evening and consumed two cocktails each night and more on weekend evenings.

Six months prior to referral to our clinic, Marquise had a myocardial infarction. He had a stent placed and began cardiac rehabilitation, but he did not complete the program. Marquise tended to compare himself to others and make negative judgments about his perceived capability in comparison to others' competence. Watching other patients walk briskly around the track without any evidence of fatigue while he struggled was intolerable. In addition, his team of physicians and exercise specialists contained not a single person of color, and this bothered him greatly.

Marquise was interviewed in May, after tax season. On assessment, Marquise reported a family history of heart disease, diabetes, and obesity. Marquise demonstrated several unhealthy behaviors, including using alcohol as a self soothing agent, lack of exercise and maladaptive interpretations of stressful work situations. Marquise was the first person in his family to complete college and become a professional. In school he was calmed by the stability and reproducibility of mathematics, but in the actual world of accounting, clients frequently asked for exemptions, begged him to look for tax loopholes, and challenged Marquise when he disallowed deductions. He felt angry and resentful and emotionally unprepared for these client demands.

Marquise endorsed feelings of sadness and hopelessness about his physical condition and feared a second heart attack. He worried about the increases in heart rate that he experienced while exercising and during work stress. His scores on the psychological inventories were 16 (Beck Depression Inventory) and 22 (Beck Anxiety Inventory) indicating moderate depression and significant anxiety.

Level One interventions. The Level One interventions implemented for Marquise were breathe, sleep, and move. The mindful breathing technique was taught to Marquise to restore a normal respiratory rhythm, moderate anxiety, and prepare him for the Level Three intervention, HRV feedback. Marquise was instructed to practice the breathing technique first for 2–3 min a day and then to increase the time to 5 min per day. Since his sleep was not usually restful and he was waking up fatigued almost every morning, sleep hygiene recommendations were provided. A regular bedtime was established for weekdays and weekends. He was instructed to avoid caffeine after 6 pm and to eat a light meal in the evening. He was to use the bedroom for sleep, for intimacy, and not for watching television, reading accounting document, or other activities that are not conducive to facilitating initiation of sleep. During this discussion, Marquise revealed that he and Chantal had not been intimate since his heart attack; he felt that he was damaged and also greatly feared the sensations of rapid heart rate and flushing that occurred during sex.

The issue of possible substance abuse was addressed early in therapy. It was determined that Marquise's use of alcohol was overuse and occasional abuse but not dependence. Marquise readily understood that he was using alcohol as a stress management technique and that it basically was not working very well. It was explained to Marquise that alcohol interfered with sleep, and sleep is one of the basic rhythms that needed to be reestablished. This plan was devised: Marquise was to dilute the alcohol in each of his two drinks that he had in the evening, and he was to use a sugar free mix to decrease calories. Once that routine was established, Marquise was instructed to eliminate the alcohol from one drink and continue with the alcohol in the second drink. He was to drink the nonalcoholic beverage first and the alcoholic beverage second, again with the same dilution as before. After 1 month, Marquise reported that he preferred to have one full strength alcoholic beverage than two weaker ones and this is what he continued with for the remainder of treatment.

Thirdly, Marquise was instructed to begin to move, slowly increasing the amount of movement that he performed each day. The word "exercise" was not used because of the negative connotations to this word for Marquise, in particular his "failure" at cardiac rehabilitation. So emphasis was placed on movement, for example, taking a short walk in his neighborhood and climbing the stairs at his office.

Level Two interventions. The Level Two interventions consisted of relaxation skill building and a return to cardiac rehabilitation. The physician in charge of cardiac rehabilitation was contacted and was willing to accommodate Marquise's concerns. Marquise was assigned a time for rehabilitation when most of the other patients were in early recovery from a cardiac event. Instead of facilitating comparison between Marquise's capability and that of patients who had been in rehab for several months, Marquise now saw patients closer to his stage of progress. Nothing could be done about the lack of diversity in the rehab staff, but there were other patients in the program who were African American.

Marquise reported that the mindful breathing techniques were helpful to him, resulting in reduced physiological tension and greater calm. Progressive relaxation was introduced next and daily practice recommended. Initially, Marquise's practice of PR was carefully monitored to ensure that he was doing the exercise correctly and not over-tensing the muscles or holding his breath. Marquise was also taught the pause technique, an intervention that is particularly appropriate for patients who react very quickly or overreact to stressful stimuli. For example, during work, Marquise's coworkers were sometimes hesitant to bring any problem to him, so, Marquise was instructed to pause before acknowledging the person who came to his door. Then, before answering a question, he was again to pause and breathe slowly twice. At first, Marquise reported that he was not able to do this, so he was instructed to practice this technique when an immediate response was not required, such as email. Marquise was to refrain from responding to email for 5 s, even if he was very sure of his reply, crafting a methodical way to develop the habit of pausing before reacting.

Level Three interventions. Level Three interventions consisted of psychotherapy (cognitive behavioral therapy, CBT), advanced relaxation, and psychophysiological skills, specifically HRV biofeedback. After the technique of HRV was explained and demonstrated, Marquise became fascinated by the technology and the opportunity to watch his breathing and heart rate on the computer screen. He quickly improved his ability to generate coherence and high variability. When he requested other training techniques, he was offered the Stress Eraser (Muench, 2008) and then the Respirate device (Elliott et al., 2004) and mastered them. During this phase of treatment, ambulatory blood pressure monitoring (AMBP) was implemented and the printouts reviewed with Marquise including the evidence for nighttime dipping (Pickering, Shimbo, & Haas, 2006). His memories of highly stressful situations did not coincide with dangerous elevations in BP or heart rate, and the normal exercise or stress induced increases in BP were observed to quickly recover.

By the end of 10 weeks of treatment, BPs at rest had decreased by 10 mmHg SBP and 8 mmHg DBP. Marquise was gently encouraged to resume intimacy with his wife and soon suggested that he had done so. CBT techniques emphasized countering negative attitudes about exercise, changing beliefs about "failure," and altering all or none thinking. Reversal of such negative cognitive patterns is known to decrease risk for recurrence of heart attack (Guilliksson et al., 2011; Witkower & Rosado, 2005). Marquise's successes with his HRV biofeedback were used as examples for CBT, highlighting his mastery of the biofeedback techniques and control over his physiology. In addition, his fascination with precision and accuracy facilitated his belief in CBT and cardiac rehab, as evidenced-based therapies to regain and maintain cardiovascular health. His CBT progressed more quickly than predicted.

The outcome of Marquise's case was very positive. He completed cardiac rehabilitation within 6 months, improving his performance on the 12 min walk test from 3,000 steps to 3,300 steps, a good response (Badenhop, Chapman, Fraker, & Smith, 1999). He decreased his alcohol consumption by 50%. His BP decreased and he lost 10 lb. His mood improved, such that his score on the Beck Depression Inventory decreased from 16 to 6 and his Beck Anxiety score was reduced from 22 to 8. His positive response to the portable physiological monitoring and feedback devices facilitated his continued practice of the relaxation techniques. At 1 year follow-up, Marquise said that his work stress had significantly lessened or "maybe I am different and the stress is the same." Counseling clients and mentoring peers were not his top priority, but he only rarely experienced anger towards the clients who asked questions or colleagues who needed assistance.

Case Summary

Marquise presented with medical, emotional, and behavioral problems, complicated by his highly stressful occupation, substance overuse, and low sense of self-efficacy. Depression and anxiety made it difficult for him to practice self-care and to meet the demands of cardiac rehabilitation. Mindful breathing provided the initial platform in treatment (Mourya, Mahajan, Singh, & Jain, 2009; Schneider et al., 2005) followed by specific relaxation techniques, biofeedback, and CBT (Rainforth et al., 2007). HRV biofeedback was the key intervention because of the evidence supporting interdependency between cardiac health and respiration (Lehrer, 2007; McCraty, Atkinson, & Tomasino, 2003; Purcell et al., 2010). The encouragement provided by the cardiac rehab staff, the other patients in rehab, and the mental health provider seemed to increase Marquise's capacity to manage stress, while frequent positive reinforcement gradually built his confidence (Matthews, Gallo, Raikkonen, & Kuller, 2008; Schwerdtfer & Friedrich-Mai, 2009). Stress management effects on BP have been supported by controlled studies and meta-analysis (Linden, Phillips, & Leclerc, 2007; Linden et al., 2001; McGrady, 2005; McGrady & Linden, 2003). Finally, the Pathways Model provided methods of intervention for each aspect of the client's malfunctioning cardiovascular system.

Dysautonomia: Autonomic Nervous System Disorders

Etiology of ANS Disorders

The ANS disorders comprise a multitude of problems including pure autonomic failure, neurocardiogenic syncope, and postural orthostatic tachycardia syndrome, among others, which present clinically as hypotension, light-headedness, dizziness, or repeated fainting (Grubb, Kanjwal, Karabin, & Imran, 2008). The two main causes of syncope are cardiac arrhythmias and neurocardiogenic (vasovagal) syndromes, the latter being the most common. In both of these conditions cerebral blood flow is compromised, resulting in short-term loss of consciousness followed by spontaneous recovery. Frequent syncopal episodes are disruptive to lifestyle, clearly distressing to the client and others in the family and social network (Byars, Brown, Campbell, & Hobbs, 2000; Shaffer, Jackson, & Jarecki, 2001). Mechanisms underlying syncope are complex and involve increased sympathetic activity and decreased parasympathetic tone. Diagnosis of neurocardiogenic syncope is obtained by history and physical examination and confirmed by head-up tilt table testing (ESC, 2009; Grubb, 2005a, 2005b).

Although psychiatric comorbidity with NCS is very common and estimated at 25%, Kanjwal, Kanjwal, Karabin, and Grubb (2009) caution against rapid conclusions that syncopal episodes are "psychogenic" and recommend a thorough evaluation. The most common disorders correlated with NCS are those in the mood, anxiety, and somatoform categories (McGrady & McGinnis, 2005; Cohen, Thayapran, Ibrahim, Quan, & von zur Muhlen, 2000). It is reasonable to suggest that treatment of syncope should combine medical and psychotherapeutic/behavioral interventions. Client compliance to therapy recommendations is crucial, since those suffering from NCS may be asked to modify fluid intake, diet, sleep/wake schedule, exercise, work, and school hours; take medication; and participate in mental health interventions (ESC, 2009).

Case of Gabriella (Gaby)

Gaby was a 16-year-old tenth grade girl, who came to the clinic accompanied by both parents. She described current frequent dizziness, repeated syncopal episodes, rapid heart rate, severe neck tension, and occasional headaches. Gaby described warning signals of impending syncope as light-headedness, lessening visual field, and fear. She had daytime panic attacks several times a month, which sometimes resulted in fainting and other times resolved on their own. Symptoms began around the time of puberty and had worsened during the past 6 months. She underwent a complete cardiovascular examination, including testing by tilt table which was positive for neurocardiogenic syncope (NCS). Medical management consisted of an SSRI (paroxetine), fludrocortisone, and instructions to increase fluid and salt intake (Grubb, 2005a, 2005b; Olshansky, 2005). Childhood medical history was unremarkable. However, when Gaby was 5 years old, there were several incidents of sexual abuse by an uncle (touching of genitals). Gaby reported this to her mother who confronted the uncle; shortly thereafter, he moved out of the city and was no longer in contact with the family.

As Gaby's capacity to regularly attend school lessened, an Individualized Educational Plan (IEP) was designed that allowed Gaby to receive tutoring at home. She was highly intelligent and based on standardized tests was 2 years beyond grade level in math. In her other subjects, she was at grade level or a few months beyond grade level. Gaby had three younger siblings, for which she had many responsibilities, including preparing the evening meal, helping the kids with their homework and doing some of the laundry. Both parents were employed so her mother believed that "since Gaby is sitting home all day, she can help."

Social interactions were limited for Gaby; there was a male friend (Kevin) who was also a gifted mathematician, and one neighborhood friend who came to visit when she wasn't too busy. Gaby was not allowed to go out with other teenagers because, as her father said, "If she is so sick she can't go to school, she can't go out and party either." Gaby had dropped out of drama club because she had trouble maintaining upright posture and rarely attended church because services were crowded and she was sensitive to noise and excessive heat. Exercise also produced symptom of dizziness and excessive fatigue.

After her parents left the room, Gaby reported that she felt disconnected from her school and her friends and overwhelmed with her responsibilities for the younger siblings. She craved social interactions and wanted to "be like other teens." She saw her gift in mathematics as a potential way out of the house and into college, but she also felt dependent on her parents for everything. During this part of the conversation, Gaby hyperventilated and experienced high anxiety, which slowly resolved with the help of the therapist.

Level One interventions. The Level One interventions for Gaby were soothing and breathing. She was instructed in the mindful breath exercise and asked to practice every day. The soothing exercise that she chose was prayer, since her faith was important to her, despite her reluctance to attend church. Gaby was willing to practice her breathing and to continue to pray and made the commitment to engage in treatment. When the Pathways Model was explained to her parents, they were skeptical, but at least committed to bringing Gaby to our clinic weekly for a few weeks.

Level Two interventions. The Level Two interventions began only 2 weeks later, because we did not know how many times Gaby's parents would drive her to sessions. Progressive relaxation, postural counter-maneuvers, and physical exercise were recommended. Her treatment team modified the progressive relaxation technique for Gaby, to incorporate proportionally more time in the tensing phase (McGrady, Bush, & Grubb, 1997). In addition to daily practice, we encouraged Gaby to use her modified progressive relaxation whenever she felt dizzy or light-headed. Postural manipulations of leg crossing and tensing were taught and daily use encouraged (Krediet, van Dijk, Linzer, van Lieshout, & Wieling, 2002). Short periods of walking, with gradually increasing distance and speed, were also advised. Gaby began to improve; specifically the incidence of syncope decreased and so did the number of panic attacks. However, Gaby's parents were unwilling to modify their parenting style until there was more evidence of improvement. After 8 weeks, her father finally admitted that they had treated Gaby like "Cinderella" and persuaded her mother to decrease the number of daily household tasks.

An opportunity was available for Gaby and her friend Kevin to participate in a state sponsored math contest. A major goal was for her to complete the 3-h exam, without becoming so symptomatic with dizziness or presyncope that she had to leave. During one evening of study for the test, Gaby became light-headed and dizzy and fainted. Kevin put his arms around her to lower her onto the couch and called for help. When Gaby's 8-year-old brother came into the room, he yelled that Gaby and Kevin were "touching"; this event produced an extreme reaction in Gaby's parents and resulted in dismissal of Kevin from the home and an increase in the number of syncopal episodes. Gaby reported these events at the next available session, crying bitterly about her feelings of isolation and helplessness. The therapist listened empathically and encouraged Gaby to continue to study on her own and practice with electronic resources. Additionally, the parents were invited to come in for discussion, an opportunity that they declined

Level Three interventions. The Level Three intervention consisted of psychodynamic psychotherapy, which provided Gaby with a platform to understand her parents' actions, and the paradox of overprotectiveness and excessive responsibility. Her parents' reaction to the "touching" incident with Kevin was related to their desire to protect her from further abuse, and they had believed the interpretation of an 8 years old. Gaby still remembered the abuse by her uncle, but the memories were not intrusive; she thought that her parents believed her and had done what they could. Muscle biofeedback (SEMG) and thermal biofeedback complimented by Autogenic Training were implemented to facilitate general relaxation and loosening of the neck muscles. Gaby responded well to the biofeedback sessions and consistently demonstrated lower forehead and neck tensions levels and the ability to warm her hands over 90°F. Autogenic Training seemed to be effective in stabilization of the ANS, similarly to its application in motion sickness (Cowings et al., 1994). The number of syncopal episodes decreased to almost zero during the next month.

Treatment continued on a bimonthly basis through Gaby's last year of high school. Gaby returned to school full-time the last semester of her senior year and was able to drive with her physician's approval. She scored in the top 1% of math students in the state contest and obtained a full scholarship to a major university. Her fainting episodes did not recur. Dizziness and light-headedness were significantly reduced and Gaby was able to manage them using progressive relaxation and by dietary changes during hot weather. Incidents of panic attacks were reduced to zero and overall anxiety levels were considered manageable. Two years later, Gaby came to visit and reported that college was "awesome" and her grades were all honors. She was participating in one of the faith-based student organizations and had an active social life.

Case Summary

Application of the Pathways Model to clients who are underage or unable to come to appointments on their own is challenging and often requires the therapist to engage significant family members. The case of Gaby illustrated the need to involve parents in obtaining the history, seeking commitments for appointment keeping, and eventually facilitating changes in parental attitudes towards the teenager's illness. Gaby's presentation was not unusual; the medical condition—neurocardiogenic syncope—was complicated by an anxiety disorder (Kouakam et al., 2002). Although her current lifestyle was significantly compromised, Gaby was highly intelligent and could verbalize goals for the future. The Pathways Model Level One and Two interventions included breathing, soothing, modified progressive relaxation, postural counteractions, and exercise. The Level Three interventions—biofeedback and psychotherapy—produced the most benefits because they allowed Gaby to understand and regain control over her reactions to stress. Medications were gradually tapered and discontinued in accordance with medical advice. Gaby continued to utilize the diet modification, postural changes, and relaxation techniques for at least 2 years after conclusion of therapy.

References

Badenhop, D., Chapman, B., Fraker, T., & Smith, I. (1999). Performance and improvement on 12 minute walk distance during phase II cardiac rehabilitation [Abstract]. *Journal of Cardiopulmonary Rehabilitation, 19*, 309.

Bigger, J. T., & Glassman, A. H. (2010). The American Heart Association science advisory on depression and coronary heart disease: An exploration of the issues raised. *Cleveland Clinic Journal of Medicine, 77*(3), S12–S19.

Bonnet, F., Irving, K., Terra, J. L., & Berthez, N. P. (2005). Anxiety and depression are associated with unhealthy life style in patients at risk of cardiovascular disease. *Atherosclerosis, 178*, 339–344.

Brook, R. D., & Julius, S. (2000). Autonomic imbalance, hypertension, and cardiovascular risk. *American Journal of Hypertension, 13*, 112S–122S.

Byars, K., Brown, R., Campbell, R., & Hobbs, S. (2000). Psychological adjustment and coping in a population of children with recurrent syncope. *Journal of Developmental and Behavioral Pediatrics, 21*(3), 189–197.

Carney, R. M., Freedland, K. E., & Veith, R. C. (2005). Depression, the autonomic nervous system, and coronary heart disease. *Psychosomatic Medicine, 67*(Suppl 1), S29–S33.

Chobanian, A. V., Bakris, G. L., Black, H. R., Cushman, W. C., Green, L. A., & Izzo, J. L. (2003). Seventh report of the Joint National Committee on prevention, detection, evaluation, and treatment of high blood pressure. *Hypertension, 42*(6), 1206–1252.

Cohen, T., Thayapran, N., Ibrahim, B., Quan, C., Quan, W., & Von Zur Muhlen, F. (2000). An association between anxiety and neurocardiogenic syncope during head-up tilt table testing. *Pacing and Clinical Electrophysiology, 23*, 837–841.

Cowings, P., Toscano, W., Miller, N., Pickering, T., Shapiro, D., Stevenson, J., et al. (1994). Autogenic-feedback training: A potential treatment for orthostatic intolerance in aerospace crews. *The Journal of Clinical Pharmacology, 34*, 599–608.

Das, S., & O-Keefe, J. H. (2006). Behavioral cardiology: Recognizing and addressing the profound impact of psychosocial stress on cardiovascular health. *Cancer Atherosclerosis Report, 8*, 111–118.

Davies, J. C., Hood, S. D., Christmas, D., & Nutt, D. J. (2008). Psychiatric disorders and cardiovascular disease: Anxiety, depression and hypertension. In L. Sher (Ed.), *Psychological factors and cardiovascular disorders: The role of psychiatric pathology and maladaptive personality features* (pp. 69–89). New York: Nova Biomedical Books.

Dimsdale, J. E. (2008). Psychological stress and cardiovascular disease. *Journal of the American College of Cardiology, 51*(13), 1237–1246.

Elliott, W., Izzo, J., Jr., White, W. B., Rosing, D., Snyder, C. S., Alter, A., et al. (2004). Graded blood pressure reduction in hypertensive outpatients associated with use of a device to assist with slow breathing. *Journal of Clinical Hypertension, 6*(10), 553–559.

European Society of Cardiology (ESC). (2009). Guidelines for the diagnosis and management of syncope (version 2009). *European Heart Journal, 30*, 2631–2671.

Force, T. (1996). Heart rate variability: Standards of measurement, physiological interpretation, and clinical use. *Circulation, 93*, 11043–11065.

Ganong, W. F. (2005). *Review of medical physiology* (22nd ed.). New York: Lange Medical Publications.

Grubb, B. P. (2005a). Neurocardiogenic syncope. *The New England Journal of Medicine, 352*(10), 1004–1010.

Grubb, B. P. (2005b). Neurocardiogenic syncope. In B. P. Grubb (Ed.), *Syncope: Mechanisms and management* (pp. 47–71). Malden, MA: Blackwell.

Grubb, B. P., Kanjwal, Y., Karabin, B., & Imran, N. (2008). Orthostatic hypotension, and autonomic failure: A concise guide to diagnosis and management. *Clinical Medicine: Cardiology, 2*, 279–291.

Guilliksson, M., Burell, G., Vessby, B., Lundin, L., Toss, H., & Svardsudd, K. (2011). Randomized controlled trial of cognitive behavioral therapy vs. standard treatment to prevent recurrent cardiovascular events in patients with coronary heart disease. *Archives of Internal Medicine, 171*(2), 134–140.

Holt-Lunstad, J., Smith, T. W., & Uchino, B. N. (2008). Can hostility interfere with the health benefits of giving and receiving social support? The impact of cynical hostility on cardiovascular reactivity during social support interactions among friends. *Annals of Behavioral Medicine, 35*, 319–330.

Hughes, J. W., & Stoney, C. M. (2000). Depressed mood is related to high-frequency heart rate variability during stressors. *Psychosomatic Medicine, 62*, 796–803.

Kanjwal, K., Kanjwal, Y., Karabin, B., & Grubb, (2009). Psychogenic syncope? A cautionary note. *Pacing and Clinical Electrophysiology, 32*, 862–865.

Kaplan, M. S., & Nunes, A. (2003). The psychosocial determinants of hypertension. *Nutrition, Metabolism and Cardiovascular Disease, 13*(1), 52–59.

Kario, K., Schwartz, J. E., Davidson, K. W., & Pickering, T. G. (2001). Gender differences in associations of diurnal blood pressures variation, awake physical activity, and sleep quality with negative affect. *Hypertension, 38*, 997–1002.

Khawaja, I. S., Westermeyer, J. J., Gajwani, P., & Feinstein, R. E. (2009). Depression and coronary artery disease: The association, mechanisms, and therapeutic implications. *Psychiatry, 8*(1), 38–51.

Kop, W. J., Kuhl, E. A., Barasch, E., Jenny, N. S., & Gottlieb, S. S. (2010). Association between depressive symptoms and fibrosis markers: The cardiovascular health study. *Brain, Behavior, and Immunity, 24*, 229–235.

Kouakam, C., Locroix, D., Klug, D., Baux, P., Marquie, C., & Kacet, S. (2002). Prevalence and prognostic significance of psychiatric disorders in patients evaluated for recurrent unexplained syncope. *The American Journal of Cardiology, 89*, 530–535.

Krediet, C., van Dijk, N., Linzer, M., van Lieshout, J., & Wieling, W. (2002). Management of vasovagal syncope: Controlling or aborting faints by leg crossing and muscle tensing. *Circulation, 10*, 1684–1689.

Kubansky, L. D., Davidson, K. W., & Rozanski, A. (2005). The clinical impact of negative psychological states: Expanding the spectrum of risk for coronary artery disease. *Psychosomatic Medicine, 67*(S1), S10–S14.

Lehman, B. J., Kiefe, C. I., Taylor, S. E., & Seeman, T. E. (2009). Relationship of early life stress and psychological functioning to blood pressure in the CARDIA study. *Health Psychology, 28*(3), 338–346.

Lehrer, P. (2007). Biofeedback training to increase heart rate variability. In P. Lehrer, R. Woolfolk, & W. Sime (Eds.), *Principles and practice of stress management* (pp. 227–248). New York: Guilford Press.

Linden, W., Klassen, B. A., & Phillips, M. (2008). Can psychological factors account for a lack of nocturnal blood pressure dipping? *Annals of Behavioral Medicine, 36*, 253–258.

Linden, W., Lenz, J. W., & Con, A. H. (2001). Individualized stress management for primary hypertension: A controlled trial. *Archives of Internal Medicine, 161*, 1071–1080.

Linden, W., Phillips, M. J., & Leclerc, J. (2007). Psychological treatment of cardiac patients: A meta-analysis. *European Heart Journal, 28*(24), 2972–2984.

Luke, R. G., (1996). Evaluation of the patient with hypertension. In J.S. Alpert (Ed.) Cardiology for the primary care physician St. Louis, MO: Morby.

Matthews, K. A., Gallo, L., Raikkonen, K., & Kuller, L. H. (2008). Association between socioeconomic status and metabolic syndrome in women: Testing the reserve capacity model. *Health Psychology, 27*, 576–583.

McCraty, R., Atkinson, M., & Tomasino, D. (2003). Impact of a workplace stress reduction program on blood pressure and emotional health in hypertensive employees. *Journal of Alternative and Complementary Medicine, 9*(3), 355–369.

McGrady, A. (2005). Biofeedback in cardiovascular disease. In W. Frishman, M. I. Weintraub, & M. Micozzi (Eds.), *Complementary and integrative therapies for cardiovascular disease* (pp. 143–144). St. Louis, MO: Elsevier Mosby.McGrady, A. V., Bush, E. G., & Grubb, B. P. (1997). Outcome of biofeedback-assisted relaxation for neurocardiogenic syncope and headache: A clinical replication series. *Applied Psychophysiology and Biofeedback, 22*(1), 63–72.

McGrady, A., & Linden, W. (2003). Hypertension. In M. S. Schwartz & F. Andrasik (Eds.), *Biofeedback: A practitioner's handbook* (pp. 382–408). New York: Guilford Press.

McGrady, A., & McGinnis, R. (2005). Psychiatric disorders in patients with syncope. In B. Grubb (Ed.), *Syncope: Mechanisms and management* (pp. 214–224). Malden, MA: Blackwell.

McGrady, A., McGinnis, R., Badenhop, D., Bentle, M., & Rajput, M. (2009). Effects of depression and anxiety on adherence to cardiac rehabilitation. *Journal of Cardiopulmonary Rehabilitation and Prevention, 29*, 358–364.

Mezick, E., Matthews, K. A., Hall, M., Kamarck, T. W., Strollo, P. J., Buysse, D. J., et al. (2010). Low life purpose and high hostility are related to an attenuated decline in nocturnal blood pressure. *Health Psychology, 29*(2), 196–204.

Muench, F. (2008). HRV: The manufacturers and vendors speak: The portable StressEraser heart rate variability biofeedback device: Background and research. *Biofeedback, 36*(1), 35–39.

Olshansky, B. (2005). Syncope: Overview and approach to management. In B. Grubb (Ed.), *Syncope: Mechanisms and management* (pp. 1–46). Malden, MA: Blackwell.

Park, K. E., & Pepine, C. J. (2010). Pathophysiologic mechanisms linking impaired cardiovascular health and neurologic dysfunction: The year in review. *Cleveland Clinic Journal of Medicine, 77*(S3), S40.

Pickering, T. G., Shimbo, D., & Haas, D. (2006). Ambulatory blood-pressure monitoring. *The New England Journal of Medicine, 354*(22), 2368–2374.

Purcell, E., Urlakis, M., & Shaffer, F. (2010). Physiological and emotional effects of resonant diaphragmatic breathing. Presentation to the annual meeting of the Association for Applied Psychophysiology and Biofeedback, San Diego, CA.

Rainforth, M. V., Schneider, R. H., Nidich, S. I., Gaylord-King, C., Salerno, J. W., & Anderson, J. W. (2007). Stress reduction programs in patients with elevated blood pressure: A systematic review and meta-analysis. *Current Hypertension Report, 9*(6), 520–528.

Randall, G., Bhattacharyya, M. R., & Steptoe, A. (2009). Marital status and heart rate variability in patients with suspected coronary artery disease. *Annals of Behavioral Medicine, 38*, 115–123.

Reckelhoff, J. F. (2001). Gender differences in the regulation of blood pressure. *Hypertension, 37*, 1199–1208.

Rozanski, A., Blumenthal, J. A., Davidson, K. W., Saah, P. G., & Kubzansky, L. (2005). The epidemiology, pathophysiology and management of psychosocial risk factors in cardiac practice: The emerging field of behavioral cardiology. *Journal of the American College of Cardiology, 45*, 637–651.

Sakakibara, M., & Hayano, J. (1996). Effect of slowed respiration on cardiac parasympathetic response to threat. *Psychosomatic Medicine, 58*, 32–37.

Sakakibara, M., Takeuchi, S., & Hayano, J. (1994). Effect of relaxation training on cardiac sympathetic tone. *Psychophysiology, 31*, 223–228.

Salomon, K., Clift, A., Karlsdottir, M., & Rottenberg, J. (2009). Major depressive disorder is associated with attenuated cardiovascular reactivity and impaired recovery among those free of cardiovascular disease. *Health Psychology, 28*(2), 157–165.

Sarkar, U., Ali, S., & Whooley, M. A. (2007). Self-efficacy and health status in patients with coronary heart disease: Findings from the heart and soul study. *Psychosomatic Medicine, 69*, 306–312.

Schneider, R. H., Alexander, C. N., Staggers, F., Rainforth, M., Salerno, J. W., Hartz, A., et al. (2005). Long-term effects of stress reduction on mortality in persons ≥ 55 years of age with systemic hypertension. *The American Journal of Cardiology, 95*, 1060–1064.

Schwerdtfer, A., & Friedrich-Mai, P. (2009). Social interaction moderates the relationship between depressive mood and heart rate variability: Evidence from an ambulatory monitoring study. *Health Psychology, 28*(4), 501–509.

Shaffer, C., Jackson, L., & Jarecki, S. (2001). Characteristics, perceived stressors, and coping strategies of patients who experience neurally mediated syncope. *Heart & Lung, 30*(4), 244–249.

Sher, L. (2001). Effects of seasonal mood changes on seasonal variations in coronary heart disease: Role of immune system, infection, and inflammation. *Medical Hypothesis, 56*(1), 104–106.

Surtees, P. G., Wainwright, W. J., Luben, R., Wareham, N. J., Bingham, S. A., & Khaw, K. (2008). Depression and ischemic heart disease mortality: Evidence from the EPIC-Norfolk United Kingdom prospective cohort study. *The American Journal of Psychiatry, 165*, 515–523.

Surtees, P. G., Wainwright, W. J., Luben, R., Wareham, N. J., Bingham, S. A., & Khaw, K. (2010). Mastery is associated with cardiovascular disease mortality in men and women at apparently low risk. *Health Psychology, 29*(4), 412–420.

Vella, E. J., Kamarck, T. W., & Shiffman, S. (2008). Hostility moderates the effects of social support and intimacy on blood pressure in daily social interactions. *Health Psychology, 27*(2), 5133–5162.

Vijayvergiya, R. (2008). Role of psychological risk factors in pathogenesis of coronary artery disease. In L. Sher (Ed.), *Psychological factors and cardiovascular disorders: The role of psychiatric pathology and maladaptive personality features* (pp. 1–11). New York: Nova Biomedical Books.

Whooley, M. A., de Jonge, P., Vittinghoff, E., Otte, C., & Moos, R. (2008). Depressive symptoms, health behaviors, and risk of cardiovascular events in patients with coronary heart disease. *Journal of the American Medical Association, 300*(20), 2379–2388.

Widmaier, E. P., Raff, Hershel, R., & Strang, K. T. (2006). *Vander's human physiology: The mechanisms of body function* (10th ed.). New York: McGraw-Hill.

Winkleby, M. A., Kraemer, H. C., Ahn, D. K., & Warady, A. N. (1998). Ethnic and socioeconomic differences in cardiovascular disease risk factors. *Journal of American Medical Association, 280*, 356–362.

Witkower, A., & Rosado, J. (2005). Cognitive-behavioral therapy in cardiac illness. In W. Frishman (Ed.), *Complementary and integrative therapies for cardiovascular disease* (pp. 151–166). St. Louis, MO: Elsevier Mosby.

Wright, J. T., Harris-Haywood, S., Pressel, S., Barzilay, J., Baimbridge, C., Bareis, C. J., et al. (2008). Clinical outcomes by race in hypertensive patients with and without the metabolic syndrome. *Archives of Internal Medicine, 168*(2), 207–217.

Yan, L. I., Liu, K., Matthews, K. A., Daviglus, M. L., Ferguson, T. F., & Kiefe, C. I. (2003). Psychosocial factors and risk of hypertension: The coronary artery risk development in young adults (CARDIA) study. *Journal of the American Medical Association, 290*(16), 2138–2148.

Chapter 12
Headache and Back Pain

Abstract Chronic pain is a complex psychobiological condition that creates personal suffering and disability. Chronic pain disorders are often associated with mood, anxiety, and somatoform disorders. Two types of chronic pain are discussed in this chapter: headache and back pain. The Pathways Model is applied to two patient cases, each with their own life stories and unique psychological issues that required treatment with multilevel interventions.

Keywords Chronic pain • Migraine • Tension headache • Back pain • Relaxation • Imagery • Cognitive behavioral therapy

Chronic Pain and Quality of Life

About 30% of the US population suffers from chronic pain, and millions of physician visits are made each year by persons with pain complaints. Low back pain and headache are the most common of the chronic pain conditions (Bonica & Loeser, 2000). Migraine and tension-type headache (TTH) are the most frequently diagnosed types of headache (Penzien, Rains, & Andrasik, 2002). The 1-year prevalence of episodic headache is about 38% and that of chronic TTH, at least 15 days per month of pain, is 2–3%. Migraine headache is diagnosed in 12–14% of the US population; eighteen percent of women and 7% of men experience migraine-type headaches (Lawler & Cameron, 2006; Lipton, Stewart, Diamond, Diamond, & Reed, 2001). In the elderly population, nonmalignant chronic pain is associated with functional impairments and poor quality of life, compounding the effects of other chronic medical and psychiatric conditions (Morone & Greco, 2007).

Common problems of patients with chronic pain include psychological suffering, sleep disorders, and emotional problems, particularly anxiety and depression (Arnow et al., 2006; Roy-Byrne et al., 2008). Persons in pain may feel hopeless about the future if they anticipate more weeks, months, and years of suffering. Worry and anxiety about finding pain relief and inability to function normally at work and in family relationships dominate consciousness (Strigo, Simmons, Matthews, Craig, & Paulus, 2008). Chronic pain and disrupted sleep are intercorrelated, and the person with chronic pain has fewer hours of restorative, deep sleep, resulting in fatigue and low energy during waking hours. In addition, sleep deprivation increases pain sensitivity, even in normal subjects (Roehrs, Hyde, Blaisdell, Greenwalk, & Roth, 2006). Multiple awakenings increase spontaneous pain and decrease the ability to inhibit pain signals, potentially through impaired pain inhibitory pathways (Smith, Edwards, McCann, & Haythornthwaite, 2007). As the person continues to experience pain, behavior also changes, moving more and more towards the dependent sick role and away from a personal empowerment perspective (McGrady, 2002). The severity of comorbid psychiatric disorders not only makes treatment decisions more complex but also moderates treatment success (Holroyd, Labus, & Carlson, 2009).

The burden of illness due to headache was estimated from a survey of people with migraine, TTH, and combined types. The latter had poorer mental, physical, and social functioning. In women there was a negative association between headache and income. That is, the more frequent and the more severe the headaches, the lower the income. In women the burden of illness was highest in those with both migraine and tension headaches, then in migraine, and then in TTH (Waldie & Poulton, 2002).

Migraine Headache

Migraine head pain is usually unilateral, throbbing, and located in the temporal or frontotemporal areas. The multiple associated symptoms that occur during onset (prodrome), pain phase, and postdrome include gastrointestinal, autonomic, and sensory disturbances. Nausea and vomiting are reported either prior or during the headache. Some individuals have aura preceding the pain phase, and the aura manifests itself as visual distortions, for example, zigzag lines or holes in the visual field (scotoma), in other sensory modalities, such as tingling of the skin, or in hemiparesis (one-sided transient paralysis) (Headache Classification Committee, 1988). Headaches cause significant losses of productivity in missed school days or lost work time, in addition to compromised social activities, which can be particularly distressing for sufferers (Lipton et al., 2001).

Migraine is believed to be due to hyperexcitability of the brain, with excessive firing of nerve cells in the brain stem and cortex, which activates the trigeminovascular system. The serotonergic neurons of the dorsal raphe initiate trigeminal nerve activity. Pain-producing peptides are emitted from the trigeminal nerve and transmit signals to other brain areas for processing of the pain information (Baskin & Weeks, 2003). According to Peroutka (2004), migraine shares characteristics with several chronic sympathetic nervous system disorders. For example, in comparison to controls, migraineurs demonstrate heightened adrenergic receptor sensitivity and orthostatic hypotension. Low levels of norepinephrine during headache-free intervals in addition to reduced responses to the cold pressor challenge and the isometric exercise (hand grip) test are presented as further evidence for the hypothesis that migraine is a type of sympathetic dysfunction.

Tension-Type Headache

TTH differ in pain quality, frequency, and duration from migraine. The pain is usually bilateral, located across the forehead, along the back of the head and neck, but not pulsating in quality, although the pain may be as severe as that of migraine (Headache Classification Committee, 1988). TTH may initially occur several times a week for a few hours, but over time, the episodic tension headache pattern converts to the chronic form in some people (Chen, 2009; Vandenheede & Schoenen, 2002). Chronic TTH differs from episodic headache in poorer treatment response, more frequent medication overuse, and lower quality of life (Mathew, 2006). Persons with chronic TTH seem to have exaggerated chronic pericranial muscle tenderness during palpation. Increases in tenderness precede the onset of pain and continue during the headache. This tenderness is postulated to be due to abnormal central pain modulation (Neufeld, Holroyd, & Lipchik, 2000). Over time, central sensitization and hyperalgesia develop (Bezov, Ashina, Jensen, & Bendtsen, 2011); these changes may result from frequent overactivation of stress responses coupled with weak coping resources (Lee, Zambreanu, Menon, & Tracey, 2008). Similarities between migraine and TTH are suggested, in that hypersensitivity and lack of resilience exists in both, although the pathophysiological mechanisms are different.

Assessment of the Patient with Chronic Pain

The evaluation of the patient with chronic pain includes both a self-evaluation and the professional assessment. A daily pain log should be kept for 2 weeks so that the times of most severe pain, partially remitted pain, and pain-free times can be identified. The patient should also keep a diary of hours of sleep and number of awakenings and a mood log. This information assists the clinician in identifying associations between sleep disruption, mood, and pain. The clinician then institutes a full psychological evaluation. The patient undergoes an automated psychophysiological assessment, including surface electromyography (SEMG), heart rate variability, and skin temperature. Potential targets for intervention are identified after the psychophysiological assessments and a psychological screening.

The Case of Melinda

Melinda (Mandy) was a 19-year-old female with migraine since age 12 and chronic daily headaches for the past 3 years. The daily pain was described as varying in intensity, all over her head, with no nausea or other gastrointestinal symptoms. The migraines occurred monthly at the time of her period. Mandy revealed that she has always been a worrier. Her mother, who participated in the interview, confirmed this statement. In addition, when Mandy had severe pain, she was also very irritable and prone to anger. As a child, she chewed her nails relentlessly and pulled on her hair. At the time of evaluation, Mandy lived with her mother and father, both of whom were employed. The father had coronary artery disease and had suffered two prior heart attacks, one of which occurred in Mandy's presence when she was 10 years old. Although mom's health was good, Mandy worried because her mom drove about 60 miles round trip to work every day. A history of depression and anxiety existed on the paternal side of the family. There were no reports of abuse or traumatic experiences. Mandy's neurologist had conducted a complete exam and it was unremarkable. Trials of the triptan family of drugs produced no benefit. Zoloft™ had a temporary positive effect, but Mandy was subsequently weaned off of this medicine because of the side effects of tingling in the extremities.

Mandy was in her first year at a division III college and walked on to the basketball team. She was intelligent and did extremely well in school. She had made friends in college, particularly other women on the team. At the team meals, Mandy was too nervous to eat, as the conversation turned to the next practice or upcoming games. She was concerned about the headaches interfering with her dream of continuing to play at the college level. Sometimes, during competition, Mandy became extremely angry and frustrated with her teammates' mistakes or her own, and these anger episodes caused the coach to bench her. Mandy discussed her worries about her father's health status and her mother's difficult drive to work.

Mandy's diagnoses included generalized anxiety disorder, migraine, and TTH. Based on the Pathways Model, genetic predisposition intersected with environmental stressors and an anxious personality type. Educating Mandy about the hypothesized relationship between her pain and stress and anxiety was not challenging. Her intelligence and motivation to "get this mess figured out" produced a cooperative patient.

Level One interventions. The first Level One intervention, breathing, produced the beginning of a calming effect, and she began to engage in daily mindful breathing practice. The second appropriate Level One intervention was "feeding." Mandy was instructed in the mindful eating procedure and learned to appreciate her food and to eat slowly. She also learned to direct the conversation away from the sport during the beginning of the meal since the soup and salad were the most difficult for her. As she continued to eat, her anxiety levels decreased, and she could tolerate some discussion of the next game.

Level Two interventions. Progressive relaxation was introduced as the first Level Two intervention. Mandy began daily practice of the slow tense-relax sequence and was instructed to use this technique before practice and before games. She found this technique very helpful and observed that it reduced her anxiety significantly. Some decrease in daily pain, approximately 25%, was reported after 4 weeks, but the monthly migraine occurred on schedule. Mandy's second Level Two intervention consisted of "cognitive renewal." During this time, Mandy described her anxious thoughts and "catastrophic thinking" about her mother and father. Sometimes, she could not get the thoughts out of her mind, picturing her dad crumpling to the floor with a heart attack or her mom crashing her car on her way to work.

Level Three interventions. Level Three interventions consisted of a total of 20 sessions of biofeedback, relaxation therapy, and cognitive behavioral therapy (CBT). Muscle tension levels in the forehead were moderately elevated, and her finger temperature was 75°F at rest (optimal finger temperature is 94–96°F, when the autonomic nervous system is relaxed and in balance, and the circulation to the fingers is enhanced). CBT began by addressing the obsessive ruminations about the health and safety of her parents. She was taught the thought-stopping technique. At the end of 3 months of therapy, the daily headaches were improved by 50% and the negative thinking and worry about her parents were significantly decreased. The monthly migraine continued to appear on schedule.

The fourth month of treatment began at the same time as the basketball season. Mandy's description of her posture and facial expression during games seemed to indicate extremely high muscle tension in the face, the neck, and shoulders. Her mother traveled to the college campus to videotape Mandy during competition, which corroborated our impression. Long discussions took place about the perceived need to maintain a "game face" on and off the court. During training, her muscle tension levels decreased significantly, and Mandy instituted relaxation of her face and neck during every small break in the game. Thermal biofeedback training facilitated Mandy's learning of the autonomic relaxation response. She was able to warm her hands with thermal feedback and warmth-related imagery. After 1 year of intervention, the daily headaches were reduced by 75%, and the frequency of her migraines decreased to one every 3–4 months. Anxious rumination was controlled by thought stopping and general anxiety was estimated to be 50% decreased. Interestingly, Mandy reported that the next basketball season was her most successful and that she found competition more enjoyable while maintaining excellent performance.

Case Summary

Mandy initially presented with a 7-year history of both migraine and TTH, which had evolved into a chronic daily headache pattern. She also displayed a pattern of irritability and frequent frustration with herself and others, and anxiety episodes, especially around the basketball games. Mandy enthusiastically implemented her Level One interventions, including mindful diaphragmatic breathing and mindful eating. Her Level Two interventions comprised progressive muscle relaxation and cognitive renewal. Her Level Three treatments included muscle and thermal biofeedback, passive relaxation exercises, and CBT. After 1 year of treatment, her headaches and anxiety episodes were significantly reduced in frequency.

Research Support for Case Interventions

A meta-analysis of biofeedback treatments in headache was conducted by Nestoriuc, Martin, Rief, and Andrasik (2008). Medium to large effect sizes were found for adult migraine and TTH, and benefits were stable on average for 14 months. Headache frequency was the main variable, with information gathered from structured headache log. In addition to pain, anxiety, perceived self-efficacy, depression, and consumption of medicine were also improved. Facial pain, temporomandibular disorders, and teeth clenching were especially relevant to Mandy's case. Parafunctional activities are movements of the jaw and mastication muscles that do not coincide with talking, chewing, or swallowing. Repeated tightening of the jaw muscles, in addition to simple tooth contact, increased tension significantly and increased headache severity. When Mandy became aware of her almost constant "game face," she learned to relax her jaw, a substitute for the unwanted behavior (habit reversal) (Glaros, 2008). During massage sessions, persons in one study showed less anxiety, lower heart rates, and decrease in salivary cortisol. Reductions in migraine frequency persisted for at least the 3 weeks of follow-up. Massage may help both migraine and TTH headaches through reduction in muscle tension, improved circulation of blood and lymph, and a reduction in substance P in the saliva and presumably in the bloodstream (Lawler & Cameron, 2006). In most cases, medication and behavioral approaches must be combined for long-term success (Flor & Diers, 2007; Holroyd & Drew, 2006).

Psychophysiological Basis for Transition from Acute to Chronic Pain

Some individuals sustain an injury, experience pain ranging from mild to very severe pain, heal physically, and then suffer no more. In contrast, others may have a similar injury, experience mild or moderate pain, but develop chronic pain, despite healing of the physical injury. Pain responses vary among babies and young children as evidenced by wide variations in the length of crying after an injection. Genetic predisposition increases the risks of chronic pain, particularly migraine headache (Diatchenko & Slade, 2005). The pain pathways that normally function to protect the individual from physical damage are hypersensitive and respond to even small pain signals. The neurons show exaggerated responses to stimuli that are usually too weak to reach threshold. When there is actual injury, hormones or inflammatory molecules are released which may sensitize nociceptors. After the original injury has healed, the pain processing pathways continue to send impulses, resulting in the experience of pain (Lipton et al., 2001). Neuroticism is a personality trait manifesting as anxious, depressed, hostile, high arousal, and variable emotionality. This trait has been suggested to mediate physiological responses to nociceptive stimuli. Higher scores on scales measuring neuroticism were correlated with greater pain sensitivity (Charles, Gatz, Kato, & Pedersen, 2008).

The fear-avoidance model has been proposed as a possible explanation for the persistence of pain (Vlaeyen & Linton, 2000). Anxious fear affects the experience of pain and the patient's decisions when experiencing pain. Patients who are hurting develop negative beliefs and tend to catastrophize even small problems. Imagining negative consequences of activity, for example, increases the likelihood that moving the body will be avoided or that actions will be stiff and guarded. Those with higher anxiety expect more pain and stop movement sooner than they are actually physically capable of doing (Strigo et al., 2008). Bodily sensations such as pressure or touch may be misinterpreted as pain.

Pain and disability are themselves chronic stressors, affecting a person's ability to perform daily tasks at home or at the workplace. Family criticism is also relevant if the person with pain is compared to other family members and found to be less efficient and less productive. The patient experiences isolation from the peer group because of the need for more rest or the time taken up by physical therapy and doctor's appointments.

Cognitive factors, such as perception and concentration, affect processing of the pain signal. For example, attention can increase and distraction can decrease brain activation related to pain (Villemure & Bushnell, 2002). In addition to anxious and depressive *thoughts*, feelings also affect the intensity of pain. For example, in low back pain patients, higher levels of "anger in" and "anger out" are correlated with greater sensitivity to acute and chronic pain stimuli ("Anger in" refers to suppressed or internalized anger and "anger out" refers to expressed anger). Anger results from the experience of being hurt, similarly to the person's reactions to intended harm by another person (Bruehl, Burns, Chung, & Quartana, 2008). Anger is related to increased sensitivity to pain. Suppression of emotion is an active process requiring recruitment of inhibitory processes, which then compete for attention against cognitive or behavioral activities. If patients think that it is inappropriate to feel, let along express anger at their doctors, the emotion will be suppressed, and this will later lead to over-experiencing of other negative emotions (Burns et al., 2008). Further, pain anticipation may enhance the experience of pain, whether the pain occurs as expected from a medical procedure, physical therapy, or in situations where pain is not explainable by any physiological insult (Bensten, Rustoen, Wahl, & Miaskowski, 2008).

The Case of Peter

Peter was a 55-year-old married man with severe, chronic pain of the hip and leg. He arrived in a wheel chair, pushed by his wife, since the distance from the elevator to the clinic was too far for him to walk. Peter had a 10-year history of back and hip pain and had delayed surgery to try medical management and physical therapy. Four months prior to the evaluation, Peter had surgery, but the pain did not remit and actually intensified. Two months later, at a follow-up appointment, he was told that the surgery had failed, and that was the reason for the severe pain. He underwent a second surgery, resulting in some relief, but he still experienced pain every day, now compounded by anxiety. The patient had a history of anxiety since young adulthood, which had been successfully managed with relatively low doses of Klonopin prior to the first surgery. At the time of the evaluation, he reported severe anxiety and almost daily episodes of panic. During the attacks, he shook and had trouble getting his breath. Whenever he sat still, he focused on the pain and on the failed first surgery; he worried that the second surgery was not a success either, and that he was not being told about its failure. He became depressed and tearful. He admitted suicidal thoughts but denied any plan or intent to commit suicide. Peter often had trouble getting to sleep and woke up early. There was a history of anxiety disorder in both of his parents and depression on his father's side. One uncle committed suicide because he had terminal cancer and severe pain. Peter had been prescribed Klonopin for the anxiety, Vicodin and tramadol for the pain, Ativan as needed for anxiety, and Elavil for mood and sleep. He had a college degree and was employed full time in a very responsible position. At the time of evaluation, he was on medical leave from work.

Pathways Interventions in the Case of Peter

Education. First, Peter was educated about chronic pain, with an emphasis on the psychophysiological links among mood, anxiety, anger, sleep quality, stress, and pain. The pain pathways are hard wired in our central and autonomic nervous systems, such that Peter was responding to the chronic pain signal as if it were an acute pain signal, resulting in an overactivity of the hypothalamic pituitary axis (HPA). The self-defeating, fearful, and hopeless thoughts resulted in an avoidance of activity, which in turn reinforced his depression. Peter thought he had no control over his situation, except to take medication when the pain was worse. Goals were set for treatment and the initial emphasis was placed on the short-term goals of learning simple relaxation techniques and experiencing intermittent pain relief. The long-term goal was to decrease pain and improve functionality so that Peter could return to work. It was important to begin intervention slowly but firmly for Peter. Because his fear of further pain was so high and his thoughts of betrayal by the surgeon so ever present, explanations of all interventions needed to be detailed and logical. But since Peter desperately wanted to obtain relief, the team judged his readiness for change to be high (Kerns & Habib, 2004). He committed to active participation in therapy, including home practice of relaxation techniques.

Level One interventions. The Level One interventions instituted for Peter were mindful breathing, self-soothing, sleeping, and moving. The premise for a breathing-based relaxation therapy was that Peter exhibited rapid, shallow breathing patterns when the pain was severe and when he felt anxious. Many individuals with chronic pain exhibit maladaptive breathing patterns, and in many cases, a capnometer will show deficient CO_2 levels in the airways. Certainly for Peter, hyperventilation during panic attacks escalated his anxiety and further intensified uncomfortable sensations of loss of control. Peter had a positive response to mindful breathing practice, so he was advised to practice twice daily at home, increasing the length of the breathing exercises to 5 min. It was important to avoid overwhelming Peter with instructions and to reinforce each small effort that he made in his own behalf.

The second Level One intervention to reestablish normal rhythms was self-soothing. Peter's ability to quiet himself when he had anxious thoughts or severe pain was minimal, so he was instructed to sit in a comfortable rocking recliner, rocking gently and practicing mindful breathing during rocking. Soothing motions to decrease anxiety overlapped with the necessity to move his body. Although Peter had been told by the surgeon to "get out of the wheelchair, throw away those crutches, and walk," fear and negative emotions prevented him from trusting the doctor's recommendations. Peter did agree to use the crutches more often at home and to do some mild stretching of the arms every day. He began to report slight decreases in anxiety, with panic attacks decreasing from daily to four per week. Sleep onset insomnia decreased on most nights; however, early morning awakening continued.

Level Two interventions. The Level Two interventions for Peter were progressive relaxation, exercise, and communication. The premise of progressive relaxation is that people with chronic pain have high levels of arousal and muscle tension, so the goal is to gain control over the tension in the body and eventually to achieve control over pain. During clinic sessions, Peter's anger at the surgeon and his fatalistic thinking were explored. His communication with his wife began to improve. His conversations with his wife about his fears finally clarified for her why Peter was so reluctant to take what she considered minor risks of getting around the house. Physical therapy began during this phase of treatment and slow progress was made in strengthening Peter's leg and back muscles. Reports of pain decreased by about 30% and panic attacks were reduced to one per week.

Level Three interventions. The goals of the Level Three interventions were to reestablish control over muscle tension, decrease generalized anxiety, and improve mood by interactive guided imagery, SEMG biofeedback, and CBT. The most successful therapy was interactive guided imagery. Peter was highly visual and could describe the appearance of his hip and back in both the painful and pain-free, healed conditions. Imagining the healing process not only produced pain relief but also improved mood. Practice recommendations for relaxation with imagery were increased from one per day to three times per day, and he implemented this plan without complaint. It is possible that the success of imagery depended on relaxation and on changing stimulus quality and quantity. The images of the painful areas were transformed into those of healing and tissue health.

Biofeedback, relaxation training, and imagery helped Peter to relax his muscles during clinic sessions, at home, and after challenging physical therapy sessions. CBT addressed the need for adaptive coping. Fear and hopelessness were replaced by a more positive attitude towards self-efficacy. Each indication of progress was praised and reinforced, leaning on the client's intrinsic desire to get well. Peter began working from home via computer, then going to his office for a few hours at a time. Gradually, he worked 20, then 30, and finally 40 h per week. His employer was very supportive of Peter's efforts to return to work full time and thus allowed him to initially work from home or attend meetings by speaker phone.

At the end of 18 months of weekly, then bimonthly sessions, and 6 months of monthly follow-up, goals had been reached. Pain logs showed a reduction of approximately 80%. There were no panic attacks in a 6-month period. Peter progressed from wheelchair/crutches, to a walker, to a cane, and finally to walking unassisted. He returned to work full time. During weeks of seasonally heavy workload, he was able to perform at a high level. Medication reductions consisted of elimination of Vicodin and Tramadol, use of Tylenol as needed, continuation of Elavil, and occasional use of Ativan or Xanax. There were no suicidal thoughts. A maintenance plan was developed for the use of the mind-body skills long term. Long-term management of chronic pain requires the patient to continue practice of relaxation and to continue to use the new coping strategies. Peter committed to the basic self-care principles based on the Pathways Model and promised to contact the clinic should any further problems arise.

Case Summary

Peter presented initially with chronic disabling pain of the hip and leg, aggravated by failed spinal surgeries, and accompanied by almost daily panic attacks. Peter benefitted from Level One interventions including mindful breathing, self-soothing, sleep modification, and movement. He cooperated willingly with the Level Two interventions: progressive muscle relaxation, physical exercise, and communication. He also utilized three Level Three interventions: interactive guided imagery, SEMG biofeedback, and CBT.

The course of treatment for Peter was long and complicated, spanning approximately 20 sessions in the first year and an additional ten sessions in the second year of treatment. Several crises occurred during the treatment, in particular a serious problem with one of Peter's sons and a necessity to work 60 h per week for a month during a work emergency. Although pain and anxiety increased during both of these situations, Peter verbalized an understanding of why stress increased pain and negative mood. He tolerated the uncomfortable feelings and sensations without experiencing any panic episodes. Increasing relaxation and imagery practice reestablished control during those times. Contact between the therapist and the surgeon was used to reinforce Peter's motivation to get well and to indirectly suggest to the surgeon that Peter was not considering litigation.

Chronic pain is complex and multidimensional. It consists of both sensory and cognitive components with the added dimension of suffering. Based on the Pathways Model, the etiology of chronic pain is genetic, physiological, emotional, and behavioral.

The assessment process identifies the problem and the client's motivation to change, goals are set, and the desired outcomes are captured in detail. Intervention considers both the experience of pain at the cognitive level and peripheral, sensory components (Baskin & Weeks, 2003). Therapy combines physiological, behavioral, and psychological elements with the client actively engaged throughout (Holroyd, 2002). More advanced age does not seem to be a contraindication to psychophysiological therapies. Middaugh and Pawlick (2002) reported that older adults with headache had similar success rates compared to younger adults in behavioral treatment and had higher treatment compliance, although treatment protocols may need to be simplified. The meta-analysis by Hoffman, Papas, Chatkoff, and Kerns (2007) supported using multidisciplinary treatments to reduce self-reported pain, moderate disability, and improve quality of life in persons with chronic low back pain. CBT and self-regulation therapies (SRT), including biofeedback and relaxation, were found to demonstrate moderate to large positive effect sizes. SRT produced particularly impressive results for depression in persons with low back pain. This observation intuitively makes sense since SRT return control to the person, instead of promoting dependence on providers or medicine for relief. Although neural mechanisms underlying relaxation and imagery are not completely understood, it has been suggested that endogenous opioids modulate pain sensations in a manner similar to exogenous opioids like morphine (Bruehl et al., 2008).

For some patients, like Peter, who are gifted in visualization, guided, interactive imagery can produce significant benefits (Birklein & Maihöfner, 2006). After active treatment is complete, maintenance of the sense of self-efficacy and mastery over physiological reactions to stress will allow the patient to deal with temporary setbacks. Promising new therapies for complex pain syndromes, such as motor imagery or mirror therapy, give hope to suffering patients and the clinicians who treat them.

References

Arnow, B. A., Hunkeler, E. M., Blasey, C., Lee, J., Constantino, M. J., Fireman, B., et al. (2006). Comorbid depression, chronic pain and disability in primary care. *Psychosomatic Medicine, 68*, 262–268.

Baskin, S. M., & Weeks, R. E. (2003). The biobehavioral treatment of headache. In D. Moss, A. McGrady, T. C. Davies, & I. Wickramasekera (Eds.), *Handbook of mind-body medicine for primary care* (pp. 205–222). Thousand Oaks: Sage.

Bensten, S. B., Rustoen, T., Wahl, A. K., & Miaskowski, C. (2008). The pain experience and future expectation of chronic low back pain patients following spinal fusion. *Journal of Clinical Nursing, 17*, 153–159.

Bezov, D., Ashina, S., Jensen, R., & Bendtsen, J. (2011). Pain perception studies in tension headache. *Headache, 51*(2), 262–271.

Birklein, F., & Maihöfner, C. (2006). Use your imagination: Training the brain and not the body to improve chronic pain and restore function. *Neurology, 67*, 2115–2116.

Bonica, J. J., & Loeser, J. D. (2000). History of pain concepts and therapies. In J. D. Loeser, S. H. Butler, C. R. Chapman, & D. C. Turk (Eds.), *Bonica's management of pain* (pp. 3–16). Philadelphia: Lippincott, Williams & Wilkins.

Bruehl, S., Burns, J., Chung, O. Y., & Quartana, P. (2008). Anger management style and emotional reactivity to noxious stimuli among chronic pain patients and health controls: The role of endogenous opioids. *Health Psychology, 27*(2), 204–214.

Burns, J. W., Quartana, P., Gilliam, W., Gray, E., Matsuura, J., et al. (2008). Effects of anger suppression on pain severity and pain behaviors among chronic pain patients: Evaluation of an ironic process model. *Health Psychology, 27*, 645–652.

Charles, S. T., Gatz, M., Kato, K., & Pedersen, N. L. (2008). Physical health 25 years later: The predictive ability of neuroticism. *Health Psychology, 27*(3), 369–378.

Chen, Y. (2009). Advances in the pathophysiology of tension-type headache: From stress to central sensitization. *Current Pain and Headache Report, 13*(6), 484–494.

Diatchenko, L., & Slade, G. D. (2005). Human molecular genetics. *Human Molecular Genetics, 14*, 135–143.

Flor, H., & Diers, M. (2007). Limitations of pharmacotherapy: Behavioral approach to chronic pain. *Handbook of Experimental Pharmacology, 177*, 415–427.

Glaros, A. (2008). Temporomandibular disorders and facial pain: A psychophysiological perspective. *Applied Psychophysiology and Biofeedback, 33*, 161–171.

Headache Classification Committee of the International Headache Society. (1988). Classification and diagnostic criteria for headache disorders, cranial neuralgias, and facial pain. *Cephalalgia 8* (suppl 7), 1–96.

Hoffman, B. M., Papas, R. K., Chatkoff, D. K., & Kerns, R. D. (2007). Meta-analysis of psychological interventions for chronic low back pain. *Health Psychology, 26*(1), 1–9.

Holroyd, K. A. (2002). Assessment and psychological management of recurrent headache disorders. *Journal of Consulting and Clinical Psychology, 70*(3), 656–677.

Holroyd, K. A., & Drew, J. B. (2006). Behavioral approaches to the treatment of migraine. *Seminars in Neurology, 26*(2), 199–207.

Holroyd, K. A., Labus, J. S., & Carlson, B. (2009). Moderation and meditation in the psychological and drug treatment of chronic tension-type headache: The role of disorder severity and psychiatric comorbidity. *Pain, 143*(3), 213–222.

Kerns, R. D., & Habib, S. (2004). A critical review of the pain readiness to change model. *The Journal of Pain, 5*, 357–367.

Lawler, S. P., & Cameron, L. D. (2006). A randomized controlled trial of massage therapy as a treatment for migraine. *Annals of Behavioral Medicine, 32*(1), 50–59.

Lee, M. C., Zambreanu, L., Menon, D. K., & Tracey, I. (2008). Identifying brain activity specifically related to the maintenance and perceptual consequence of central sensitization in humans. *The Journal of Neuroscience, 28*(45), 11642–11649.

Lipton, R. B., Stewart, W. F., Diamond, S., Diamond, M. L., & Reed, M. (2001). Prevalence and burden of migraine in the United States: Data from the American Migraine Study II. *Headache, 41*, 646–657.

Mathew, N. T. (2006). Tension-type headache. *Current Neurological and Neuroscience Report, 6*(2), 100–105.

McGrady, A. (2002). Psychophysiological foundations of the mind-body therapies. In D. Moss, A. McGrady, T. C. Davies, & I. Wickramasekera (Eds.), *Handbook of mind-body medicine for primary care* (pp. 43–55). Thousand Oaks: Sage.

Middaugh, S. J., & Pawlick, K. (2002). Biofeedback and behavioral treatment of persistent pain in the older adult; a review and a study. *Applied Psychophysiology and Biofeedback, 27*(3), 185–202.

Morone, N. E., & Greco, C. M. (2007). Mind-body interventions for chronic pain in older adults: A structured review. *Pain Medicine, 8*(4), 359–375.

Nestoriuc, Y., Martin, A., Rief, W., & Andrasik, F. (2008). Biofeedback treatment for headache disorders: A comprehensive efficacy review. *Applied Psychophysiology and Biofeedback, 33*, 125–140.

Neufeld, J. D., Holroyd, K. A., & Lipchik, G. L. (2000). Dynamic assessment of abnormalities in central pain transmission and modulation in tension-type headache sufferers. *Headache, 40*, 142–151.

Penzien, D. B., Rains, J. C., & Andrasik, F. (2002). Behavioral management of recurrent headache: Three decades of experience and empiricism. *Applied Psychophysiology and Biofeedback, 27*(2), 163–181.

Peroutka, S. J. (2004). Migraine: A chronic sympathetic nervous system disorder. *Headache, 44*, 53–64.

Roehrs, T., Hyde, M., Blaisdell, B., Greenwalk, D. M., & Roth, T. (2006). Sleep loss and REM sleep loss are hyperalgesic. *Sleep, 29*(2), 145–151.

Roy-Byrne, P. P., Davidson, K. W., Kessler, R. C., Gordon, J. G., Asmundson, G. J. G., Goodwin, R. D., et al. (2008). Anxiety disorders and comorbid medical illness. *Focus, 6*, 467–485.

Smith, M. T., Edwards, R. R., McCann, U. D., & Haythornthwaite, J. A. (2007). The effects of sleep deprivation on pain inhibition and spontaneous pain in women. *Sleep, 30*(4), 494–505.

Strigo, I. A., Simmons, A. N., Matthews, S. C., Craig, A. D., & Paulus, M. P. (2008). Association of major depressive disorder with altered functional brain response during anticipation and processing of heat pain. *Archives of General Psychiatry, 65*(11), 1275–1285.

Vandenheede, M., & Schoenen, J. (2002). Central mechanisms in tension-type headaches. *Current Pain and Headache Report, 6*(5), 392–400.

Villemure, C., & Bushnell, M. C. (2002). Cognitive modulation of pain: How do attention and emotion influence pain processing? *Pain, 95*, 195–199.

Vlaeyen, J. S., & Linton, S. J. (2000). Fear-avoidance and its consequences in chronic musculoskeletal pain: A state of the art. *Pain, 85*, 317–332.

Waldie, K. E., & Poulton, R. (2002). The burden of illness associated with headache disorders among young adults in a representative cohort study. *Headache, 42*, 612–619.

Chapter 13
Fibromyalgia Syndrome

Abstract Fibromyalgia is a medical syndrome first described 200 years ago, but only recently officially recognized by medical science. The patient with fibromyalgia experiences widespread pain, often burning, in all four quadrants of the body. Fibromyalgia is often accompanied by additional symptoms, including fatigue, low energy, sleep disturbance, morning stiffness, depression, anxiety, and cognitive deficits. Fibromyalgia is best understood as a "pain amplification disorder," accompanied by allodynia and hyperalgesia. A variety of lifestyle and self-care interventions can be useful in moderating the patient's symptoms and improving quality of life. A case study illustrates the Pathways Model guided treatment program for a 34-year-old female with fibromyalgia.

Keywords FIbromyalgia • Allodynia • Hyperalgesia • Lifestyle and self-care • Graded interventions

Understanding the Fibromyalgia Syndrome

Definition of the Fibromyalgia Syndrome

The patient with fibromyalgia experiences widespread muscle pain, often burning, either constant or recurrent, and varying in severity. The muscle pain is often confusing to the patient and the health practitioner, because the pain fades or intensifies and changes location within the body, without a clear trigger. The pain often (not always) begins at the site of an injury, but becomes systemic, spreading around the entire musculoskeletal system. Over time the entire musculature shows changes, including *allodynia*—extreme sensitivity to exertion, strain, or trauma, with many routine activities triggering intense and severe pain.

In order to be medically diagnosed, the patient must meet the international classification criteria adopted in the Copenhagen Declaration (Quintner, 1992).

To be diagnosed with fibromyalgia syndrome, the patient must report the presence of "unexplained widespread pain or aching, persistent fatigue, generalized (morning) stiffness, non-refreshing sleep, and multiple tender points" (Quintner, 1992). The clinician will manually palpate the musculature bilaterally at 18 specified points. Patients with fibromyalgia will typically report pain on palpation at 11 or more tender points, although occasionally the diagnosis will be made in the presence of less than 11 tender points.

In addition, the muscle pain is often accompanied by a confusing variety of seemingly unrelated symptoms. Patients frequently report fatigue, low energy, sleep disturbance, morning stiffness, symptoms of irritable bowel syndrome, emotional symptoms such as depression and anxiety, and cognitive deficits such as poor concentration, impaired memory, and a clouding of their consciousness ("fibro fog") (Glass, 2006; Russell, 2001).

Prevalence of the Disorder

Fibromyalgia affects at least five million persons in the USA and approximately 3–6% of the population worldwide. The National Fibromyalgia Association estimates the fibromyalgia sufferers in the USA at ten million, and a National Arthritis Data Workgroup, drawing on available national surveys, estimated five million (Lawrence et al., 2008; National Fibromyalgia Association, 2009). Fibromyalgia is more likely to occur in females, with a recent large-scale study by Weir et al. (2006) reporting that females were 1.64 times more likely to be diagnosed by their physician with fibromyalgia. Previous research has estimated that women constituted as high as 75–90% of fibromyalgia patients (National Fibromyalgia Association, 2009). The incidence of fibromyalgia increases with age. Approximately 1% of women ages 18–29 suffer with fibromyalgia, but about 7% of women ages 70–79 suffer from fibromyalgia (Neumann, & Buskila, 2003).

In addition, patients with fibromyalgia suffer from many other disorders—"comorbidities." Recent research by Weir et al. (2006) showed that patients with a fibromyalgia diagnosis were anywhere from 2.14 times to 7.05 times more likely to suffer with depression, anxiety, headache, irritable bowel syndrome, chronic fatigue syndrome, systemic lupus erythematosus, and rheumatoid arthritis. In particular, the experience of chronic, daily pain is strongly associated with subsyndromal or clinical mood disturbances (Benjamin, Morris, McBeth, Macfarlane, & Silman, 2000).

Fibromyalgia is much more likely to afflict patients who are already ill with another disorder, especially rheumatic disorders, viral infections, and systemic illnesses. While about 0.5–5% of the general population in the USA suffers with fibromyalgia, up to 15.7% of clinic populations suffer with fibromyalgia. At the extreme, 65% of clinic patients with lupus erythematosus suffer with fibromyalgia (Neumann & Buskila, 2003).

Fibromyalgia is not a psychosomatic disorder. It can occur in individuals who are in full psychological health. Nevertheless, a history of traumatic life events, prolonged stress, and negative emotion increases the risk for fibromyalgia (Boisset-Pioro, Esdaile, & Fitzcharles, 1995; Ellis, 2008; Goldberg, Pachas, & Keith, 1999).

Economic Burden. Fibromyalgia presents a tremendous economic burden for the individual and for the larger society. The total economic burden of fibromyalgia consists of underemployment, disability payments, lost work hours, direct medical care costs for treatment of fibromyalgia specifically, and increased costs for all medical care. Patients with fibromyalgia frequently reduce work hours or accept less demanding work because of their condition (Russell, 2001). A 1997 US study reported that 16% of patients with fibromyalgia qualified for Social Security disability status, and 26.5% reported receiving at least one type of disability benefit (Wolfe et al., 1997). A recent US study calculated mean health care costs three times higher for a group of patients with any health care visits for fibromyalgia in a 3-year period, compared with a comparison group with no medical visits for fibromyalgia in the same period. The median costs for the fibromyalgia group were five times higher (Berger, Dukes, Martin, Edelsberg, & Oster, 2007). A study by Robinson et al. (2003) examined the claims data for employees of a Fortune 100 manufacturer and showed that fibromyalgia patients had many comorbid conditions and health care costs three times higher than the comparison group. The prevalence of disability was twice as high in the fibromyalgia group as in the total employee group.

As recently as the 1980s, many patients who presented their symptoms to physicians were diagnosed as depressed or neurotic and referred to psychologists or informed that their pain was imaginary. In 1987, however, the American Medical Association formerly recognized fibromyalgia as a medical syndrome; in 1990 the American College of Rheumatology (ACR) formulated precise diagnostic criteria, and in 1992 the international medical community formulated the Copenhagen Declaration, which adopted and refined the ACR diagnostic criteria for research and clinical practice worldwide. The "Copenhagen Declaration" document also recognized that fibromyalgia is the most common cause of widespread musculoskeletal pain. At last, the world medical community agreed that fibromyalgia is neither rare nor imaginary.

Mechanisms and Models for Fibromyalgia

The early name for this condition, fibrositis, implied an inflammation of the muscles (Smythe & Moldofsky, 1997), and rheumatology remains the medical specialty with the greatest experience in the diagnosis and treatment of fibromyalgia. However, tissue inflammation, if involved, is only one of many mechanisms relevant to fibromyalgia. Today, fibromyalgia is best understood as a "pain amplification disorder," that is, as a disorder in which allodynia and hyperalgesia are the primary mechanisms. Hyperalgesia signifies that one's body perceives a stimulus that would normally be mildly painful as severely painful. Allodynia means that a stimulus that would normally not be painful at all, such as someone brushing one's arm, is now perceived as painful (Staud, Vierck, Cannon, Mauderli, & Price, 2001). Fibromyalgia may begin with a specific injury producing tissue trauma and pain, and through a peripheral and central sensitization process, the entire system becomes highly sensitive to perceiving pain with minimal peripheral input. (Onset may also seem to come "out of the blue," without a precipitating injury or illness, and in this case the trigger for the sensitization process is less clear.) In addition, pain-related negative emotion and sleep deprivation contribute both to the pain experience and the correlated cognitive deficits (Staud, 2006a; Staud et al., 2006).

Pathophysiological changes can be measured in many physiological systems in fibromyalgia: in neuroendocrine, autonomic nervous system dysregulation, changes in brain function and activation, and muscular pathology and activation patterns. Research has provided abundant evidence that the autonomic nervous system is dysregulated in fibromyalgia, with reports of abnormal sympathovagal balance (Cohen et al., 2001), baroreflex dysfunction (Reyes Del Paso, Garrido, Pulgar, Martín-Vázquez, & Duschek, 2010), pervasive dysfunction of the autonomic nervous system (Staud, 2008), elevated heart rate, and decreased heart rate variability (HRV) (Cohen et al., 2000, 2001; Reyes Del Paso et al., 2010). There are some direct relationships suggesting the importance of autonomic regulation for fibromyalgia symptoms. For example, there is an inverse relation between baroreceptor function and pain levels in fibromyalgia (Reyes Del Paso et al., 2010).

The brain and central nervous system are dysregulated in fibromyalgia, as the frequency of cognitive deficits, such as problems with attention and concentration suggests. Geenan and Bijlsma (2010, p. 98) discussed "structural and functional changes in the brain." Donaldson reported on the quantitative EEGs of patients with fibromyalgia and showed a range of abnormal patterns of cortical activity, depending on the severity of the fibromyalgia symptoms (Donaldson, Donaldson, Mueller, & Sella, 2003). The disorganization of normal brain activation patterns in the EEG appeared to correlate with patient reports of cognitive deficits.

Donaldson also identified several abnormalities in the muscles of fibromyalgia patients (Donaldson & Sella, 2003; Donaldson, Sella, & Mueller, 1998). High basal levels of muscle tension, even at rest, asymmetries (higher levels of muscle tension in the same muscle on one side of the body than on the other), co-activations (muscles that are not functionally involved in a movement tense anyway during activity), failure to recover after exertion (muscles do not relax again following use), and long-term atrophy of muscle tissue, with shortening of muscle fibers and increased sensitivity. These muscular patterns are similar to those seen in myofascial pain and may result from postural bracing in the presence of pain and from inactivity following the onset of pain. Staud (2006b) also reported pathology in the muscles at a microscopic level, including changes in muscle acid-base balance due to ischemia and the appearance of jagged red fibers, inflammatory infiltrates, and "moth-eaten fibers."

Treatment of fibromyalgia presents many challenges to medical and mental health providers. After a meta-analysis of clinical trials, Goldenberg, Burckhardt, and Crofford (2004) recommended a stepwise program, which combined educational, pharmacological, psychological, and behavioral therapies. Targeted psychological intervention can moderate the intensity of fibromyalgia symptoms. Bennett and Nelson (2006, p. 416) reviewed the outcome data provided by 13 cognitive behavioral therapy (CBT) programs for fibromyalgia patients and reported "worthwhile improvements in pain-related behaviors, self-efficacy, coping strategies, and overall physical function." But CBT did not produce sustained pain relief. The outcomes were best when CBT was applied to adolescent patients with fibromyalgia. Bennett and Nelson (2006) concluded that CBT should be regarded as an adjunctive treatment, most helpful for those patients with prominent emotional distress and dysfunctional thinking and behavior, but potentially helpful for others as well.

The Case of Elizabeth

Elizabeth was a 34-year-old high school teacher, married, and the mother of three, referred by her primary care physician for psychological treatment of depression accompanying fibromyalgia. Elizabeth resented her physician for the referral, because she believed she needed better medical care, and insisted that her depression was a normal emotional reaction to her medical problems.

Elizabeth slipped on a wet floor at her school in October and fell into a row of lockers. She experienced sharp pain in her left shoulder, but still had full use of her arm and hand, so she continued working. She filed an "Incident Report" at school, only because several students had seen her fall and summoned the principal. She sought no medical care, although her employer encouraged her to see an occupational physician under contract to the school system.

Elizabeth's pain initially receded and then worsened over the next several weeks. She tried to "work it out," by swimming daily after school and doing some stretching exercises. In January, she began to experience an "achy soreness" through her shoulders, neck, and arms. The soreness became a burning sensation and became more bothersome, so she reduced her swimming and began using a heating pad on her shoulders and arms. Although the pain receded in the upper body, she experienced similar aching and burning in her lower back, buttocks, and legs. By the end of January, she noticed the quality of her sleep declining with delayed onset and frequent awakenings. She found herself drowsy at work and experienced poor concentration and short-term memory lapses.

The following April she was scheduled for an annual physical and asked her physician to evaluate the baffling pattern of wandering pain. She wondered if she had done some kind of spinal or nerve damage. Her primary care physician referred her to an orthopedic specialist, who ordered an X-ray of the upper torso and an upper body MRI. There were no positive findings on the X-ray or MRI, and the orthopedic specialist assessed her problem as "slow healing" and "soft tissue damage" from the original injury. He encouraged her to "give her body time to heal" and "avoid exertion." He prescribed a pain medication, Flexeril, for pain control and relief of muscle tension and spasm. Unfortunately, the pain medication seemed to worsen her sleep problems and increase the drowsiness during the work day. Elizabeth found it increasingly difficult to complete paperwork such as grade sheets at school. She became more edgy, irritable, and moody and began skipping the medication whenever she could tolerate the pain. She reduced activities and began to spend much of her nonwork time resting in a recliner, which was uncharacteristic for this previously athletic and active woman.

In July, Elizabeth's sister commented to Elizabeth that her symptoms resembled those of a close friend with fibromyalgia. Elizabeth's sister provided the name of the friend's rheumatologist, who saw Elizabeth, and conducted a screening for fibromyalgia, including identification of 13 tender points, the palpation of which elicited sharp pain. The pain occurred in all four quadrants of her body, with enough tender points to meet the ACR criteria for fibromyalgia. The rheumatologist diagnosed Elizabeth with posttraumatic fibromyalgia, secondary to her original worksite injury. He recommended she begin a gentle exercise program and suggested the medication Amitryptaline to help her mood and sleep. Based on research evidence, he explained that this medication, originally marketed as an antidepressant, also sometimes moderated the intensity of pain and improved sleep (O'Malley et al., 2000). He advised Elizabeth that fibromyalgia was a real disorder, sometimes disabling, with few effective treatments. He recommended that she get 8 or more hours of sleep per night, since sleep deprivation seems to exacerbate many of the secondary symptoms of fibromyalgia. He also offered to complete a social security disability application for her, if she found it difficult to do her job.

Elizabeth was relieved to have a diagnosis, and her mood actually lifted in the weeks following her diagnosis, until her primary care physician informed her that the fibromyalgia label was just the rheumatologist's way of labeling depression and suggested she seek psychotherapy. This frustrated her further, because she had begun to read about fibromyalgia online, and did not accept her primary care physician's dismissal of fibromyalgia as a psychosomatic illness.

Elizabeth attempted running and provoked a severe episode of burning and debilitating pain. She tried to get more regular sleep and found herself awakening several times a night in pain, and her daytime drowsiness and cognitive lethargy worsened. The Amitryptaline seemed to help her sleep onset, but she continued to awaken frequently through the night.

When the next school year began in August, her principal announced a new accelerated math program, effective immediately, and distributed study materials for all high school math and homeroom teachers. Elizabeth found she could not focus her mind on the study guides and became irritable, displaying anger outbursts at school. The mild cognitive deficits that she had noticed early in the onset of fibromyalgia now seemed much more severe. She requested a 6-week leave, and the rheumatologist provided a disability letter, with an indefinite time line. Seeing the letter elicited an episode of intense sobbing. Her spouse drove her to the primary care physician's office, who for the second time referred her to a behavioral medicine clinic for treatment of depression and for pain management.

Pathways Treatment for Elizabeth: Education. The first step in Elizabeth's treatment was to assure her that her pain was real and that fibromyalgia syndrome is an actual disorder, documented by thousands of research studies worldwide. The message to Elizabeth was as follows:

> We recognize the diagnostic signs here of fibromyalgia syndrome. This is a real medical disorder. Many people suffer a similar pain disorder; you are not alone. Help is available,

and many people can live more fully again. We can recommend life style changes, and teach you skills and provide information that will help you to manage this condition. If that isn't enough help, we can give you the names of group-based programs and other fibromyalgia specialists, who will help you to manage your condition.

Elizabeth broke down and sobbed profusely on hearing these words. She had begun to question her sanity, especially since her long-term and trusted physician said that her pain was just a symptom of depression. In contrast, one member of her treatment team had contributed to a book for patients on self-care for fibromyalgia (Moss, 2007), and she was given a copy and encouraged to read the introductory sections, which describe the realities of fibromyalgia and an orientation to self-care.

Elizabeth was clinically depressed at the time of the initial evaluation, yet careful interview found no past history of traumatic experiences, prolonged life stress, or recurrent depressive episodes. The current health crisis and progressive disability were the most stressful events in her life to date, and the current depression appeared to be a consequence of, rather than a contributor to, the onset of her fibromyalgia. Elizabeth cooperated with requests for a daily pain log and a diary of physical activity. In the first week of record keeping, her fibromyalgia pain reached at least 8–9 daily on a 10-point scale, and her activity diary was nearly empty. She had learned to avoid activity, because it hurts.

Level One Interventions. Elizabeth's Level One interventions began with movement. Her rheumatologist had recommended mild exercise, and she had responded by overexerting. The Pathways team discussed pleasurable movement and encouraged her to enjoy gentle motions, to pace herself, and particularly to not overexert. Emphasis was placed on "movement" and not "exercise," because to her exercise meant 10 K runs and freestyle sprints in the pool. She came up with the idea of doing slow dancing with her preschool daughter, using graceful swaying movement. She tried some slow movements from side to side in the clinic with music. Although the body motion felt good, she could feel the muscle soreness more acutely, which is an example of the allodynia that accompanies fibromyalgia. Elizabeth's nervous system had become so sensitized that even swaying motion was initially experienced as painful soreness. She was encouraged to be very gentle and do only short periods of movement; she also decided to walk her daughter two blocks to the nearby park.

Elizabeth's second Level One intervention was mindful breathing. She was so worried about her health problems and so preoccupied with her pain and limitations, that her tenseness and vigilance were visible. She was taught mindful diaphragmatic breathing in her second session and initially had some difficulty with pacing her breathing. She found that she was alternately breath holding and breathing very rapidly. Her therapist introduced her to the EZ-Air Plus™, a downloadable breath pacer available at www.bfe.org. Elizabeth found that by watching the EZ-Air Plus and simultaneously monitoring the movement of her abdomen with her hand, she could breathe comfortably and smoothly. Initially we set the EZ-Air Plus at nine breaths a minute, because even this seemed almost too slow for her. Later she was slowly shaped to six breaths a minute, using the EZ-Air Plus.

After the first 2 weeks of therapy, Elizabeth reported that she found the movement enjoyable, but had to talk to herself about pacing and not pushing too hard.

Her choices of music with a fast hard rock beat led to harsher, jerky movement which then exacerbated her pain. As long as she kept the music soft and slow paced, the movement felt good to her, although she experienced some tingling in her musculature that confused her. She also found the breathing soothing and within 1 week had the pacer set at six breaths per minute. She reported less of an edgy, irritable feeling and reported that both of her daughters (ages 4 and 8) were joining her in the EZ-Air Plus sessions.

Level Two Interventions. Elizabeth's first Level Two intervention was Aquatherapy, a gentle-graded exercise, three times a week, in a therapeutic pool with water temperature in the mid-90s (Houglum, 2010, pp. 383–413). The warmth of the water soothes and relaxes the muscles, facilitating movement with less muscle complaint, while the buoyancy of the water reduces physical impact and lessens pain. The Aquatherapy sessions were conducted by a physical therapist and designed for individuals with fibromyalgia, arthritis, and myofascial pain, beginning with range of motion and gentle flexibility exercises and proceeding slowly into muscle stretch exercises tailored to each person's condition. An initial PT evaluation by the Aquatherapy team showed some upper body bracing and a mild twisting in her posture, with left-sided tensing, and restricted range of motion in all quadrants. Even in the warm water, Elizabeth found that she needed to stop and rest after 10 min of exercise, because of increasing soreness and burning.

Elizabeth's second Level Two intervention was "gentle yoga." Elizabeth began the gentle yoga only after 6 weeks of Aquatherapy. The yoga trainer placed significant emphasis on an initial meditation, with yogic breathing. This reinforced the practice that Elizabeth was already doing with the EZ-Air Plus. Then the instructor added only one to two Hatha yoga asanas each week—the traditional postures which comprise the yogic tradition. Elizabeth was encouraged to accept the slow pace and enjoy the process of re-acquaintance with her body and musculature. She began with standing asanas and found that she could tolerate the yoga as long as she took rest breaks intermittently.

Elizabeth had been a natural athlete in high school and was a dual sport athlete in college (volleyball and tennis). The slow pace of both the Aquatherapy and the Extra Gentle Yoga frustrated her. However, when she bought a yoga DVD and tried to move ahead faster, she triggered a flare up of fibromyalgia pain, and a worsening of irritability and depressed mood. During this time, her rheumatologist added an additional medication, Lyrica, to moderate her pain and assist sleep. She complained that it made her drowsy during the day, but the Lyrica seemed to moderate her pain and improved her ability to tolerate both water-based exercise and yoga.

Level Three Interventions. Elizabeth's Level Three interventions included two forms of biofeedback, the first being HRV biofeedback. We referred earlier to the dysregulation of the autonomic nervous system in fibromyalgia and the reduction in HRV. Research shows an inverse relation between baroreceptor function and pain levels in fibromyalgia (Reyes Del Paso et al., 2010). In addition, Hassett et al. (2007) have shown that HRV biofeedback reduced pain and depression and improved functioning, in a study of 12 women with fibromyalgia. Hence, HRV biofeedback was provided for Elizabeth, in hopes of restoring autonomic regulation. It was also hoped that HRV biofeedback would moderate depressed mood, as suggested in the study by Karavidas et al. (2007).

The short story on HRV biofeedback is that healthy human beings have higher variability in their heart rate. Many medical and emotional disorders are associated with lowered HRV, and it has become an index in medical research for healthy autonomic function, cardiovascular health, and emotional health. Research in the past 15 years, especially a stream of research following the publication of a treatment protocol by Lehrer, Vaschillo, and Vaschillo (2000), has shown therapeutic benefit for a wide range of clinical disorders, including asthma (Lehrer et al., 2004), posttraumatic stress disorder (Zucker, Samuelson, Muench, Greenberg, & Gevirtz, 2009), fibromyalgia (Hassett et al., 2007), cardiovascular illness (DelPozo, Gevirtz, Scher, & Guarneri, 2004), and other disorders.

Elizabeth's HRV biofeedback began with an assessment session, identifying baseline patterns in respiration and HRV. Elizabeth's overall HRV was low for a 34-year-old woman, who had been athletic and active until recently. Her "SDNN"—the standard deviation of the interbeat interval of her heart beat—was 44 ms. This is medically an indication of poor health and low vitality (Kleiger, Miller, Bigger, Moss, & The Multicenter Post-Infarction Research Group, 1987). The mean oscillation in her heart rate, the "HeartRateMaximum minus the HeartRateMinimum," was only five beats, which is very low for her age.

Elizabeth had already engaged in several weeks of practice of mindful breathing and yoga, before beginning biofeedback, and she showed a good ability to maintain smooth diaphragmatic breathing. An initial assessment showed that her optimal breathing rate for producing higher HRV was 5.5 breaths per minute. We guided Elizabeth in the office, to practice breathing now exactly at 5.5 breaths a minute, and taught her a number of strategies to increase her HRV. In one exercise, she watched the fluctuation of her heart rate and breathing on the computer screen and began her inhalation each time the heart rate began to move up. She also was trained to increase the % of her total HRV in the low frequency range and reached levels in the 80% range within three sessions. She liked this HRV training process and at the 12-week point, was able to produce 14 point oscillations in heart rate and SDNN indices during the training session of 110–120 ms range. Her baseline HRV slowly improved, although remaining in the "compromised health range."

Elizabeth's second form of biofeedback training—muscle biofeedback (sEMG)—began in her fourth week of HRV biofeedback. Her initial evaluation had showed some abnormal patterns in muscle tension, similar to those described by Donaldson et al. (1998). Elizabeth showed asymmetry in muscle tension between the muscles along the right of her spine and those on the left, with the left side showing substantially greater elevation in muscle tension. (Her physical therapist had found the same phenomenon several weeks prior). She showed the following co-activation patterns: When she turned her head, there was a recruitment of muscle activation in the lumbar paraspinal muscles, which are functionally not assistive for this movement. The muscles of the shoulder and neck showed severe elevation in muscle tension readings (at some sites greater than 30 microvolts, while a relaxed muscle carries less than one microvolt) while standing and failed to relax significantly when she returned to a seated position.

Elizabeth began using muscle biofeedback to learn greater awareness and control over the musculature of her body, as described in Drexler, Mur, and Gunther (2002). She was already doing extensive muscle stretching in Aquatherapy and yoga, and she was encouraged to gently and then more strenuously stretch and tense muscles and then gradually relax them. During this stage of treatment, she found that several components of her Pathways program reinforced one another. She learned to recognize the sensations of tense and relaxed muscles through her muscle biofeedback and then noticed tensing reactions in her back when yoga elicited a burning sensation. She began to countermand such spontaneous tensing reactions and took pleasure in her increased flexibility and skills in yoga.

Clinically, Elizabeth showed significant improvement in her fibromyalgia pain levels. Her pain log showed many days in which the pain levels never exceeded 4 or 5 on a 10-point scale, yet her activity diary showed a return to more normal levels, including walking, Aquatherapy, and yoga, and an increased facility in household tasks. She was still on disability leave from work, but at this point spoke with her school principal about a graduated return, beginning with part-time work. There were some initial problems with the school requiring that she be 100% recovered prior to return, but her teacher's union intervened and negotiated a step-wise return, which is more optimal for any patient with chronic pain and fatigue. She eventually returned to full-time work.

Emotionally, Elizabeth felt more like herself. She took pride in the various strands of her rehabilitation plan and became a missionary preaching to her friends and colleagues about self-efficacy, self-regulation, and active engagement in one's own health care. The initial period of her fibromyalgia, especially the medical message that her disorder was somehow either imaginary or a mental health problem, had been destructive for her. The development of the Pathways treatment plan, with the emphasis on acquisition of skills and pursuit of specific objectives, restored her self-confidence and hope. Since elements of CBT had been interspersed with her biofeedback sessions, she took great pride in re-languaging her pain, announcing that she observed no pain today but mild "discomfort" in several areas.

Case Summary

Fibromyalgia is a syndrome marked by the presence of pain throughout the musculature and often accompanied by a variety of other seemingly unrelated symptoms, including fatigue, low energy, sleep disturbance, morning stiffness, symptoms of irritable bowel syndrome, emotional symptoms such as depression and anxiety, and cognitive deficits. Fibromyalgia is a disorder of pain amplification, which often follows a specific injury or illness. Many ordinary activities and sensations are experienced as painful. Research suggests both central and peripheral processes of sensitization with changes taking place in the individual's biochemistry, autonomic nervous regulation, central nervous system, and musculature. A history of traumatic life events, prolonged stress, and negative emotion increases the risk for fibromyalgia.

Case Summary

Elizabeth was a 34-year-old married mother of three, and a high school teacher. She was injured in a fall at her worksite, and over a period of weeks, the initial localized pain transformed into a systemic pain process with aching and burning pain throughout much of her musculature. She reported sleep disturbances and mild cognitive deficits, which progressed to a severe level overtime. She was initially treated with a muscle relaxant, Flexeril, then with a tricyclic antidepressant (Amitryptaline) for sleep and pain management, and eventually with Lyrica, a neuromodulator that lessened pain and enhanced sleep.

Elizabeth's Level One interventions included movement and mindful breathing. Although Elizabeth had attempted to increase her movement before, she commonly overexerted, triggering severe pain and inactivity. Based on the Pathways Model, she accepted gentle movement with music and a short walk to the park with her daughter. Her mindful breathing was aided by the use of a downloadable breath pacer, the EZ-Air Plus™, and the breathwork served to calm the agitation and edgy irritability she had experienced.

The Level Two recommendations for Elizabeth were Aquatherapy and gentle yoga. The Aquatherapy built on her Level One gentle movement experiences. The warm water soothed her, and her instructor introduced gradual range of motion and flexibility exercises followed by gentle muscle stretch exercises. Elizabeth felt a tingling and burning intermittently during the Aquatherapy, but was encouraged to stop and enjoy the water whenever the discomfort grew more intense. She began gentle yoga after 6 weeks of Aquatherapy, first with meditation and yogic breathing and later adding the standing asanas. Her ability to continue in yoga encouraged her, and she tried briefly to accelerate her yoga progress, but a return of intense burning pain persuaded her to accept the instructor's slower timetable.

Elizabeth agreed to accept two forms of biofeedback for her Level Three interventions. The initial biofeedback modality, HRV biofeedback, seemed a natural choice for her, because the training rests strongly on further refinement of breathing skills. Elizabeth's HRV assessment showed indications of very low HRV, but she progressed in the first 4 weeks. As soon as she showed some mastery in HRV biofeedback, a second form of biofeedback training was added—sEMG muscle biofeedback. Elizabeth's initial biofeedback assessment showed several patterns often associated with chronic pain. Elizabeth became excited about achieving muscle awareness and muscle control and began utilizing her new muscle relaxation skills whenever she experienced discomfort in her yoga and Aquatherapy sessions. She also took pride in relabeling her pain as "discomfort," and announced milestones in her returns to normal activities in weekly emails to friends and family.

Elizabeth was a good example of a patient doing well with the Pathways approach to both chronic pain and fibromyalgia. First, each element in her Pathways treatment plan interacted with each other element, reinforcing her gains and her sense of self-efficacy. Second, her condition was a chronic one. She experienced considerable progress during her 6 months of Pathways consultations and treatment. She understood, however, that her fibromyalgia syndrome was still present, but remained determined to continue setting new activity goals and coping positively with setbacks.

References

Benjamin, S., Morris, S., McBeth, J., Macfarlane, G., & Silman, A. (2000). The association between chronic widespread pain and mental disorder. *Arthritis and Rheumatism, 43*(3), 561–567.

Bennett, R., & Nelson, D. (2006). Cognitive behavioral therapy for fibromyalgia. *Nature Clinical Practice. Rheumatology, 2*(8), 416–424.

Berger, A., Dukes, E., Martin, S., Edelsberg, J., & Oster, G. (2007). Characteristics and healthcare costs of patients with fibromyalgia syndrome. *International Journal of Clinical Practice, 61*, 1498–1508.

Boisset-Pioro, M. H., Esdaile, J. M., & Fitzcharles, M. A. (1995). Sexual and physical abuse in women with fibromyalgia syndrome. *Arthritis and Rheumatism, 38*(2), 235–241.

Cohen, H., Neumann, L., Alhosshle, A., Kotler, M., Abu-Shakra, M., & Buskila, D. (2001). Abnormal sympathovagal balance in men with fibromyalgia. *Journal of Rheumatology, 28*(3), 581–589.

Cohen, H., Neumann, L., Shore, M., Amir, M., Cassuto, Y., & Buskila, D. (2000). Autonomic dysfunction in patients with fibromyalgia: Application of power spectral analysis of heart rate variability. *Seminars in Arthritis and Rheumatism, 29*(4), 217–227.

DelPozo, J., Gevirtz, R. N., Scher, B., & Guarneri, E. (2004). Biofeedback treatment increases heart rate variability in patients with known coronary artery disease. *American Heart Journal, 147*(3), E11.

Donaldson, M., Donaldson, C. C. S., Mueller, H. H., & Sella, G. (2003). QEEG patterns, psychological status and pain reports of fibromyalgia sufferers. *American Journal of Pain Management, 13*(2), 1–27.

Donaldson, C. C. S., & Sella, G. (2003). Fibromyalgia. In D. Moss, A. McGrady, T. Davies, & I. Wickramasekera (Eds.), *Handbook of mind body medicine for primary care* (pp. 323–332). Thousand Oaks, CA: Sage.

Donaldson, C. C. S., Sella, G. E., & Mueller, H. H. (1998). Fibromyalgia: A retrospective study of 252 consecutive referrals. *Canadian Journal of Clinical Medicine, 5*(6), 116–127.

Drexler, A. R., Mur, E. J., & Gunther, V. C. (2002). Efficacy of an EMG-biofeedback therapy in fibromyalgia patients. A comparative study of patients with and without abnormality in (MMPI) psychological scales. *Clinical and Experimental Rheumatology, 20*, 677–682.

Ellis, L. E. (2008). Etiology, diagnosis and treatment of fibromyalgia: A practical and effective approach. In G. R. Walz, J. C. Bleuer, & R. K. Yep (Eds.), *Compelling counseling interventions* (pp. 161–171). Ann Arbor, MI: Counseling Outfitters, LLC.

Geenan, R., & Bijlsma, J. W. (2010). Deviations in the endocrine system and brain of patients with fibromyalgia: Cause or consequence of pain and associated features. *Annals of the New York Academy of Sciences, 1193*, 98–110.

Glass, J. M. (2006). Cognitive dysfunction in fibromyalgia and chronic fatigue syndrome: New trends and future directions. *Current Rheumatology Reports, 8*(6), 425–429.

Goldberg, R. T., Pachas, W. N., & Keith, D. (1999). Relationship between traumatic events in childhood and chronic pain. *Journal of Disability and Rehabilitation, 21*(1), 23–30.

Goldenberg, D. I., Burckhardt, C., & Crofford, L. (2004). Management of fibromyalgia syndrome. *Journal of the American Medical Association, 292*(19), 2388–2395.

Hassett, A. L., Radvanski, D. C., Vaschillo, E. G., Vaschillo, B., Sigal, L. H., Buyske, S., et al. (2007). A pilot study of the efficacy of heart rate variability (HRV) biofeedback in patients with fibromyalgia. *Applied Psychophysiology and Biofeedback, 32*, 1–10. doi:10.1007/s10484-006-9028-0.

Houglum, P. A. (2010). *Therapeutic exercise for musculoskeletal injuries* (3rd ed.). Champagne, IL: Human Kinetics.

Karavidas, M. K., Lehrer, P. M., Vaschillo, E., Vaschillo, B., Marin, H., Buyske, S., et al. (2007). Preliminary results of an open label study of heart rate variability biofeedback for the treatment of major depression. *Applied Psychophysiology and Biofeedback, 32*, 19–30.

Kleiger, R. E., Miller, J. P., Bigger, J. T., Moss, A. J., & The Multicenter Post-Infarction Research Group. (1987). Decreased heart rate variability and its association with increased mortality after acute myocardial infarction. *The American Journal of Cardiology, 59*, 256–262.

References

Lawrence, R. C., Felson, D. T., Helmick, C. G., Srnold, L. M., Choi, H., Deyo, R., et al. (2008). Estimates of the prevalence of arthritis and other rheumatic conditions in the United States: Part II. *Arthritis and Rheumatism, 58*(1), 15–25.

Lehrer, P. M., Vaschillo, E., & Vaschillo, B. (2000). Resonant frequency biofeedback training to increase cardiac variability. Rationale and manual for training. *Applied Psychophysiology and Biofeedback, 25*(3), 177–191.

Lehrer, P., Vaschillo, E., Vaschillo, B., Lu, S., Scardella, A., Siddique, M., et al. (2004). Biofeedback treatment for asthma. *Chest, 126*, 352–361.

Moss, D. (2007). Behaviorally reconnecting mind and body. In S. Ostalecki (Ed.), *Fibromyalgia: The complete guide from medical experts and patients* (pp. 273–288). Boston: Jones and Bartlett.

National Fibromyalgia Association. (2009). *About fibromyalgia*. Retrieved from, http://www.fmaware.org/site/PageServer.

Neumann, L., & Buskila, D. (2003). Epidemiology of fibromyalgia. *Current Pain and Headache Reports, 7*, 362–368.

O'Malley, P. G., Balden, E., Tomkins, G., Santoro, J., Kroenke, K., & Jackson, J. L. (2000). Treatment of fibromyalgia with antidepressants: A meta-analysis. *Journal of Internal Medicine, 15*(9), 659–666.

Quintner, J. (1992). Fibromyalgia: The Copenhagen declaration. *Lancet, 340*(8827), 663–664.

Reyes Del Paso, G. A., Garrido, S., Pulgar, A., Martín-Vázquez, M., & Duschek, S. (2010). Aberrances in autonomic cardiovascular regulation in fibromyalgia syndrome and their relevance for clinical pain reports. *Psychosomatic Medicine, 72*(5), 462–470.

Robinson, R. L., Birnbaum, H. G., Morley, M. A., Sisitsky, T., Greenberg, P. E., & Claxton, A. J. (2003). Economic cost and epidemiological characteristics of patients with fibromyalgia claims. *Journal of Rheumatology, 30*(6), 1318–1325.

Russell, I. J. (2001). Fibromyalgia syndrome. In S. Mense, D. G. Simon, & I. J. Russell (Eds.), *Muscle pain: Understanding its nature, diagnosis and treatment* (pp. 289–352). Philadelphia: Lippincott Williams & Wilkins.

Smythe, H. A., & Moldofsky, H. (1977). Two contributions to understanding the "fibrositis syndrome". *Bulletin on the Rheumatic Diseases, 28*, 928–931.

Staud, R. (2006a). Biology and therapy of fibromyalgia: Pain in fibromyalgia syndrome. *Arthritis Research and Therapy, 8*(3), Epub April 24.

Staud, R. (2006b). Fibromyalgia syndrome: Mechanisms of abnormal pain processing. *Primary Psychiatry, 13*(9), 66–71.

Staud, R. (2008). Heart rate variability as a biomarker of fibromyalgia syndrome. *Future Rheumatology, 3*(5), 475–483.

Staud, R., Vierck, C. J., Cannon, R. L., Mauderli, A. P., & Price, D. D. (2001). Abnormal sensitization and temporal summation of second pain (wind-up) in patients with fibromyalgia syndrome. *Pain, 91*(1), 165–175.

Staud, R., Vierck, C. J., Robinson, M. E., & Price, D. D. (2006). Overall fibromyalgia pain is predicted by ratings of local pain and pain-related negative affect–possible role of peripheral tissues. *Rheumatology, 45*(11), 1409–1415.

Weir, P. T., Harlan, G. A., Nkoy, F. L., Jones, S. S., Hegman, K. T., Gren, L. H., et al. (2006). The incidence of fibromyalgia and its associated comorbidities: A population based retrospective cohort study based on International Classification of Diseases, 9th Revision Codes. *Journal of Clinical Rheumatology, 12*(3), 124–128.

Wolfe, F., Anderson, J., Harkness, D., Bennett, R. M., Caro, X. J., Goldenberg, D. L., et al. (1997). Work and disability status of persons with fibromyalgia. *Journal of Rheumatology, 24*(6), 1171–1178.

Zucker, T. L., Samuelson, K. W., Muench, F., Greenberg, M. A., & Gevirtz, R. N. (2009). The effects of respiratory sinus arrhythmia biofeedback on heart rate variability and post traumatic stress: A pilot study. *Applied Psychophysiology and Biofeedback, 34*(2), 135–143.

Chapter 14
Gastrointestinal Disorders

Abstract This chapter begins with a brief description of the processes of digestion and absorption in the gastrointestinal tract and then follows with a discussion of the effects of psychological and behavioral factors on gastrointestinal function. Medical, psychotherapeutic, and psychophysiological interventions applicable to functional gastrointestinal disorders are described. The case study presents the Pathways Model in a young adult male with irritable bowel syndrome (IBS).

Keywords Gastrointestinal disorders • Digestive processes • Irritable bowel syndrome • Case study

Overview of Gastrointestinal Function

The gastrointestinal (GI) system moves solids and liquids taken from the external environment through the mouth into the internal environment through a highly organized system of tubular structures. The following is a brief description of the functions of the GI system, summarized from Widmaier, Raff, and Strang (2001) and Guyton and Hall (2000). Four processes (digestion, secretion, absorption, and motility) operate to accomplish the main function of the GI system, which is to absorb nutrients. Regulation of these GI processes is based within the GI system itself, in addition to neural and endocrine influences, further modified by behavioral and psychological factors.

The presence of food in the mouth stimulates chewing to break up food into smaller particles and secretion of saliva to moisten the contents. The bolus of food moves into the esophagus and further into the stomach. All along this process, the parasympathetic and sympathetic branches of the autonomic nervous system control the rates of motility, while the strength of the contraction (peristaltic waves) is influenced largely by distention.

The enteric nervous system is located entirely in the walls of the esophagus, stomach, and intestine to regulate motility (the myenteric nervous plexus), secretions, and blood flow (the submucosal plexus). Both divisions of the autonomic nervous system have important influences on these two plexi and GI function; the parasympathetic system, mainly through the vagus nerve, acts to increase activity of the enteric nervous system and thereby enhances GI functions. In contrast, the sympathetic nervous system inhibits smooth muscle contraction, thereby decreasing movements of the tract. These autonomic nervous patterns in GI function represent a reversal of that in most physiological systems. For example, in the cardiovascular system the sympathetic system increases heart rate, and the parasympathetic system brakes the heart rate. We will return to this paradoxical autonomic pattern later, when we examine the GI system and its stress response.

The endocrine system is another major controller of GI function. Throughout the tract, secretory glands promote two major outcomes. First is the release of digestive enzymes, from the mouth to the distal end of the ileum; second is the production of mucous to provide for lubrication to aid in the passage of food through the tract and protection of the walls of each portion of the GI system.

In the mouth, saliva mixes with food and moistens it for easier swallowing. The stomach mucosa contains the oxyntic (acid forming) glands and the pyloric glands, which release mucus, pepsinogen, and the hormone gastrin. In concert with the pancreatic and intestinal enzymes, proteins are broken down into small peptides and eventually to amino acids, which are easily absorbed. The acid in the stomach must be neutralized by bicarbonate in the small intestine so that highly acidic contents do not continue to pass through the rest of the GI system. Fat globules that pass into the intestine are first emulsified (made soluble) and then digested by lipase from the pancreas, resulting in fatty acids and monoglycerides. Bile is secreted by the liver and its main function is to solubilize and facilitate digestion of fats. Finally, starch is digested by amylases (contained in saliva and pancreatic secretions) and other enzymes in the intestine to form smaller molecules of monosaccharides. Undigested food moves to the large intestine, where fecal matter is formed and stored until defecation takes place.

From the brief description above, it is clear that GI function is dependent on behavior, beginning with the initial act of ingesting liquids and solids through the final expelling of liquid and solid by-products of digestion. As discussed in the chapter on obesity, appetite for food, choice of what foods to eat, preparation of food, and the timing of eating and quantity of food and drink consumed are all within conscious control. Furthermore, the involvement of the autonomic nervous system at every stage of the digestive process highlights the relevance of psychological processes to GI function. For example, the effects of stress can be manifested in pain from distention of the stomach or intestine; pain can also result from rapid passage of food throughout the tract and frequent bowel movements. Conversely, pain can also be caused by lack of food or by food with little fiber and constipation.

Functional GI Disorders

The functional GI disorders include a wide spectrum of problems whose diagnoses are based on symptoms and not on the detection of organic disease. The disorders include irritable bowel syndrome (IBS), functional dyspepsia, and Functional Abdominal Pain Syndrome (FAPS). Because of the absence of organic findings, diagnoses are based on the Rome criteria of symptoms and chronicity (Thompson et al., 1999).

Patients with functional GI disorders demonstrate increased sensitivity of their visceral pain receptors, resulting in sensations of discomfort from normal contractions or distensions of the gut. Stress sensitivity is another shared feature among the functional GI disorders. The neural pathways that transmit visceral pain signals also regulate the stress response (Mayer & Wong, 2010). When there is excess reactivity, corticotrophin-releasing factor and the hypothalamic–pituitary–adrenal axis maintain stress responses, despite the actual end of the stressful situation. Continued release of stress mediators, such as pro-inflammatory cytokines and catecholamines, results in inappropriate (for the stimulus) inflammation (Roy-Byrne, Davidson, Kessler, Asmundson, & Goodwin, 2008). In a study of children with functional abdominal pain, autonomic dysregulation was identified as a possible mechanism. But instead of excessive sympathetic drive being conceptualized as the major imbalance, vagal withdrawal may be the major mediator of the functional GI disorders (Sowder, Gevirtz, Shapiro, & Ebert, 2010).

Psychological stress influences on functional GI disorders have been explored in greatest detail in patients with IBS. The prevalence of stressful life events in patients with IBS is consistently greater than control subjects, and stressful life events intensify existing symptoms of IBS. Suarez, Mayer, Ehlert, and Nater (2010) explored the relationship of stress to GI functional disturbances in a large questionnaire-based study. Perceived chronic stress, greater stress reactivity, and use of maladaptive coping strategies predicted symptoms of functional gastrointestinal disorders. In fact, half of patients who received the diagnosis of IBS reported stressful life circumstances prior to the onset of symptoms. In particular, a history of sexual abuse was more common in patients with IBS (Creed et al., 2005; Talley, Fett, & Zinsmeister, 1994).

Crane and Martin (2004) studied the use of types of coping strategies in patients with one of two functional disorders (irritable bowel and inflammatory bowel disease). Emotional passive coping was correlated in both groups with higher levels of anxiety and depression. The authors also suggested that illness-related social learning that occurs during childhood influences the development of the sick role and illness-related behaviors in adulthood. Since tracing patterns of behavior from infancy to adulthood is difficult, researchers relied on subjects' memories of past experience and current patterns of behavior. Two hundred eighteen women participated in a study that sought to correlate severity and frequency of symptoms of inflammatory bowel disease and attachment style. Results showed that the anxious and avoidant attachment styles were positively correlated with disease severity and negative effect. In addition, low social support and low coping efficacy predicted disease status for the anxious attachment group (Gick & Sirois, 2010).

Not surprisingly, a strong association exists between IBS and some psychiatric disorders, in particular anxiety and mood disorders. Overall, rates of psychiatric disorders in treatment seeking IBS patients ranged from 50 to 90 % (Roy-Byrne et al., 2008). Lackner, Quigley, and Blanchard (2004) questioned whether the relationship between depression and abdominal pain in patients with IBS was linear. Patients' beliefs about their GI disorder and their pain, in particular the tendency to catastrophize and maintain feelings of helplessness, link symptoms with depression (Kovacs & Kovacs, 2007). In a large study conducted in 15 primary care practices, patient attitudes, particularly those associated with depression, escalated the number of GI symptoms (Mussell et al., 2008). These findings are important because patients' beliefs regarding their pain lead them to make behavioral choices affect adherence to medical recommendations. Patients suffering with IBS overreacted to mild symptoms, feared sensations emanating from the visceral areas, and also underestimated their capabilities to cope. Due to the nature of the symptoms of the functional GI disorders, patients tend to withdraw from or become reluctant to engage in social activities, further increasing the risk for depressive symptoms.

Irritable Bowel Syndrome

IBS is a functional gastrointestinal disorder, which is characterized by pain in the abdominal region, bloating or distension of the abdomen, and bowel function abnormalities (frequency and consistency). IBS affects women three times more frequently than men. Approximately 9–10 % of the US population is affected, accounting for approximately three million doctor visits a year (Talley, 2006). The diagnosis of IBS depends on negative physical findings (physical examination, standard blood analysis, stool tests, colonoscopy as indicated) and meeting the Rome criteria: at least 3 months of symptoms, including abdominal pain accompanied by change in frequency of the stool and disturbed defecation at least 25 % of the time. The disturbance is defined as altered frequency of bowel movements, passage of mucous, altered consistency of feces, and distention of the abdomen (Thompson et al., 1999).

Medical treatment of IBS is challenging since there is no one dietary recommendation or medication that consistently improves the overall symptom picture. One of the first clinical tasks is to explain to the patient the mechanisms of food movement, processing through the gastrointestinal tract, and regulation by the nervous system. Often printed materials and diagrams of the GI system are used for educational purposes and to diagram the potential effects of stress on digestion and absorption. Many practitioners use visual displays of the enteric and the autonomic nervous systems to elucidate the role of psychological influences on GI function. Based on the hypersensitivity hypotheses described above, careful explanations of the recognized effects of stress on GI activity are necessary without implying either blame or psychopathology where it does not exist (Suarez et al., 2010). Reassurance should be provided so that the patient does not equate the severity of the pain with organicity. A collaborative, problem-solving, supportive relationship between the primary care physician and the patient should be cultivated (Fink, Rosendal, & Toft, 2002).

One traditional intervention for IBS consists of regulating diet, depending on whether the patient complains of diarrhea or constipation (Watson & Smith, 2003). A food diary provides information about the patient's food intolerance or sensitivity to substances such as lactose, fructose, or wheat-containing products. Addition of fiber may resolve constipation, but in contrast can also worsen bloating and distention (Lacy, 2006). Antispasmodics relax the smooth muscle of the intestine, thereby relieving excessive contractility and decreasing the speed of transit in the GI tract. However, controlled studies of this class of medicines are few, and supportive evidence for benefit is not strong (Mayer & Wong, 2010).

Psychopharmacological treatment of IBS is varied and includes antianxiety agents and tricyclic antidepressants, in addition to the serotonin reuptake inhibitors. Benzodiazepines are sometimes used if anxiety is prominent; however, long-term treatment with this class of drugs is not recommended due to the potential for addiction (Talley, 2006). Regarding the antidepressant class of medicines, the tricyclic antidepressants were associated with reductions in abdominal pain and improved quality of life in patients with functional GI disorders, but the efficacy of the SSRIs has not been proven in patients with GI problems without psychiatric comorbidity (Mayer & Wong, 2010).

Psychotherapeutic, behavioral, and applied psychophysiological therapies have been implemented in patients with functional GI disorders, IBS. After medical evaluation, nutritional assessment, and medical management, patients with psychiatric comorbidity or those in whom stress was identified as a symptom trigger are referred to mental health providers (Herschbach et al., 1999). Symptom logging is necessary to establish the baseline and to track progress over time. The criteria for improvement are less severe abdominal pain, fewer episodes of bowel dysfunction, and improved ability to function in the social and work setting.

Hypnotherapy is another mind–body therapy that has been studied as an intervention for IBS (Gholamrezaei, Ardestani, & Emami, 2006; Palsson & Collins, 2003). The standard protocol consisted of seven 45-min biweekly hypnosis sessions, and patients were recommended to practice at home daily using recorded hypnotic suggestions. Clinically and statistically significant improvements were recorded in abdominal pain, bloating, and abnormal bowel movements (Palsson, Turner, Johnson, Burnett, & Whitehead, 2002). Subsequently, the protocol was expanded to a home-based intervention, using educational resources and CDs. Patients improved in symptoms of IBS, but less dramatically than patients treated in clinic. Anxiety predicted poor treatment response in this group, which raises intriguing questions about mediation of the treatment effects (Palsson, Turner, & Whitehead, 2006).

Cognitive behavioral-type interventions have also been successfully used in patients with IBS. Twelve weeks of Cognitive Behavior Therapy (CBT) produced improvement in IBS symptom severity and improved quality of life in 74 patients with IBS (Lackner et al., 2008). However, there was no improvement in psychological distress as measured by the Brief Symptom Inventory scale. In a primary care practice, a CBT-based self-management intervention produced significant relief of symptoms in 76 % of treated patients in contrast to 21 % of usual care patients (Moss-Morris, McAlpine, Didsbury, & Spence, 2010). Blanchard et al. (2007) conducted a large-scale study of group cognitive therapy in comparison to a psychoeducational support group and a third group who monitored symptoms. Both CBT and the psychoeducational support group produced significant improvements in symptoms in comparison to the monitoring group alone. Abdominal pain, tenderness, and gas were decreased. At 3 months follow-up, the patients sustained the improvements that occurred during active treatment.

The effects of interventions based on relaxation have also been studied in patients with functional GI disorders. In a controlled outcome study, Benson's Relaxation Response Meditation was found superior to wait-list control in reducing abdominal pain, bloating, belching, and gas (Keefer & Blanchard, 2001). At 1-year follow-up of this group of patients (wait-listed were treated also), additional improvements were noted in pain and bloating if patients continued to practice the meditation technique (Keefer & Blanchard, 2002). In another study, a program of autogenic training (8 weekly sessions) was provided to patients with IBS while a control group participated in group discussions about meal habits and lifestyles. This type of relaxation was based on the original method of Schultz, comprising the repetition of simple specific phrases emphasizing heaviness and warmth in the arms and legs, cool sensations in the forehead, and regular heart rate. At the end of training, patients in the autogenic group reported significant relief in symptoms and lessening of bodily pain. No differences were observed in anxiety or SF-36 scores (Shinozaki et al., 2010).

Functional Dyspepsia

Diagnosis of FD is based on the Rome criteria of 3 months of symptoms (epigastric pain, burning, fullness after meals, or early satiation, with possible bloating and nausea) and no evidence of organic disease. Forty percent of FD patients show some impairment in gastric accommodation so that food rapidly moves out of the proximal stomach and remains in the distal areas of the stomach, which may explain the sensations of excessive fullness after a meal. FD and IBS are so frequently comorbid that definition of two separate disorders has been questioned. Psychiatric comorbidity, particularly anxiety and depression, is also shared between FD and IBS. There are no well-controlled mind–body clinical trials that guide the treatment of FAPS (Mayer & Wong, 2010).

Functional Abdominal Pain Syndrome

FAPS is characterized by at least three episodes of abdominal pain during at least 3 months, unrelated to GI function, which are associated with some loss of daily function. The patient does not meet criteria for another functional GI disorder that would explain the pain. Although medical management has not produced impressive results, patients treated with mind–body therapies such as CBT, hypnotherapy, and biofeedback have shown improvements. In a study of children and adolescents with FAPS, heart rate variability biofeedback produced improvements in pain severity and frequency (Sowder et al., 2010). Humphreys and Gevirtz (2000) also reported significant reductions in recurrent abdominal pain after treatment with breathing training and thermal biofeedback.

The Case of Rod

Rod was a 28-year-old married male who presented with GI symptoms, primarily abdominal pain, bloating, gas, and diarrhea. During college, the symptoms were intermittent, but worsening had occurred during the past 3 years. His primary care physician diagnosed him with IBS of moderate severity, based on the Rome criteria. A food elimination strategy had only revealed very mild reactions to caffeine and carbonated beverages and he easily stayed away from those substances. Rod was referred to a gastroenterologist who first treated Rod with the antispasmodic medication mebeverine, which produced only slight improvements and then a tricyclic antidepressant (nortriptyline), resulting in a brief reduction in abdominal pain. But the gastroenterologist subsequently recommended our practice because he suspected that stress was a major contributor to Rod's symptoms.

Rod came to his first appointment accompanied by his wife of 3 years, Bethany. Their appearance as a couple was striking; both were tall and attractive. During the interview, Rod described the actual onset of symptoms in high school, but these were attributed by his mother to "upset stomach." In college, Rod majored in finance and information systems and played tennis for the school. Prior to highly competitive matches, his symptoms increased and he used antidiarrheal medicine to control his bowels. He met Bethany in his senior year of college and they married 3 years later. At the time of the interview, Rod worked as a financial analyst in the tax department for a Midwestern city government. He received good evaluations from his boss who praised Rod's attention to detail and dedication to his job. During busy work periods, Rod described his reactions as, "My gut is furious with me and I can't do anything about it." Occasionally, Rod was asked to make presentations to the city staff regarding budget projections based on tax revenue. As soon as Rod was informed that he had to speak to a group of people, he became symptomatic and worried about having to leave quickly during his talk. So, he skipped meals before the presentation. If someone asked a question about his calculations, Rod felt like he "had been punched in the gut," although he knew the answer and was actually very good at explaining difficult concepts in simple language. After a presentation, it took several days for the symptoms to ameliorate.

When Bethany was asked for comment, she stated that she was worried about Rod and the effect of the symptoms on Rod personally as well as the impact of IBS on their shared interests. When Bethany and Rod dated, they were very active; hiking and biking were some of their favorite hobbies. But lately, Rod was more preoccupied with the locations of the nearest rest rooms than enjoying the scenery. Bethany also thought that Rod's job was too stressful. In the current (at the time) financial environment, Rod had to present people with bad news about investments and increasing taxes. Bethany said that Rod would be better off starting his own business where he could be his own boss. There was a trust fund started by Bethany's grandmother that could be used for that purpose.

Pathways Level One: Soothe and Mindful Breathing. The pathways concepts were explained to Rod and Bethany, and Rod verbalized understanding and willingness to begin. The Level One interventions were Soothe and Mindful Breathing (Keefer & Blanchard, 2001). Rod was to concentrate on calming and soothing his "angry" gut. He was instructed to sit in his rocking chair, breathing into his abdominal area as follows, "I take a deep breath in and direct that breath to my abdomen, calming whatever is angry and upset." "I give my GI system a chance to respond and I give it my permission to relax." After 2 weeks, Rod returned to the clinic and reported that although this exercise felt good, it was not effective. He was agitated and angry during this appointment, insulting his own body, calling himself a baby, a weakling, and disgusting. "I can't control my own bowels and I wish that I could rip them out." "You've seen Bethany—she is gorgeous and smart." "She could have any man in the city and she won't stay with a man who may soil himself at any time." (This had never happened.) "I can't take any pressure, like talking in front of a few people on information that I know or my gut blows up." During this appointment, most of the time was spent on providing empathetic and active listening. Then, educational materials were provided demonstrating that indeed the gut does have a mind of its own (the enteric nervous system), but the brain can exert control through the autonomic nervous system (Watson & Smith, 2003). Looking at the diagrams of the digestive process and the neural control centers was helpful to Rod. He agreed to continue in treatment and to try the Level Two interventions.

Level Two: Progressive Relaxation. Rod was taught progressive muscle relaxation and recommended to add this relaxation technique to his breathing practice. Rod was instructed to be mindful about each muscle group in both the tense and the relaxed conditions and during the exercise to emphasize a sense of control over physiological responses. Two weeks later, Rod reported slight improvement, but he remained pessimistic about his progress and himself. A recent experience where he was on the interview team for a job candidate resulted in his feeling "choked up," like he had a lump in his throat, and this had unnerved him. "My other end is screwed up too." Rod also revealed that a stressful conversation had taken place with Bethany regarding finances and the idea of Rod starting his own business. The therapy team began to realize that Bethany's financial status was hard for Rod to understand. Their wedding had cost $75,000, more than both of Rod's parents made in a year. Bethany spoke about money as if it was nothing, saying "we have it" or "that's what money is for—to be used for advancement in careers, or to support worthy organizations." But Rod could not accept this because he had watched his parents' careful money management during his youth and continued the same budgetary practices during college. It was decided that a joint session with Rod and Bethany would be held in order to explore the financial issues.

In subsequent weeks, Rod continued the practice of progressive relaxation, and finally he reported that progress was slow, but steady; he felt that the tensing and subsequent release of tension helped him feel more in control. He realized that the mindful focus on individual muscle groups released his mind from constantly thinking about sensations in his abdomen. He also told us that Bethany had readily agreed to the joint session.

Level Three: Hypnosis, Cognitive Behavior Therapy, and Joint Psychotherapy: The joint session with Rod and Bethany was long and intense. Rod expressed his fear of leaving his job to start a business. He would have to hire a staff and interact with potential customers on a daily basis. In addition, he conceived of the trust fund as "not his money," despite Bethany's assurances. Rod also verbalized his "terror" of worsening symptoms resulting from work stress. He fantasized that he would need surgery and then would have "a bag for a gut" the rest of his life. Bethany was stunned by these statements. She saw her husband as a man of exceptional financial acumen, but thought that the potential for advancement in the municipal office of taxation was limited. Rod explained that he was still growing at this job and his boss had discussed future promotions with him. Bethany cried when Rod talked about his gut as the enemy, saying that she loved his body and then said, "your gut is my gut too." This statement brought Rod to tears as he finally believed that Bethany did not find him disgusting.

Bethany reminded Rod of a situation that happened while they were in college, when they barely knew each other. Bethany had been given a date rape drug. Rod had walked into the fraternity house, saw what was happening, and had gotten Bethany to the emergency room and stayed with her while they pumped her stomach. She had been disgusted with herself, but Rod had not blinked and had never blamed her. She, Bethany, was not leaving Rod over "a mad gut." She wanted to do anything she could to help him. By the end of this session, Rod admitted that psychological factors had a significant impact on his symptoms, so he was going to stay in the Pathways Interventions Program. Bethany agreed that she would not mention "new business" to Rod until we could meet again.

CBT was used to counter Rod's negative self-statements about his gut, his future health, and the imagined reactions of people to him. The treating therapist became aware of how often Rod would reference his gut in his communication. "I had a gut feeling" was a statement about projected tax revenue. "This gal is going to be a pain in the gut" referred to a new coworker that Rod had to train. And the therapist's personal favorite, "The head economist came over today and twisted all the tax people's guts into knots." Homework assignments consisted of Rod identifying and documenting these negative phrases and other automatic thoughts and countering these self-statements with more positive interpretations. He developed *Personal Coping Cards* to increase his confidence at work. Soon, Rod had ten coping cards for various situations at work that could create anxiety, but none of the new coping strategies mentioned his gut. The focus was on countering negative, particularly "gut-relevant" terminology with positive self-confidence-building statements.

The two additional joint sessions were used to help Rod and Bethany dialogue about the meaning of money, Rod's career goals (which did not include owning a financial services business), and Bethany's dreams for the future. She and Rod agreed to make financial decisions together, so that Rod could appreciate the levels of risk and benefits of their spending as well as their philanthropy. It was agreed that since Rod and Bethany wanted children, a stable job was necessary to maintain health insurance and other benefits. In contrast, Bethany was a talented artist who took lessons weekly and occasionally displayed her work. However, there was little income from her art, so the recommendation was made that the money from the trust fund be used to enhance Bethany's career, renting better space, and obtaining additional art lessons as needed.

The hypnosis protocol was implemented for Rod according to guidelines provided by Palsson et al., (2002). Palsson et al. provide a highly scripted program of hypnosis in seven 45-min sessions. Some of the CBT interventions described above were conducted in the same session as the hypnosis. Rod demonstrated an excellent response to the hypnotic procedure and willingly practiced at home with the CD provided. Each week, his symptom logs showed improvements in abdominal pain, bloating, and urgency or frequency of bowel movements.

At the end of 20 weeks of treatment, Rod reported significant improvements in all symptom categories. Abdominal pain no longer occurred daily; mild discomfort was experienced once or twice a week. Bloating and diarrhea were reduced by 80 %. Rod's most disturbing symptom, urgency, was rarely experienced. Rod considered his anxiety to be decreased significantly at home and at work. He anticipated work responsibilities and relied on the progressive relaxation exercise as part of his preparation for potentially anxiety-producing situations. The keywords "control" and "calm gut" cued Rod to relax his GI system, clearing his mind for intellectual work. He reported that the coping cards stayed in his desk drawer most of the time because he instinctively knew how to cope with most situations. When something new was presented to Rod at work, he did not react immediately, but gave himself a chance to think through the challenge and then formulate a coping plan.

Two years after the end of active treatment, the team received an invitation to a gallery opening featuring works of local artists, including Bethany, so one staff member attended. Bethany, who was obviously pregnant, graciously accepted the Best of Show Award. She attributed her success to her wonderful husband, who "not only encouraged her in her art but managed all the finances" so she could concentrate on creating her watercolors. In the end, Bethany had created a business model for herself similar to what she had tried to persuade Rod to adopt. Rod whispered to the therapist that he was doing "terrific" and had just received a promotion at his job. The increased responsibilities meant, "More tax issues, more complicated software, but no punches in the gut."

Case Summary

The case of Rod presented several unique challenges to the Pathways Model. First, the client was unresponsive to the Level One intervention, so the team moved quickly to Level Two. Frequent encouragement was necessary to keep Rod in the program. Second, Rod's language and modes of expression were permeated with negative references to the GI system. Rod had to learn to replace that language with other verbiage. Third, Rod and Bethany's patterns of interaction about finances and health were dysfunctional. Bethany truly believed that Rod was capable of great success in the financial world, but did not hear or understand Rod's fears of self-employment. Rod interpreted Bethany's concern for him as disappointment or disgust about his problem. Fourth, multiple higher level interventions were required to meet outcome goals. The most effective interventions were progressive relaxation, which allowed Rod to feel more in control of his symptoms; hypnosis, which directly impacted the GI system; and joint psychotherapy sessions with Rod and Bethany.

References

Blanchard, E. B., Lackner, J. M., Sanders, K., Krasner, S., Keefer, L., Payne, A., et al. (2007). A controlled evaluation of group cognitive therapy in the treatment of irritable bowel syndrome. *Behaviour Research and Therapy, 45*, 633–648.

Crane, C., & Martin, M. (2004). Social learning, affective state and passive coping in irritable bowel syndrome and inflammatory bowel disease. *General Hospital Psychiatry, 26*, 50–58.

Creed, F., Guthrie, E., Ratcliffe, J., Fernandes, L., Rigby, C., Tomenson, B., et al. (2005). Reported sexual abuse predicts impaired functioning but a good response to psychological treatments in patients with severe irritable bowel syndrome. *Psychosomatic Medicine, 67*(3), 490–499.

Fink, P., Rosendal, M., & Toft, T. (2002). Assessment and treatment of functional disorders in general practice: The extended reattribution and management model and advanced educational program for non-psychiatric doctors. *Psychosomatics, 43*(2), 93–131.

Gholamrezaei, A., Ardestani, S. K., & Emami, M. H. (2006). Where does hypnotherapy stand in the management of irritable bowel syndrome? A systematic review. *Journal of Alternative and Complementary Medicine, 12*(6), 517–527.

Gick, M. L., & Sirois, F. M. (2010). Insecure attachment moderates women's adjustment to inflammatory bowel disease severity. *Rehabilitation Psychology, 55*(2), 170–179.

Guyton, A. C., & Hall, J. E. (2000). *Textbook of medical physiology*. Philadelphia: W.B. Saunders Company.

Herschbach, P., Henrich, G., & von Rad, M. (1999). Psychological factors in functional gastrointestinal disorders: Characteristics of the disorder or of the illness behavior? *Psychosomatic Medicine, 61*, 148–153.

Humphreys, P. A., & Gevirtz, R. N. (2000). Treatment of recurrent abdominal pain: Components analysis of four treatment protocols. *Journal of Pediatric Gastroenterology and Nutrition, 31*(1), 47–51.

Keefer, L., & Blanchard, E. B. (2001). The effects of relaxation response meditation on the symptoms of irritable bowel syndrome: Results of a controlled treatment study. *Behaviour Research and Therapy, 39*, 801–811.

Keefer, L., & Blanchard, E. B. (2002). A one year follow-up of relaxation response meditation as a treatment for irritable bowel syndrome. *Behaviour Research and Therapy, 40*(5), 541–546.

Kovacs, Z., & Kovacs, F. (2007). Depressive and anxiety symptoms, dysfunctional attitudes and social aspects in irritable bowel syndrome and inflammatory bowel disease. *International Journal of Psychiatry in Medicine, 37*(3), 245–255.

Lackner, J. M., Jaccard, J., Krasner, S. S., Katz, L. A., Gudleski, G. D., & Holroyd, K. (2008). Self-administered cognitive behavior therapy for moderate to severe irritable bowel syndrome: Clinical efficacy, tolerability, feasibility. *Clinical Gastroenterology and Hepatology, 6*(8), 899–906.

Lackner, J. M., Quigley, B. M., & Blanchard, E. B. (2004). Depression and abdominal pain in IBS patients: The mediating role of catastrophizing. *Psychosomatic Medicine, 66*, 435–441.

Lacy, B. E. (2006). *Making sense of IBS*. Baltimore, MD: The Johns Hopkins University Press.
Mayer, E., & Wong, H. (2010). Abdominal, peritoneal, and retroperitoneal pain. In S. M. Fishman, J. C. Ballantyne, & J. P. Rathmell (Eds.), *Bonica's management of pain* (pp. 899–925). Philadelphia: Lippincott Williams & Wilkins.
Moss-Morris, R., McAlpine, L., Didsbury, L. P., & Spence, M. J. (2010). A randomized controlled trial of a cognitive behavioural therapy-based self-management intervention for irritable bowel syndrome in primary care. *Psychological Medicine, 40*, 85–94.
Mussell, M., Kroenke, K., Spitzer, R. L., Williams, J. B., Herzog, W., & Lowe, B. (2008). Gastrointestinal symptoms in primary care: Prevalence and association with depression and anxiety. *Journal of Psychosomatic Research, 64*(6), 605–612.
Palsson, O. S., & Collins, R. W. (2003). Functional bowel and anorectal disorders. In D. Moss, A. McGrady, T. Davies, & I. Wickramasera (Eds.), *Handbook of mind-body medicine in primary care* (pp. 299–311). Thousand Oaks, CA: Sage.
Palsson, O. S., Turner, M. J., Johnson, D. A., Burnett, C. B., & Whitehead, W. E. (2002). Hypnosis treatment for severe irritable bowel syndrome: Investigation of mechanism and effects on symptoms. *Digestive Diseases and Sciences, 47*(11), 2605–2614.
Palsson, O. S., Turner, M. J., & Whitehead, W. E. (2006). Hypnosis home treatment for irritable bowel syndrome: A pilot study. *International Journal of Clinical and Experimental Hypnosis, 54*(1), 85–99.
Roy-Byrne, P. P., Davidson, K. W., Kessler, R. C., Asmundson, G. J. G., & Goodwin, R. D. (2008). Anxiety disorders and comorbid medical illness. *Focus, 6*, 467–485.
Shinozaki, M., Kanazawa, M., Kano, M., Endo, Y., Nakaya, N., Hongo, M., et al. (2010). Effect of autogenic training on general improvement in patients with irritable bowel syndrome: A randomized controlled trial. *Applied Psychophysiology and Biofeedback, 35*(3), 189–198.
Sowder, E., Gevirtz, R., Shapiro, W., & Ebert, C. (2010). Restoration of vagal tone: A possible mechanism for functional abdominal pain. *Applied Psychophysiology and Biofeedback, 35*(3), 199–206.
Suarez, K., Mayer, C., Ehlert, U., & Nater, U. M. (2010). Psychological stress and self-reported functional gastrointestinal disorders. *The Journal of Nervous and Mental Disease, 198*(3), 226–229.
Talley, N. J. (2006). *Conquering irritable bowel syndrome: A guide to liberating those suffering with chronic stomach or bowel problems*. Philadelphia, PA: B.C. Decker.
Talley, N. J., Fett, S. L., & Zinsmeister, A. R. (1994). Gastrointestinal tract symptoms and self-reported abuse: A population based study. *Gastroenterology, 107*(4), 1040–1049.
Thompson, W. G., Longstreth, G. F., Drossman, D. A., Heaton, K. W., Irvine, E. J., & Muller-Lissner, S. A. (1999). Functional bowel disorders and functional abdominal pain. *Gut, 45*, 43–47.
Watson, B., & Smith, L. (2003). *Gut solutions*. Clearwater, FL: Renew Life Press and Information Services.
Widmaier, E. P., Raff, H., & Strang, K. T. (2001). *Vander, Sherman, & Luciano human physiology: The mechanisms of body function*. Boston: McGraw Hill.

Chapter 15
Sleep Disorders

Abstract Sleep is a natural, repetitive function of the brain that restores energy and partially maintains mental and physical health. Disruptions in sleep, particularly slow-wave sleep, are associated with mood disturbance, decreased function, and physical illness. The Pathways Model is useful in understanding sleep disorders, whether they be primary or secondary to depression or anxiety. Two examples are presented in this chapter to elucidate the three levels of interventions as applied to one case of primary and one case of secondary sleep disorder.

Keywords Sleep/wake cycle • Sleep disorders • Interventions • Sleep hygiene

Introduction: Normal Sleep

Humans sleep to conserve energy, to control body temperature, and to maintain physical and emotional health. The necessary length of a person's sleep is determined by their ability to function during the day without feeling drowsy. Alert people will not become sleepy because they are sitting still or bored. Some adults need up to 8–9 h of sleep in a 24-h period; others can function quite well on 5–6 h of sleep. Variation also exists in the timing of optimal functioning, whether early morning or evening (Aeschbach et al., 2003).

All mammals that have been studied demonstrate regular sleep patterns and suffer consequences of sleep deprivation. In humans, the sleep rhythm develops during the first 2 years of life and follows a 24-h cycle. During a normal night, about 75% of the time consists of slow-wave, restorative sleep, characterized by high-amplitude, low-frequency brain waves, and 25% is rapid eye movement (REM) or dream sleep (Sadock & Sadock, 2008).

Sleep length is influenced by many factors, including heredity, age, need for vigilance, number of hours of awake time, stimulation, social learning, conditioning, and daily routine. If the person needs to be vigilant or there is too much noise or light, falling asleep will be more difficult, whereas long hours of wakefulness speed sleep onset. The sleep–wake cycle is primarily controlled by the circadian clock, which is influenced by a complicated network of molecular clocks in the brain and regulatory genes, which in turn control oscillations of neurons and other peripheral clocks in the body (Hamet & Tremblay, 2006).

In order to effectively assist patients with sleep disorders, it is important to understand the interrelationships among the sleep–wake cycle and other biological rhythms. These include body temperature, appetite, and hormone levels, particularly of cortisol, epinephrine, and growth hormone. The lowest body temperature usually occurs in the early morning hours, and the highest occurs during early evening. Appetite and satiety are controlled by neuronal centers in the hypothalamus, which are linked to the internal time-keeping clocks (Froy, 2010). Leptin, a neurochemical that decreases appetite, is suppressed during short sleep and other hormones that stimulate the desire to eat are increased. Finally, the hypothalamic–pituitary–adrenal (HPA) axis is involved in both the stress response and the sleep–wake cycle, and thus, these two physiological cycles interact within a multidimensional framework (Buckley & Schatzberg, 2005).

Sleep Deprivation and Its Effects

Sleep deprivation can be classified in two ways: the number of hours of missed sleep or the duration of deprivation, i.e., the number of days. Total sleep deprivation, a rare phenomenon, is defined as complete lack of sleep; partial deprivation refers to less sleep than usual. A few days of partial or total sleep deprivation is labeled as acute, whereas chronic deprivation refers to partial deprivation for years. After prolonged wakefulness, the drive to sleep is so strong that sometimes despite the person's best efforts to stay awake, a microsleep (20- to 30-s doze) occurs. Microsleeps can have severe consequences if they happen during potentially dangerous activities, such as driving or using machinery (Woodward, 2003).

Insufficient sleep or multiple awakenings during the night are associated with mood disruption, particularly irritability, anxiety, and depression (Hamilton, Catley, & Karlson, 2007; Zohar, Tzischinsky, Epstein, & Lavie, 2005). Evidence is building that misalignment between the sleep–wake cycle and the circadian rhythm oscillators in the brain contributes to clinical-level psychopathology (Kripke, Nievergelt, Joo, Shekhtman, & Kelsoe, 2009). For example, patients with depression complain of early morning awakenings (terminal insomnia) while anxious patients often have difficulties with first sleep onset (onset insomnia). Although specific evidence that supports clock genes' role in anxiety and depression is lacking, a stronger case can be made for mistiming of the brain clocks in bipolar disorder and dementia (Hamet & Tremblay, 2006; Lamont, Legault-Coutu, Cermakian, & Boivin, 2007).

The relationship among poor sleep quality, fewer hours of sleep, and worsening pain is well established (Hamilton et al., 2007). In healthy normal sleepers, as little as 4 h of sleep deficit produced hyperalgesia the following day (Roehrs, Hyde, Blaisdell, Greenwald, & Roth, 2006). Another example of the importance of restorative sleep is in fibromyalgia, a pain condition discussed in detail in an earlier chapter. Patients reporting continuous, high-quality sleep suffer less intense pain and are also able to cope more effectively with negative life events (Hamilton et al., 2008).

The HPA axis has multiple effects on sleep quality and quantity (Buckley & Schatzberg, 2005). A rise in cortisol must occur to prepare the person for morning wakefulness, stimulate the appetite, and increase blood pressure and heart rate in anticipation of physical activity. In contrast, hyperactivity in HPA activity has multiple negative effects. Slow-wave sleep decreases, cortisol levels increase at inappropriate times, and sleep is disrupted. The vicious cycle of broken sleep, increased arousal, and insomnia continues, since sleep deprivation is associated with further activation of the hypothalamic–pituitary axis.

The internal body clock is located in the part of the brain called the suprachiasmatic nucleus (SCN). Although light sets the main clock in the SCN, there are also oscillators—peripheral clocks in other cells and tissues in the body. In addition to light, shift work, lack of sleep, and anxiety affect the internal clocks. Disruption in sleep can block the body's normal circadian rhythm, alter insulin production, and change the levels of other hormones that are important to weight control. Sleep-deprived people produce more of the hormone that promotes hunger (ghrelin) and less of the hormone that suppresses appetite (leptin). To emphasize this point, medically healthy individuals who had their sleep disrupted for several consecutive nights had elevated blood glucose and elevated insulin after the sixth consecutive night of disruption. After a big meal, the increase in glucose levels in the blood turns off the neurons that produce orexin, making people feel sleepy. Daytime fatigue is partially explained by the change in the normal rhythm of fatigue-producing cytokines, such as IL-6. These substances can be conceptualized as primordial signals to the human brain to conserve energy after eating (Froy, 2010).

The Case of Brandon

Brandon was a 23-year-old in his second year of law school who presented with complaints of onset insomnia and terminal insomnia for the past month. It was taking him more than an hour to fall asleep several times a week. His daytime fatigue was described as "exhaustion." Brandon was worried about completing his class requirements and thought that maybe he had chosen the wrong profession. He was attending class every day, but it was a struggle to stay awake. His daily consumption of caffeine was 4–6 cups of coffee per day, a pattern that began when he started school 8 months ago. Brandon had no time for exercise, nor was he eating a balanced diet. He was on no medication and had no medical diagnoses. Alcohol consumption, mainly on the weekends, was described as 3 or 4 beers with law school friends.

The assessment process began with Brandon keeping a 2-weeks sleep and activity log prior to his first appointment. A careful history revealed that as a child, Brandon had sleep problems; he was a hard child to get to sleep and then he woke up once or twice a night until he was almost 3. During his teenage years, Brandon stayed up until midnight on school nights and had great difficulty getting up in the morning.

The most likely diagnosis for Brandon was primary insomnia. Although he was anxious and worried, he did not meet the criteria for generalized anxiety disorder. At times, he experienced sadness and became hopeless about his progress in law school, but he did not fulfill diagnostic criteria for any mood disorder.

Insomnia is one of the dyssomnias and is the most common sleep disruption among adults. Patients commonly complain about problems initiating and maintaining sleep or feeling fatigued during the day. Primary insomnia occurs without medical or psychiatric cause and cannot be due to substance use or medication (Morin et al., 2006).

Management of insomnia relies on multiple options, which include the benzodiazepines or the non-benzodiazepine classes of medicine, melatonin, light therapy, or one of several behavioral interventions (Buscemi et al., 2004; Morgenthaler et al., 2006).

According to the Pathways Model, Brandon's sleep problems were partially genetic in origin, later influenced by social learning and modified by current stressors. Intervention for Brandon began with education about the natural need for sleep and the relationship among disrupted sleep patterns and other circadian rhythms, such as appetite/satiety, temperature regulation, and mood. Brandon's onset insomnia and early awakenings short-circuited his restorative, slow-wave sleep and led to fatigue during the day. This information helped Brandon to understand why he was sleepy when he should be alert and sometimes very hungry at 2 am.

Level One interventions. The Level One interventions of self-soothing and mindful breathing were recommended for Brandon. He was taught mindful breathing and encouraged to use this technique every day and at bedtime. The recommended soothing technique was listening to repetitive sounds, such as music with a repeating pattern or ocean waves. We also recommended some of the sleep hygiene recommendations for Brandon (see the Box 15.1 for typical sleep hygiene recommendations) (CCI, 2013; Sadock & Sadock, 2008). These included discontinuing stimulants after 6 pm and regulating food intake so that the largest meal was not within 2 h of bedtime. Abstinence from alcohol was important; alcohol does put people to sleep, but the sleep is disrupted and fragmented, containing fewer minutes of slow-wave sleep (Morin et al., 2006). Brandon was advised to take a hot bath or shower near bedtime. When the brain cools after the bath, it will facilitate sleep, since there is a natural tendency to fall asleep when the brain is losing heat.

In summary, Brandon's habits of drinking a cup of coffee in the evening, eating his biggest meal around 7–8 pm, and studying in bed were discontinued. He could take a nap during the day if he felt sleepy but not for longer than 45 min and not within 4 h of planned bedtime. Brandon was willing to make these adjustments in his schedule. He changed his larger meal to noon and ate two smaller meals, one at 6 pm and one at 10 pm, the latter a complex carbohydrate meal. The typical sleep hygiene recommendation of going to bed and waking up at the same time every day was not realistic for Brandon. His classes were at different times from Monday to Friday and his part-time job required him to work weekends from 3 to 11 pm.

> **Box 15.1** Sleep Hygiene: Good Habits for Better Sleep
>
> 1. Have a routine. Go to bed and wake up at about the same times, even on weekends.
> 2. Keep room temperature comfortable; limit light and noise.
> 3. Avoid heavy exercise within 3 h of bedtime.
> 4. Avoid large meals within 3 h of bedtime. A light snack containing carbohydrate before going to bed is appropriate.
> 5. Limit caffeine consumption to the morning hours.
> 6. Do not watch TV, read stimulating books, or listen to loud music at bedtime.
> 7. If you do not fall asleep within 30 min, get up and do something until you feel sleepy. Do not linger in bed awake during the night or in the morning.
>
> Adapted from http://www.cci.health.wa.gov.au

Level Two interventions. Brandon began the breathing and soothing exercises and returned in 2 weeks. He reported some improvement in feelings of anxiety during the day, but sleep was still compromised. The Level Two intervention was progressive relaxation, based on the premise that Brandon's difficulties in going to sleep and maintaining sleep were due to excessive muscle tension. This made intellectual sense to Brandon, because he described tense muscles in his neck and shoulders, particularly after long hours at the computer. He was also instructed to clear the bedroom of study materials in order to recondition the bed and bedroom with the onset of sleep, instead of with stimulating activities (this strategy is called sleep control therapy) (Giardino, McGrady, & Andrasik, 2007). In addition, he was encouraged to limit activities in the bedroom to sleep and sex, in keeping with the guidelines of sleep hygiene. Watching television, engaging in conversation (or worse, arguing), and extensive reading can all elicit arousal rather than physiological relaxation (Stepanski & Wyatt, 2003).

The decision to proceed through Level One and Two platforms before beginning his Level Three intervention of cognitive behavioral therapy (CBT) was carefully considered and negotiated with Brandon. Although his self-doubts about becoming a lawyer were major issues, insomnia and anxiety were what brought Brandon to therapy. So the presenting problems had to be addressed first. CBT (Jacobs, Pace-Schott, Stickgold, & Otto, 2004; Jansson & Linton, 2005) targeted the negative thoughts that Brandon held about his inability to fall asleep as well as deeper issues about his choice of profession. Dysfunctional cognitions and distress about sleep needed to be identified, countered, and finally replaced with more positive thoughts about the ability to get to sleep. Brandon's statement: "when I sleep badly, I cannot do any studying" was challenged by the therapist. This cognitive strategy, called "hypothesis testing," was successful since on that particular day, Brandon had already completed one class assignment. He felt sleepy during the day, but he could accomplish *some* studying (Edinger et al., 2001).

After 6 weeks, Brandon reported a significant improvement in sleep. Because he was less fatigued, his studies did not seem as overwhelming and he became less anxious. He no longer noticed any microsleeps. Now, CBT was applied to his concerns about his law career. When Brandon was in his first year of law school, he was fascinated by the courses on Criminal Justice. In his second year, the professor teaching Commercial Paper was not engaging and the subject matter was of less interest. The volume of required reading on this topic and the competition with other students increased his self-doubts and worry. Brandon began to wonder if he had made a mistake in choosing law as a profession. Negative thoughts became more frequent and soon he questioned his ability to successfully complete the courses. Brandon's older brother had begun law school and flunked out, to the great disappointment of their parents. Throughout therapy, he worked to counter the negative, catastrophic thoughts of flunking out "just like big brother" and labeling a wrong career choice as a "failure" with more reality-based thinking patterns.

Case Summary

Although Brandon briefly considered dropping out of school, he realized that extreme fatigue and anxiety had negatively colored his views of law, law school, and his own performance. At the completion of therapy, Brandon was close to completing law school and had decided to specialize in criminal trial work. He continued to use the relaxation techniques and the rational thinking that he learned in CBT. He monitored his sleep quantity and quality. During stressful periods of examinations, when his hours of sleep shortened, he utilized the self-soothing and healthy sleeping techniques again with good results.

The Case of Cerise

Cerise was a 40-year-old divorced mother of a 10-year-old girl who presented with almost identical symptoms to those of Brandon. Cerise had trouble falling asleep for more than 1 month and awakened between 4:00 and 5:00 AM no matter how tired she was at bedtime. Cerise had been divorced for 2 years and had joint custody of her daughter with her ex-husband. Their daughter, Rachel, spent alternate weeks with Cerise and her father. He had already remarried and was seemingly very happy in his new relationship with his wife and his wife's two daughters by her first marriage. During the weeks that Rachel was with her father, Cerise felt sad and lonely. But when mother and daughter were together, Rachel frequently complained that the house was too quiet and that there was not enough going on. Rachel said that at her dad's house there was always something happening and her stepsiblings were fun.

When discussing her work situation, Cerise became very tearful and had difficulty describing what had happened during the past months. There was downsizing at her insurance company. Cerise retained her job for which she was very grateful, but the workload increased. Her two close friends were let go, leaving her as the only worker in a three-person office, surrounded by empty desks and idle computers. She questioned her ability to maintain productivity, but the major problem was her sense of isolation and the lack of communication with other workers.

Close examination of the contents of the interview and description of mood during the past 2 months indicated a major depressive disorder (MDD). The sleep disruption in this case was not a primary sleep disorder, like Brandon's, but a component of MDD, which is covered in detail in another chapter. Individuals with psychiatric disorders commonly have sleep disruptions of characteristic types. The person with MDD has terminal insomnia, waking up too early in the morning and not being able to get back to sleep, reduced slow-wave restorative sleep, and increased length of the dream phases of sleep (Hamilton et al., 2008). Cerise began treatment for MDD, but her insomnia also required intervention.

Cerise's pathway to illness resided in a family history of depression, a difficult break up of her marriage, and an inflexible coping style. When confronted with stressful situations, Cerise became quiet and tended to withdraw. She lacked assertiveness and clear communication skills. She became more and more isolated in all aspects of her life: home, social, and job life. Her two friends who were downsized were so angry with the company that they were not comfortable in social situations with Cerise. In addition, Cerise was prohibited to discuss the business of the office with her two friends and admittedly became tired of listening to them complain about how they were treated.

According to Hawkley, Preacher, and Cacioppo (2010), loneliness impairs daytime functioning no matter how many hours a person actually sleeps. Social isolation leads to poor sleep quality whereas social engagement during the day facilitates better slow-wave, deep sleep (Cacioppo et al., 2002). It has been suggested that loneliness and isolation bring on feelings of threat, making it difficult to go to sleep and increasing nighttime awakenings. In contrast, sleeping in a safe environment promotes restorative sleep (Cacioppo & Hawkley, 2009). In the study by Hawkley et al. (2010), persons who scored higher on a paper and pencil test of loneliness reacted to negative social words and evidenced more interference in a cognitive task than did those persons who are well integrated socially. Further, loneliness and negative attitudes and feelings impair the ability to maintain attention and concentration needed at the workplace. This research fits Cerise very closely. Since the company downsized and she was left in an office for three by herself, she had become sad and tearful and had problems concentrating, resulting in lowered motivation for her job.

Level One interventions. The Level One interventions for Cerise were communication and movement. It was recommended that Cerise step out of her office and engage in conversation with other people at her workplace. Once she did this, she realized that there were other individuals who felt as isolated as she did because of the downsizing. Cerise was also advised that during the weeks that Rachel was with her, she should find at least one activity that she and her daughter could share. The second Level One recommendation—*move*—was a prelude to recommending an exercise regimen. Since exercise can improve cognitive functions, such as memory and concentration, moving was the first step towards a regular exercise program (Ferris, Williams, & Shen, 2007; Ruscheweyh et al., 2009). Cerise and Rachel began to walk to the park that was a half mile from home where Rachel met another girl from her school.

Moving began to mobilize energy in Cerise's body and slightly improved mood. A more formal exercise program was begun later, with physician approval.

Level Two interventions. The Level Two recommendations for Cerise were progressive relaxation and exercise. This type of relaxation was chosen because it is active relaxation and serves to direct attention to the experiences of tension and relaxation (McGuigan & Lehrer, 2007). Cerise was advised to practice relaxation every day for 15 min with the CD that was provided. Within 2 weeks, Cerise noticed some improvement in sleep quality, but the early morning awakenings continued and her mood remained depressed.

Cerise told Rachel that every Wednesday that they were together, they would go to the local YMCA, where Rachel could take swimming lessons, while Cerise swam laps. Initially, low motivation made it very difficult to follow through with this part of the plan and some evenings Cerise had to "drag" herself out of the house. However, within 5 weeks of swimming 3–4 times per week, a striking and unexpected improvement in work performance, particularly in those tasks required focus and attention, was noticed during the days after swimming. Cerise reported this observation and the few pounds of exercise-associated weight loss with pride.

Level Three interventions. The Level Three interventions for Cerise were medication, CBT, and heart rate variability (HRV) feedback. The physician explained that 6–12 months of antidepressant medicine (Zoloft) could accelerate her improvement (Sadock & Sadock, 2008). CBT explored Cerise's many negative cognitions about her social interactions, work performance, mothering skills, and chances of finding a suitable partner. HRV biofeedback trains the individual to use slow diaphragmatic breathing to create larger regular oscillations in heart rate and increases overall HRV. The rationale for prescribing this form of biofeedback for Cerise, with her sleep disorder, is that HRV is more pronounced during slow-wave sleep than during REM sleep and is elevated during all sleep phases compared to wakefulness (Ebben, Kurbatov, & Pollak, 2009). A series of six sessions of HRV biofeedback helped Cerise to establish a pattern of slow breathing that she utilized each evening at bedtime.

Ten months after Cerise first came to therapy, mood and sleep were significantly improved. Early morning awakenings and daytime fatigue were rare. The exercise program was maintained whether Rachel was with her mom or not. Cerise met a woman who also swam at the YMCA and they formed a friendship, motivating each other to continue. They also talked about adding biking for outdoor exercise in the spring. Negative cognitions significantly decreased and Cerise became more skilled at identifying troublesome maladaptive thinking and countering those thoughts on her own. The physician planned to continue Zoloft for another 3 months and reevaluate at that time, with strong consideration to tapering the medicine.

Case Summary

Sleep disorders can be categorized as primary, when the sleep problem is neither part of an emotional or physical illness nor associated with the use of stimulants. Secondary sleep disorders are a component of another illness, such as depression, anxiety, or bipolar disorder. In this chapter, Brandon provided an example of a primary sleep disorder, whereas Cerise's sleep problems resulted from her MDD. Both patients' sleep disorders were addressed effectively using the Pathways Model. Brandon was treated with soothing, mindful breathing, sleep hygiene, progressive relaxation, and CBT. Cerise, whose sleep problems were secondary to MDD, began with movement and communication. These Level One interventions were followed by the Level Two interventions of progressive relaxation and physical exercise and the Level Three interventions of CBT, biofeedback, and antidepressant medication.

References

Aeschbach, D., Sher, L., Postolache, T. T., Matthews, J. R., Jackson, M. A., & Wehr, T. A. (2003). A longer biological night in long sleepers than in short sleepers. *The Journal of Clinical Endocrinology and Metabolism, 88*(1), 2–30.

Buckley, T. M., & Schatzberg, A. F. (2005). Review: On the interactions of the hypothalamic-pituitary-adrenal (HPS) axis and sleep: Normal HPA axis activity and circadian rhythm, exemplary sleep disorders. *The Journal of Clinical Endocrinology and Metabolism, 90*(5), 3106–3114.

Buscemi, N., Vandermeer, B., Pandya, R., Hooton, N., Tjosvold, L., Hartling, L., et al. (2004). Melatonin for treatment of sleep disorders. Summary, evidence report/technology assessment: Number 108. AHRQ publication number 05-E002-1. Rockville, MD: Agency for Healthcare Research and Quality. Retrieved May 26, 2009, from http://www.ahrq.gov/clinic/epcsums/melatsum.htm.

Cacioppo, J. T., & Hawkley, L. C. (2009). Perceived social isolation and cognition. *Trends in Cognitive Science, 13*, 447–454.

Cacioppo, J. T., Hawkley, L. C., Crawford, L. E., Ernst, J. M., Burleson, M. H., Kowalewski, R. B., Malarkey, W. B., Van Cauter, E., & Berntson, G. G. (2002). Loneliness and health: Potential mechanisms. *Psychosomatic Medicine, 64*, 407–417.

Centre for Clinical Interventions. (2013, accessed January 4). Sleep hygiene [On-line]. Available: http://www.cci.health.wa.gov.au/docs/Info-sleep%20hygiene.pdf.

Ebben, M. R., Kurbatov, V., & Pollak, C. P. (2009). Moderating laboratory adaptation with the use of heart rate variability biofeedback device (StressEraser). *Applied Psychophysiology and Biofeedback, 34*(4), 245–249.

Edinger, J. D., Wohlgemuth, W. K., Radtke, R. A., Marsh, G. R., & Quillian, R. E. (2001). Cognitive behavioral therapy for treatment of chronic primary insomnia. *Journal of the American Medical Association, 285*(14), 1856–1864.

Ferris, L. T., Williams, J. S., & Shen, C. L. (2007). The effect of acute exercise on serum brain-derived neurotrophic factor levels and cognitive function. *Medical and Science in Sport and Exercise, 39*(4), 728–734.

Froy, O. (2010). Metabolism and circadian rhythms–implications for obesity. *Endocrine Review, 31*(1), 1–24.

Giardino, N. D., McGrady, A., & Andrasik, F. (2007). Stress management and relaxation therapies for somatic disorders. In P. M. Lehrer, R. L. Woolfolk, & W. E. Sime (Eds.), *Principles and practice of stress management* (3rd ed., pp. 682–702). New York, NY: Guilford Press.

Hamet, P., & Tremblay, J. (2006). Genetics of the sleep-wake cycle and its disorders. *Metabolism, 10*(2), S7–S12.

Hamilton, N. A., Affleck, G., Tennen, H., Karlson, C., Luxton, D., Preacher, K. J., & Templin, J. L. (2008). Fibromyalgia: The role of sleep in affect and in negative event reactivity and recovery. *Health Psychology, 27*(4), 490–494.

Hamilton, N. A., Catley, D., & Karlson, C. (2007). Sleep and the affective response to stress and pain. *Health Psychology, 26*, 288–295.

Hawkley, L. C., Preacher, K. J., & Cacioppo, J. T. (2010). Loneliness impairs daytime functioning but not sleep duration. *Health Psychology, 29*(2), 124–129.

Jacobs, G. D., Pace-Schott, E. F., Stickgold, R., & Otto, M. W. (2004). Cognitive behavior therapy and pharmacotherapy for insomnia: A randomized controlled trial and direct comparison. *Archives of Internal Medicine, 14*(17), 1888–1896.

Jansson, M., & Linton, S. J. (2005). Cognitive-behavioral group therapy as an early intervention for insomnia: A randomized controlled trial. *Journal of Occupational Rehabilitation, 52*(2), 177–190.

Kripke, D. F., Nievergelt, C. M., Joo, E., Shekhtman, T., & Kelsoe, J. R. (2009). Circadian polymorphisms associated with affective disorders. *Journal of Circadian Rhythms, 7*, 2.

Lamont, E. W., Legault-Coutu, D., Cermakian, N., & Boivin, D. B. (2007). The role of circadian clock genes in mental disorders. *Dialogue Clinical Neuroscience, 9*(3), 333–342.

McGuigan, F. J., & Lehrer, P. M. (2007). Progressive relaxation: Origins, principles, and clinical applications. In P. M. Lehrer, R. L. Woolfolk, & W. E. Sime (Eds.), *Principles and practice of stress management* (pp. 57–87). New York: Guilford Press.

Morgenthaler, T., Kramer, M., Alessi, C., Friedman, L., Boehlecke, B., Brown, T., & Swick, T. (2006). Practice Parameters for the psychological and behavioral treatment of insomnia: An update. An American Academy of Sleep Medicine report. *Sleep, 29*(11), 1415–1419.

Morin, C. M., Rootzin, R. R., Buysse, D. J., Edinger, J. D., Espie, C. A., & Lichstein, K. L. (2006). Psychological and behavioral treatment of insomnia: update of the recent evidence (1998-2004). *Sleep, 29*(11), 1398–1414.

Roehrs, T., Hyde, M., Blaisdell, B., Greenwald, M., & Roth, T. (2006). Sleep loss and REM sleep loss are hyperalgesic. *Sleep, 29*(2), 145–151.

Ruscheweyh, R., Willemer C., Krüger, K., Duning, T., Warnecke, T., Sommer, J., et al. (2009). Physical activity and memory functions: An interventional study. *Neurobiology of Aging*.

Sadock, B. J., & Sadock, V. A. (2008). Normal sleep and sleep disorders. In B. J. Sadock & V. A. Sadock (Eds.), *Concise textbook of clinical psychiatry* (pp. 346–359). Philadelphia: Lippincott Williams & Wilkins.

Stepanski, E. J., & Wyatt, J. K. (2003). Use of sleep hygiene in the treatment of insomnia. *Sleep Medicine, 7*(3), 215–225.

Woodward, S. (2003). Sleep and sleep disorders. In D. Moss, A. McGrady, T. C. Davies, & I. Wickramasekera (Eds.), *Handbook of mind-body medicine for primary care* (pp. 393–406). Thousand Oaks, CA: Sage.

Zohar, D., Tzischinsky, O., Epstein, R., & Lavie, P. (2005). The effects of sleep loss on medical residents' emotional reactions to work events: A cognitive-energy model. *Sleep, 28*, 47–54.

Part III
Personalizing the Path to Health and Wellness

Chapter 16
Simple Pathways to Health and Wellness

Abstract Simple Pathways are user-friendly intervention strategies that can be delivered with relatively little training by the professional, and without the use of expensive instrumentation. In many cases the provider can acquire the techniques from written materials or brief instruction, and can teach clients to use the strategies for self-care. Other self-management techniques can be learned and utilized by lay persons on their own for enhancement of physical and psychological well-being. This chapter introduces the following interventions: Autogenic Training, thermal biofeedback, emotional journaling, heart rate variability biofeedback, audio-visual entrainment, mindfulness, and expressive dance. Psychoeducation is described as a component of Simple Pathways, aiding clients' understanding of the rationale and procedure for the interventions. Each of these techniques is research based and has been shown to have significant therapeutic benefits for medical and emotional disorders. The self-regulation strategies that are discussed can be utilized to enhance self-efficacy and to reinforce the individual's active role in maintaining wellness.

Keywords Low cost interventions • Autogenic training • Journaling • Biofeedback • Audio-visual entrainment • Mindfulness • Expressive movement

Introduction

The Pathways Model emphasizes the use of a wide range of interventions, from simple rocking and self-soothing to hypnosis and psychotherapy. The interventions emphasized in this book were chosen because they engage the person actively in self-care, self-regulation, and self-management. When human beings develop a plan and take action in pursuit of wellness, they experience a sense of empowerment toward their health and life decisions, whereas those who remain passive and wait for professionals to design and carry out a medical treatment often experience fear and feelings of loss of control.

The Pathways Model is an integrative health care model. It is not critical of the achievements of mainstream medical care but proposes that health care will produce healthier people and healthier communities, if lifestyle changes, wellness skills, relaxation techniques, and other Pathways Interventions are integrated into care from the beginning. For example, patients with prehypertension or with a family history of hypertension should be engaged immediately in lifestyle adjustments and wellness-oriented care before their blood pressure readings approach criteria for hypertension.

The present section is a supplement to the Pathways Interventions chapter and will emphasize techniques that a person can learn and utilize himself or herself, and interventions that almost any health professional can learn and practice with minimal cost and training. Access to health care remains a crisis both in the USA and worldwide, emphasizing the importance of lower-tech inexpensive procedures that have well-documented effectiveness. Not every community has well-trained practitioners of neurofeedback, heart rate variability biofeedback, and acceptance and commitment therapy. But any physician, nurse, pastor, psychologist, or counselor— whether in Haiti, Honduras, or Ohio—can master and teach these Simple Pathways techniques. Furthermore, with the increasing numbers of published "workbooks" for self-management of depression, anxiety, and other negative psychological states, the last section considers several examples of strategies that can be acquired and utilized by individuals without a health care provider.

Simple Pathways I: Autogenic Training

Introduction. Autogenic Training is an effective technique for personal relaxation and emotional restoration. The Autogenic Training technique is simple: A therapist speaks a series of descriptive phrases, while the client cultivates a state of openness, allowing body and mind to experience the sensations that are elicited (usually heavy and warm). The phrases can also be recorded for the client to use outside of clinic sessions. The client eventually learns the phrases and guides himself or herself in the Autogenic Training process, cultivating a passive attitude, that facilitates the effects of the repeated phrases; physiological changes indicating relaxation ensue.

Autogenic Training has been called a form of self-hypnosis (Schultz & Luthe, 1969), a type of relaxation (Stetter & Kupper, 2002) and a form of psychosomatic self-regulation (Norris, Fahrion, & Oikawa, 2007). When Autogenic Training is used to the full extent described by its founders, it is also an entire form of psychotherapy, facilitating emotional discharges in a carefully orchestrated fashion.

Historical Background. Johann Schultz (1884–1970), a German neurologist, studied hypnosis and paid close attention to his patient's experiences during hypnosis. He was determined to develop a specific technique to induce the profound state of mental and physical relaxation that patients experience in hypnosis, through the repetition of phrases designed to induce each dimension in the hypnotic experience. He drew on the research of another German physician and brain researcher Oskar Vogt. Vogt reported that his patients could voluntarily produce sensations of heaviness and warmth, and enter a self-hypnotic state. By 1926, Schultz delivered his first lecture on Autogenic Training, and in 1932, he published his first book on the subject, with the title (translated) "The Autogenic Training-Concentrative Self-Relaxation" (Schultz, 1932).

Autogenic Training remained unknown in North America, however, until another German physician, Wolfgang Luthe, published an article on Autogenic Training in English (Luthe, 1963). A collaborative book with Johann Schultz appeared in 1969, which grew into a six-volume series on Autogenic Training and its many applications. Linden (2007) published an excellent summary of the development and applications of Autogenic Training; an earlier paper presented a detailed book-length introduction to the use of Autogenic Training (Linden, 1990). Stetter and Kupper (2002) conducted a meta-analysis of 73 controlled outcome studies from 1952 to 1999 applying Autogenic Training to a variety of emotional and medical disorders. They found Autogenic Training to be as effective as other relaxation therapies for many disorders, and even more effective in combination with other therapies.

Instructions for Autogenic Training. Autogenic Training can be conducted individually or in groups. The physical environment must be comfortable and peaceful, with a warm temperature (68–75° F), a comfortable couch or mat, and quiet surroundings. The therapy and its effectiveness rest on two parallel processes. Clients are encouraged to close their eyes, and to cultivate a passive, receptive openness to the phrases, a readiness to respond mindfully, without trying to make something happen. Conversation is discouraged because it detracts from the focus and receptiveness to autogenic effects. The phrases themselves should be spoken in a soothing, quiet, yet audible fashion, in a "hypnotic voice." The phrases are organized into six exercises, following the guidelines provided by Linden (2007)[1] beginning with two autogenic phrases in each exercise, and gradually adding additional phrases for each exercise. The client will master each exercise, often practicing the newest exercise for a week, before proceeding to the next. Then each new session begins with a repetition of all exercises mastered to date, plus the newest exercise.

The reader will see that the experience builds in layers, as the client moves through the six areas or exercises. Many abbreviated forms of Autogenic Training condense the entire learning process to a 15-minutes repetition of 10–15 phrases, but as practiced by Schultz, Luthe, Linden, and many others, the Autogenic Training process is individualized and lengthy, with twice daily sessions. Several phrases in each exercise are provided below, with the understanding that they will not all be used initially, but practiced in order.

First Exercise: The Heaviness Experience
The right arm is heavy. (six repetitions)
I am very quiet. (once)
The left arm is heavy. (six repetitions)

---

[1] The language in the instructions is adapted with permission of Guilford Press from Linden (2007).

I am very quiet. (once)
The right leg is heavy. (six repetitions)
I am very quiet. (once)
The left leg is heavy. (six repetitions)
I am very quiet. (once)
The client is re-alerted after the heaviness experiences become pronounced, with an invitation to make fists repeatedly, hold the tension, let it go, bend the arms, stretch vigorously, take some long deep breaths, and open the eyes.

Second Exercise: Experience of Warmth (Vascular Dilation)
The arms are heavy. (six repetitions)
I am very quiet. (once)
The legs are heavy. (six repetitions)
I am very quiet. (once)
The right arm is pleasantly warm. (six repetitions)
I am very quiet. (once)
The left arm is pleasantly warm. (six repetitions)
I am very quiet. (once)
The right leg is pleasantly warm. (six repetitions)
I am very quiet. (once)
The left arm is pleasantly warm. (six repetitions)
I am very quiet. (once)
The client is re-alerted after the warmth experience becomes pronounced.

Third Exercise: Regulation of the Heart
In this exercise, the client is invited to attend to and focus on the beating of the heart. For individuals who are not aware of the heartbeat, several strategies are effective: The client may feel the pulse (at the carotid or in the wrist) and focus on the pulse. Alternatively, the client may lie flat on the back, with the right elbow elevated and supported so that the right hand may comfortably rest on the heart. The client is then encouraged to go into the usual experience of heaviness, warmth, and quiet, and then concentrate on sensations, including pulsing, around the heart.

Once the awareness of the heart beat is established, the instructions are:
The heart is beating calmly and regularly. (six times)
The single word—*Quiet.* (once)
The client is re-alerted after the awareness of the heart beat becomes prominent.

Fourth Exercise: Regulation of Breathing
The fourth exercise facilitates a passive awareness of breathing. The client does not exert any control over the breath to modify it.
The client goes through the previous experiences of heaviness, warmth, quiet, and the calm regular heart beat. Then the instruction is:
It breathes me. (six times)
Quiet. (once)
The unusual phrasing—it breathes me—portrays to the client that the regulation of breath will come by itself, and he or she will only experience and observe it.

Fifth Exercise: Regulation of Visceral Organs
> The fifth exercise focuses the client on the solar plexus, a location midway between the navel and the lower end of the sternum. This is a vital nerve center or plexus for internal organs. The client is invited to visualize this plexus as a sun from which warm rays emanate to all inner organs.
> *The rays of the sun are streaming and warm.* (six repetitions)
> *Quiet.* (once)

Sixth Exercise: Regulation of the Head
> The sixth exercise focuses the client on sensations of coolness in the forehead. Just as a cool cloth on the forehead is soothing, the cultivation of a sense of coolness on the forehead is usually experienced as soothing.
> The client is invited to engage in each of the first five exercises, followed by the new instruction:
> *The forehead is cool.* (six repetitions)
> *Quiet.* (once)

Once the client has mastered all six exercises, then he or she will practice all six exercises each time in a more condensed fashion:

> *The arms and legs are heavy.* (six repetitions)
> *Quiet.* (once)
> *The arms and legs are pleasantly warm.* (six repetitions)
> *Quiet.* (once)
> *The heart is breathing calmly and regularly.* (six repetitions)
> *Quiet.* (once)
> *It breathes me.* (six repetitions)
> *Quiet.* (once)
> *Sun rays are streaming and warm.* (six repetitions)
> *Quiet.* (once)
> *The forehead is cool.* (six repetitions)
> *Quiet.* (once).
> Now re-alert the client.

Simple Pathways II: Thermal Biofeedback

Biofeedback is a therapeutic technique which uses electronic instruments to monitor an individual's physiology (one function at a time) and to provide immediate information about that parameter to the trainee. The feedback facilitates awareness of bodily processes usually believed to be beyond one's control and leads to voluntary control over one's own physiology. Biofeedback was discussed in detail in the Pathways Interventions chapter, and several case studies in this book include a Level Three referral of the patient for clinical biofeedback sessions with a well-trained professional.

However, thermal or temperature biofeedback is one of the simplest forms of biofeedback, and can be learned easily with inexpensive equipment; thus thermal biofeedback is included as a simple pathway. When we provide a human being with immediate feedback on a physiological process, this enables the development of awareness and control. With the use of thermal biofeedback, the client learns to warm the extremities, usually the fingers. The warmth or coolness of the extremities then becomes a kind of spontaneous feedback to the individual about the state of relaxation or stress. *Warmer is better, showing relaxation. Cooling indicates a stress response.*

Patricia Norris, formerly at the Menninger Clinic's Voluntary Controls Clinic and one of the pioneers in biofeedback practice, recommends using thermal biofeedback and hand-warming training as an initial training phase for any individual showing signs of anxiety or life stress because of the benefits for autonomic nervous system relaxation and regulation (Norris, 2008).

The temperature biofeedback instrument uses a "thermistor"—a temperature-sensitive resistor—that is usually attached to the palmar surface of a finger. A visual display or an auditory tone communicates an increase or decrease in temperature to the trainee. Skin temperature mainly reflects arteriole diameter. Hand warming and hand cooling are produced by separate mechanisms, and their regulation involves different skills. Increased sympathetic activation associated with anxiety and hypervigilance elicits vasoconstriction and hand cooling. In contrast, hand warming involves a process of decreasing the activity of the sympathetic branch of the autonomic nervous system, enabling parasympathetic activation, and dilating the arterioles to warm the skin (Widmaier, Raff, & Strang, 2006).

In temperature biofeedback, a patient observes temperature displays with at least one-tenth of a degree resolution that are updated every few seconds. The most sophisticated and expensive thermal biofeedback instruments are sensitive to temperature changes of 1/100th of a degree Fahrenheit, and interface with a computer system so that the feedback can be provided in elaborate animations and displays. In the United States, a simple digital thermometer, with a thermistor sensitive to a tenth of a degree and an LCD visual display, can be purchased for $20.00 US. Change in peripheral temperature registers in the display every 2 seconds. This device is sensitive and fast enough for effective information transfer and feedback learning to take place.

Several other products are also available to make thermal biofeedback available at lower cost, including small alcohol thermometers, temperature-sensitive liquid crystal bands, plastic cards with temperature-sensitive surface, bio-dots, and so-called mood rings. The bands, cards, dots, and rings all have a temperature-sensitive surface that changes colors with temperature change, giving the individual at least moderately effective feedback.

The first principle of biofeedback training is that given feedback, trainees will begin to show learning. The individual is guided in the use of imagery, autogenic phrases, and mindful breathing, and each of these techniques will assist some individuals to warm their extremities. Yet, the process of feedback learning alone is powerful in itself.

Imagery of a summer day at the beach, with the warmth of the sun soaking into one's limbs and torso and with a comfortable heat radiating off the sand, will spontaneously elicit warmth in many individuals. Others will prefer an image of a warm fireplace, flickering flames, and a comfortable chair by the fire. Others will picture themselves in bed, reclining and swaddled with blankets. In each case, encourage the individual to develop the image using as many sensory modalities as possible. Feel the sun on your skin, see the heat shimmering on the sand, hear the flickering flames in the fireplace, and smell the fragrance of the wood fire. We also encourage the individual to "allow yourself to feel your body responding to the image." The process of hand warming and the process of relaxation are hindered by effortful striving and most effective when one allows the process to unfold and experiences it passively.

Autogenic Training, described in the previous section, combines very effectively with thermal biofeedback. The combination has been called Autogenic Biofeedback (Norris et al., 2007). The reader will recall that one of the physical sensations highlighted in the autogenic phrases is a comfortable flowing sensation of warmth. It follows, then, that the autogenic phrases will be effective for many clients in facilitating hand warming, especially in combination with the feedback from the biofeedback device. Mindful diaphragmatic breathing, described as another simple pathway, is also helpful for many individuals in aiding their hand warming. Relaxed, effortless breathing and a comfortable meditative state will produce spontaneous warming for many. As the breathing becomes automatic and effortless, it can also be combined with imagery of warmth.

Once the client has practiced hand warming on a repeated basis, the perception of warmth or coolness in the extremities will become more acute, and the client will become less dependent on bio-dots or the digital thermometer. The client will then develop the capacity for more rapid hand warming, as a ready strategy to relax at any time or any place, and the occasional recognition of cooling hands will become a warning of some onset of the stress response or discomfort.

The benefits of hand warming extend beyond basic relaxation to clinical conditions, particularly those in which compromise of blood flow to the extremities produces pain or slowed healing. Rice (2007a) reported on an intervention ("The WarmFeet Intervention") for clients with diabetes who have limitations in blood flow to their feet. One session of instruction followed by short periods of daily relaxation for about 2 weeks was shown to produce decreases in foot pain. The instructions can also be accessed by patients directly from a CD-ROM Rice (2007b), or can become part of diabetes education conducted by staff in a diabetes education program.

Simple Pathways III: Emotional Journaling

Sydney Jourard: Self-Disclosure and Health. Sydney Jourard, a pioneering humanistic psychologist, advocated personal transparency and self-disclosure as the pathway not only to self-discovery, but also to physical health (Moss, 1999; Rice, 1999). In the second edition of his classic, *The Transparent Self*, Jourard wrote that:

> Every maladjusted person is a person who has not made himself [or herself] known to another human being and as a consequence does not know himself ... [and] provides for

himself a cancerous kind of stress … producing the wide array of physical ills that have come to be recognized as the province of psychosomatic medicine (Jourard, 1971, p. 32).

Although Jourard believed that only in self-disclosure and dialogue does the human being come to know him or herself, he also highlighted the social pressure to conceal oneself, to suppress genuine emotional expression, and to present a façade to others. Jourard proposed that one marker of a healthy human being is the capacity to allow another person to know one fully. Alternately, he advocated that we develop the capacity to disclose fully to ourselves and to others (Jourard, 1968, 1971).

Sydney Jourard died prematurely, and his work was continued by many others. The questionnaire that he developed, the Jourard Self-Disclosure Scale, was utilized in hundreds of studies to investigate the relevance of self-disclosure for hypertension (Cumes, 1983), the counseling process (Edwards & Murdock, 1994), and the loneliness in college populations (Mahon, 1982). Today most researchers and practitioners in mind-body medicine accept that to be healthy, we must have an interpersonal connectedness and capacity to be vulnerable (Borysenko, 1988; Rice, 1999).

James Pennebaker: The Affective Journaling Research. James Pennebaker began with a fascination with self-disclosure and confession, and later developed a specific protocol that he has applied in research for 20 years (Pennebaker, 1997a, 1997b, 1999, 2002, 2004). Pennebaker instructs research participants to write freely about their deepest thoughts and feeling about some emotional issue that has affected them and their life. He encourages individuals to express themselves freely, no matter what the feeling is, and to set aside any concerns about grammar, spelling, or handwriting. Pennebaker's studies and those of many investigators who have adapted this research protocol, applied the journal model with college students, holocaust survivors, enlisted military personnel, and others. The studies have focused on many variables such as mood, feelings of well-being, blood pressure, immune function, school performance, medical visits, and absenteeism from work. In study after study, a positive therapeutic benefit has been shown (Pennebaker, 1997a, 1997b, 1999). Pennebaker (1999) specifically compared written and spoken self-disclosure about trauma, and showed that both produced more positive outcomes than writing about superficial topics.

Sheese, Brown, and Graziano (2004) conducted an emotional journaling study entirely through the internet, and found positive health enhancement effects—reduced days of illness, and a decrease in missed classes. The journaling exercise may be integrated into a positive psychology therapeutic framework with a provider or used by individuals on their own. Emmons and McCullough (2003) summarized the benefits of a gratitude exercise, where participants documented gratitude-inducing experiences; some were simple (the sun is shining) and others were more profound (growing up feeling safe). Results of this and other studies (Nelson, 2009) showed that ratings of personal well-being improved in the group given the gratitude assignment in comparison to those writing about hassles or daily events.

Smyth, Stone, Hurewitz, and Kaell (1999) applied the emotional journaling model to medical patients with asthma or rheumatoid arthritis, and carefully measured the patients' conditions prior to and following the journaling exercises. The researchers documented clinically significant improvements in the patient's medical conditions. The asthma patients reported less distress in breathing, and spirometry showed improvements in their airflow, specifically a measure called "forced expiratory volume." The patients with rheumatoid arthritis showed improved range of motion, and reduced pain and swelling. The simple activity of writing about feelings produced clinically significant objective improvements in disease status, measurable at 4 months follow-up.

A colleague, Benjamin Dominguez Trejo, of the Autonomous National University of Mexico (UNAM, Mexico City), implemented the Pennebaker emotional journaling protocol and coping skills training in interventions for large groups of survivors of Hurricane Pauline. Based on questionnaire data and salivary IgA, positive psychological and immunological outcomes of the intervention were documented (Dominquez Trejo et al. 2001). In summary, the Pennebaker emotional journal exercise is a wonderful "simple path" technique that can be used with medical patients, wellness programs, or community groups.

Pennebaker Emotional Journal: Instructions. The following instructions are adapted with permission from Moss (2005):

Each time you write in your journal, express your deepest thoughts and feelings about some important emotional event or issue that has affected you. In your writing, let go and explore your deepest emotions and thoughts. You might link your topic to your relationships with others, including parents, lovers, friends, or relatives; to your past, your present, or your future; or to who you have been, who you would like to be, or who you are now. You may write about the same general issues or experiences on all days of writing or on different topics each day. All of your writing will be completely confidential. Do not worry about spelling, sentence structure, or grammar. Journaling is most effective if you write whenever you notice that you are thinking or worrying about something too much. Set a length of time comfortable for yourself, anywhere from 10 to 20 min, and continue writing until the time is up. You do not need to feel pressured to write every day. Instead, think of expressive writing as a way to clarify your thoughts and emotions. This method is effective in helping you to get through emotional upheavals.

Simple Pathways IV: Heart Rate Variability Biofeedback

The natural state of a healthy heart is variability. One of the most prominent forms of this variability is the increase of the heart rate during inhalation and the decrease in heart rate in exhalation, that is, a constant oscillation. Young, aerobically active, and healthy persons show higher heart rate variability in contrast to people of advanced age or those with medical or psychiatric illnesses. Anxiety, depression, posttraumatic stress disorder, and fibromyalgia are examples of conditions marked by reduced heart rate variation (Nahshoni et al., 2004). Based on these findings, a measure of HRV is used as an index of illness severity and to assess the risk of sudden death, especially from cardiovascular disease (Kleiger, Miller, Bigger, & Moss, 1987). Many individuals with chronic illness maintain a sedentary lifestyle, and the lack of exercise further compromises heart rate variability, cardiovascular health, and mood.

HRV biofeedback trains the human being to increase the variability of the heart. Russian medical researchers initially developed the techniques for training patients to increase HRV, and used them to treat hundreds of children with asthma (Moss, Lehrer, & Gevirtz, 2008). American biofeedback researcher Paul Lehrer brought the Russian techniques to the USA in 1992, and working with Evgeny and Bronya Vaschiilo, developed an effective training protocol using North American biofeedback instrumentation (Lehrer, Vaschillo, & Vaschillo, 2000; Moss et al., 2008). Since that time, HRV biofeedback has been applied to asthma (Lehrer et al., 2004), depression (Karavidas et al., 2007), posttraumatic stress disorder (Zucker, Samuelson, Muench, Greenberg, & Gevirtz, 2009), fibromyalgia (Hassett et al., 2007), chronic obstructive pulmonary disorder (Giardino, Chan, & Borson, 2004), and cardiovascular disorders (DelPozo, Gevirtz, Scher, & Guarneri, 2004).

Human beings can learn to increase their heart rate variability, first of all, by practicing mindful diaphragmatic breathing at a specific "Resonance Frequency." This frequency is the breathing rate at which heart rate variability is at the highest, that is, usually between 5.5 and 7.5 breaths per minute. At this rate the process of breathing and the fluctuations in heart rate are in phase, so that at the precise end of the inhalation, the heart rate is at its peak, and at the precise end of the exhalation, the heart rate is at its nadir. The two physiological processes are completely parallel. Determining the Resonance Frequency precisely requires a sophisticated biofeedback system capable of measuring and displaying both respiration and heart rate concomitantly (Lehrer et al., 2000).

The second way to optimize heart rate variability is to use a less expensive biofeedback device, which only displays the graph of the heart rate, and to practice several strategies: (1) Begin the inhalation at the moment that a stable heart rate curve is beginning to show an increase in heart rate; then shift into exhalation the moment that the heart rate passes its peak and begins to decrease, (2) practice using one's breathing to make smooth, slow variations in the heart rate line graph (resembling a mathematical sine curve), at a rate of approximately six cycles per minute, and (3) practice breathing at a rate of six breaths per minute, while relaxing body and mind, and setting aside any distracting worries or problems. The six breaths a minute breathing rate approximates the Resonance Frequency, and will usually increase heart rate variability significantly, although not as much as breathing at the precise Resonance Frequency.

Inexpensive HRV Biofeedback Tools. The tools available for HRV biofeedback are not as inexpensive as those for thermal biofeedback. However, for between $140.00 US and $300.00 US, an individual can acquire a basic HRV monitor and feedback system. The emWave PC™ or emWave Mac™ are computer interface sensors with impressive software to acquire a heart rate signal and provide feedback to the trainee. The emWave PC™ or Mac has a breath pacer and a data screen, in addition to a variety of beautiful games and animations to guide the individual in learning to improve heart rate variability. The Healing Rhythms™ sensor and software provide mini-lectures by leaders in the mind-body health field, guiding the learning of relaxation and meditation. HRV and Galvanic Skin Response sensors, used to acquire physiological signals and provide biofeedback displays for the trainee, are also provided.

The emWave Personal Stress Reliever™ is a portable handheld device that monitors heart rate variations, and provides feedback to the trainee by means of a light bar. The individual learns to increase the size of oscillations in heart rate, and learns to produce higher coherence, which is a measure of the percentage of heart rate variability that is in the optimal frequency range. The StressEraser™ is a second portable handheld device that displays a line graph of heart rate variations on an LCD screen, and awards visible points for optimal cycles of heart rate change. The StressEraser contains a memory feature, which records the points earned for up to 999 training sessions.

Each of the devices mentioned provides feedback adequate for learning to optimize HRV. The first two systems, the emWave PC (or Mac) and the Healing Rhythms, are in the $300.00 US range, interface with a computer, and are the best inexpensive systems for in-office training or for personal training at home. The two handheld devices are optimal for portability and training in vivo—anywhere in one's life.

Another very helpful tool for training heart rate variability is a breath pacer. One of the best available breath pacers is the EZ-Air Plus™, which is available as a download from http://www.bfe.org. The software can be used free for 30 days and can then be purchased for $19.95 US. The EZ-Air Plus is a programmable breath pacer, which allows an individual to begin training at a rate near their current baseline breathing, and gradually set the pace slower to guide the individual toward the target breathing rate. If a professional has measured the individual's Resonance Frequency, the EZ-Air Plus can guide the individual to practice breathing at that precise rate. Otherwise, the individual can train at six breaths per minute. The EZ-Air Plus can also be programmed to increase the length of the exhalation relative to the inhale. Preliminary research has shown that heart rate variability is optimal when the exhalation/inhalation ratio is 2:1 (Grant, Korenfeld, Wally, & Truitt, 2010). Understanding the physiology of respiration supports this finding, since the exhalation is the time of parasympathetic dominance, and is subjectively a time of releasing and relaxing. The EZ-Air Plus can also be programmed to provide various sounds during the exhalation and inhalation phases, so that one can train with eyes closed, and continue to be guided by the pacer.

HRV biofeedback combines all of the benefits of mindful breathing, with the added value of creating a healthy heart rate rhythm and an optimal state of autonomic nervous regulation. It is important to educate individuals about the health implications of this training, and to encourage the individual to persist after the initial skills are mastered. Research shows that many individuals are able to learn the basic skill of creating a smooth, coherent variation in heart rate within four training sessions; however, the physical and emotional benefits continue to increase through at least 12 sessions of training. Thus it is like playing a musical instrument—practice over time produces more lasting effects.

Simple Pathways V: Audio-Visual Entrainment

A 57-year-old married woman, Louise, sat in a recliner in my office. During her evaluation for fibromyalgia, she mentioned her cognitive difficulties. Since the onset of her symptoms, she had gradually experienced increasing difficulty thinking clearly and solving problems. She used the popular term "fibro-fog" and observed that she really felt lost in fog at times. She suffered short-term memory deficits, poor concentration, difficulty finding words, and a loss of mental sharpness. These difficulties were worse when her sleep disturbance was worse, and she was severely sleep deprived most days.

Louise mentioned the onset of depression in her mid- to late-50s, initially reactive to chronic arthritis pain, but worsening as her fibromyalgia develops. Her Beck Depression Inventory (BDI-II) during the initial evaluation showed a score of 36, placing her in the severe range of clinical depression. She reported that she was irritable, tearful, and sad, with low energy, social withdrawal, apathy, and lethargy. She reported a gradual loss of interest and cessation of most activities outside the home. She summed up her life experience at this time as follows: "I'd just like to die and not hurt."

I began to develop a Pathways Interventions plan for Louise, but in the conversation in the first session, I mentioned that sometimes "audio-visual entrainment"—the use of sound and light stimulation—will enhance alertness and sharpen mental acuity. She jumped on this idea and begged me to schedule a second session as soon as possible, just to try the audio-visual entrainment (AVE). She promised to follow through with the rest of the Pathways plan, but she was desperate to sharpen her mind, even to a small degree. The "contraindications" for AVE, including the presence of seizure disorder, migraine, or neurological disorders, were not part of her clinical history, so I agreed to give Louise a trial session with AVE.

I placed a set of stereo earphones over Louise's ears, and a set of goggles over her eyes. I instructed her to keep her eyes closed during the light stimulation, and to speak up or remove the goggles and headphones if she became uncomfortable. The AVE system was a David™ system manufactured by Mind Alive, Inc., of Alberta, Canada. I set the system to generate a strobing light frequency beginning at 18 Hz and moving to 20 Hz, that is, 18–20 light flashes per second, and a throbbing sound at the same frequency, continuing for 20 min. This 18–20 Hz frequency corresponds to a beta range brain frequency associated with alert, awake mental processing.

Louise found the sound and light stimulation comfortable, and by the 10-min point reported that she felt her mind clearer, less tense, and restless; she had increased energy, and less pain throughout her body. After the AVE session she phoned her spouse at work, and asked him to go out to dinner. She insisted to him that she had not had an interest in activity in the past 18 months and they should take advantage of this moment. Louise continued to feel energetic, clearer in mind, with less pain until about 28 hours later and then suffered a return of pain, lethargy, and fogginess. She was able to repeat the AVE stimulation regularly thereafter and regularly achieved the improvements noted in her first trial. For a period at least until her last contact with the treatment team 2 years later, use of AVE continued to reduce systemic pain, increase alertness, energy, and motivation for Louise. She summed up her experience with AVE: "It straightens out my brain."

The History of Audio-Visual Entrainment. Siever (2007) has summarized the history of the use of light and sound stimulation, and provided an overview of research in the area. Pierre Janet, the pioneer in psychiatry, experimented with his patients at the Salpetriere Hospital around 1900. He created a flickering light by spinning a spoked wheel in front of a kerosene lantern. Janet reported that gazing into this light reduced symptoms of depression, tension, and hysteria in his patients (Pieron, 1982). Once the electroencephalograph was introduced, Adrian and Mathews conducted research showing that the alpha rhythm could be driven above or below its natural frequency through "photic stimulation" (Adrian & Mathews, 1934). In the 1950s William Kroger researched the causes by which American radar operators drifted into trance (Kroger & Schneider, 1959). Kroger collaborated with the Schneider Instrument Company and produced the first electronic photic stimulator, the "Brain Synchronizer." Kroger's research and that of others showed the powerful hypnotic effects of photic stimulation.

In 1984, David Siever released the "Digital Audio-Visual Integration Device" (David), which set a standard as a reliable source for audio-visual stimulation in the clinic. An abundance of research has followed, showing the therapeutic effects of audio-visual stimulation for sleep onset, sharpening attention in children and adults with ADHD, inducing relaxation, and increasing alertness (Collura & Siever, 2009; Siever, 2007). Additional applications have included seasonal affective disorder, dental pain disorders (including temporomandibular dysfunction), and learning disabilities (Siever, 2003a, 2003b, 2004). It might seem surprising that the AVE device could impact on so many serious disorders. However, Hammond (2006) has shown that many medical disorders are accompanied by disturbed patterns in the EEG, and related mental status effects, both of which are affected by the AVE device.

Thomas Budzynski, an early leader in the biofeedback movement, developed many creative protocols for the use of AVE, including "Brain Brightening," the use of AVE to produce cognitive improvements in elderly individuals with age-related cognitive decline (Budzynski & Budzynski, 2001). Multiuser adapters allow one to deliver AVE sessions to several individuals at once, all driven by a single DAVID™ unit. This provides the technical means to treat several children with ADHD simultaneously in a school setting, reducing the costs.

Audio-visual entrainment can "uptrain" the brain, organizing cortical activity around a faster dominant cortical frequency, thereby enhancing alertness and problem solving. AVE can also downtrain the brain, organizing cortical activity toward a slower dominant cortical frequency, facilitating relaxation or even sleep. In the case of Louise, she eventually learned to use the AVE unit in the morning for uptraining to enhance daytime alertness, and downtraining in the evening for more rapid sleep onset.

Caution: Managing Potential Adverse Effects of Audio-Visual Entrainment. It is widely known that flickering light can trigger an epileptic seizure or a migraine episode. Epilepsy is a strong contraindication for the use of AVE. Individuals with a migraine history must make a clearly informed decision whether to utilize the AVE device, knowing that onset of migraine is quite likely. If a patient is desperate enough to try the AVE with such a history, a signed informed consent is necessary. In many cases, clients will sense the onset of a headache, and by adjusting the light intensity, the sound volume, or the target frequency is able to avoid the migraine. This author has seen several patients reduce the frequency of migraines by use of the AVE device, so the benefits may outweigh the risks. It is also possible to use the sound without the light or the light without the sound when a client, with a heightened sensory sensitivity, cannot tolerate either the sound or the light or both at the same time.

Caution: Audio-Visual Entrainment Is Not Predictable in Outcomes. The response to AVE use is individualized and sometimes paradoxical. Use of a 10 Hz alpha protocol, intended to induce a relaxed yet awake state, will sometimes elicit a jittery nervous experience in a particular individual. On the other hand, occasionally a client will respond to an 18 Hz AVE session with a response of strong relaxation. To fully understand such paradoxical effects, a baseline QEEG (quantitative EEG) is helpful. The baseline cortical activation patterns of the client's brain will determine the client's response to a specific AVE protocol. Since that is often not available, the health professional is advised to carefully undertake trials in the office with several different frequencies, and carefully inquire about the client's response to each frequency. The professional should inquire about comfort with the sound volume and light intensity, since adjusting these can make the experience more effective.

Neurophysiological Mechanisms of Audio-Visual Entrainment. Light stimulation, transmitted down the optic nerve, through the optic chiasm, to the lateral geniculate of both thalami, to the visual association cortex, produces a new dominant electrical rhythm which spreads over each cortical hemisphere (Siever, 2003a). Because light is transmitted through the two thalami and into each cortical hemisphere separately, it is possible to present one frequency to the left eye, impacting on the right hemisphere, and a distinct rhythm to the right eye, impacting on the left hemisphere. Similar lateralization of stimulation is possible through the auditory systems. AVE devices are sold with many preprogrammed sessions, including more complex sessions that take advantage of such lateralization effects.

Obtaining an Audio-Visual Entrainment Device. This author has used AVE devices from several sources, but favors the DAVID™ units from Mind Alive, Inc., in Canada. Other devices are available from Sirius, Laxman, Mindlab, and Omega. AVE units generally cost between $175.00 and $400.00 US.

Simple Pathways VI: Mindfulness

Mindfulness meditation was included in our Level Three interventions as therapy for specific clinical conditions (Grossman, Nieman, Schmidt, & Walach, 2004; Kristeller, 2007). However, some aspects of mindfulness can be easily understood and then practiced by persons without supervision by a mental health provider (Benson, 1975). Mindfulness involves paying attention on purpose without judgment to whatever is going on at the time (Kabat-Zinn, 1994). The present moment may be one's breath, feeling, movement, eating, or sitting. The mind becomes quieter when only focusing on one thing, instead of rapidly changing thoughts, bodily sensations, and emotions. Learning to be mindful requires personal commitment, since initially distractions may seem impossible to overcome (McGrady, 2007). So, it is recommended that the person pick one activity, such as breathing, and be totally present for 1–2 minutes at a time, then expand the time. Walking meditation can involve paying attention to the sensations of feet hitting surface and exploring the sensations of feet on grass, sand, pavement, or snow (Jacobs-Stewart, 2003). Judgment of positive or negative leads to demands for action, in simplest terms — either approach or avoid. Therefore, giving any valence or judgment to a mindful experience defeats the purpose of being in the moment and needs to be discouraged. In summary, mindfulness can be a simple pathway to decrease stress responses and to enhance wellness. It can be combined with other Simple Pathways such as thermal biofeedback and Autogenic Training. It can stand alone as an in-depth systematic long-term intervention (Baer, 2003). Finally, mindfulness meditation is a component of other Level Three interventions, such as acceptance and commitment therapy, helpful in managing psychological and physical illnesses (Nyklicek & Kuijpers, 2008). In all applications of mindfulness, the amount of regular practice of the technique is directly correlated with improvements in physical and mental well-being (Carmody & Baer, 2008).

Simple Pathways VII: Expressive Dance

Movement is listed as a Level One intervention, and structured physical exercise is recommended as a higher level intervention in several of the patient cases described in this book. Another aspect of movement, dance, can be considered a simple pathway. Movement in dance has physical, emotional, and social aspects. Dance is an expression of feeling, whether the person is alone and moving to music or with others (Berrol, 2006). In contrast to the vegetative symptoms of depression, dance movement improves mood, but it also decreases agitation which may be paradoxically present in depressive disorders. When applied to the anxiety disorders, controlled movement instead of restless, undirected motion (tapping or fidgeting) allows the sufferer to learn to attend to physical sensations (arms and legs moving in rhythm) instead of overfocusing on uncomfortable bodily feelings (Dulicai & Hill, 2007). The physical aspects of dance sometimes constitute vigorous exercise, which not only burns calories, but improves cardiovascular health (Coccari & Weiler, 2004; Rasmussen et al., 2009). Blood flow to the brain is also enhanced by movement, thus promoting a total sense of well-being (Kramer & Erickson, 2007)

Simple Pathways VIII: Psychoeducation

Psychoeducational tools are an important component to facilitate the Simple Pathways. Each intervention listed in this chapter relies on understanding of the technique and how to implement it for personal benefit. Print media provides the therapist with suggestions on how to best educate the client, and many are also written for the intelligent lay audience. Currently in its sixth edition, the workbook by Davis, Eschelman, and McKay (2008) offers examples of relaxation scripts and worksheets that can be used as a component of therapy or by those who are interested in improving wellness.

There are many examples of audio-visual psychoeducational tools; only one will be described here. A 12-minutes video was compared to usual care in patients with whiplash who presented to an emergency room setting. The video explained in simple terms the physiology of muscle contraction, the body's normal reactions to injury and pain; demonstrations of exercises designed to relax the muscles were shown. Results showed significant benefits for the patients exposed to the video in reduced pain levels, and reduced use of narcotics up to 6 months follow-up (Oliveira, Gevirtz, & Hubbard, 2006).

Detailed self-management plans are described in Sarafino (2011). This author begins by defining behavior and explains how behaviors are learned and then progresses to applications of self-management. Data collection (such as counting minutes of exercise, logging negative thoughts, calorie counting) is emphasized before the intervention begins, during the process, and at the end. In clinical settings, the requirements for behavioral objectives in the service plan and the yearly or semiannual review of progress serve that purpose. Similarly, in the Simple Pathways paradigm, individuals are recommended to collect data themselves and refer to it in order to track progress and utilize the evidence of improvement for reinforcement of change.

Gordon (2008) published a personal guide to relieve depression, even in severely ill individuals, introducing a process he calls the seven stages of changes. The reader is led through assessment and analysis of situations that may precipitate lower mood. Recommendations for changes in cognitive processing, attitudes, and behaviors are made, and even small signs of progress are encouraged. Burns (1999) uses the cognitive behavioral model to assist persons with depression and anxiety to recognize the power of their thoughts on mood, physiology, and behavior. Some of these print media are accompanied by CDs with relaxation exercises or CD-ROM for visual as well as audio instructions.

Simple Pathways: Conclusion

There are many other "Simple Pathways" available for use by health professionals and lay people. Mindful diaphragmatic breathing is the single most powerful self-regulation strategy available to human beings. There are a variety of self-relaxation techniques, including progressive relaxation, that are useful for individuals with life stress, chronic pain, or any chronic illness. Guided imagery can be applied in a variety of ways, including the simple cultivation of a "calm scene image" for restoring a relaxed state after a collision with life stress. Hypnosis and self-hypnosis are powerful tools, useful in primary care medicine, the mental health clinic, and in everyday life. Each of these techniques was discussed in the Pathways Interventions chapter, so they were not included here.

The reader is encouraged to experiment with each of the eight Simple Pathways highlighted in this chapter, first for yourself and then for those whom you help professionally. We emphasize self-care first because it is difficult to teach self-regulation- and self-care-oriented strategies without cultivating them in oneself. Only if we know each of these strategies inwardly and personally will be able to present them credibly for the client. The first time a child asks the professional why the professionals' hands are cold, during a thermal biofeedback training session, will bring that lesson home. Each of the techniques chosen here is also empowering for the client or trainee. The client who knows how to use Autogenic Training, how to warm his/her hands, how to express emotions on paper, how to experience a moment in time, how to use breathing to optimize heart rate variability, and how to use a AVE device to facilitate the onset of sleep or an increase attentiveness is readier to cope with illness and with life. Clients who obtain educational materials in print or visual media receive reinforcement for their goals and gain confidence in their ability to achieve them.

References

Adrian, E., & Mathews, B. (1934). The Berger rhythm: Potential changes from the occipital lobes in man. *Brain, 57*, 355–384.
Baer, R. A. (2003). Mindfulness training as a clinical intervention: A conceptual and empirical review. *Clinical Psychology: Science and Practice, 10*(2), 125–143.
Benson, H. (1975). *The relaxation response*. New York: Morrow.
Berrol, C. F. (2006). Neuroscience meets dance/movement therapy: Mirror neurons and the therapeutic process and empathy. *The Arts in Psychotherapy, 33*, 302–315.
Borysenko, J. (1988). *Minding the body, mending the mind*. NY: Bantam.
Budzynski, T., & Budzynski, H. (2001). *Brain brightening—preliminary report*. Edmonton, Alberta: Mind Alive, Inc. (unpublished manuscript).
Burns, D. B. (1999). *The feeling good handbook* (rev. ed.). New York, NY: Plume.
Carmody, J., & Baer, R. A. (2008). Relationships between mindfulness practice and levels of mindfulness, medical and psychological symptoms and well-being in a mindfulness-based stress reduction program. *Journal of Behavioral Medicine, 31*(1), 23–33.
Coccari, G., & Weiler, M. (2004). Exploring the impact of dance/movement therapy on personal vitality in wellness-seeking individuals. *American Journal of Dance Therapy, 26*(1), 53–54.
Collura, T., & Siever, D. (2009). Audio-visual entrainment in relation to mental health and EEG. In J. R. Evans & A. Abarbanel (Eds.), *Quantitative EEG and neurofeedback* (2nd ed., pp. 155–183). San Diego, CA: Academic.
Cumes, D. P. (1983). Hypertension, disclosure of personal concerns, and blood pressure response. *Journal of Clinical Psychology, 39*(3), 376–381.

Davis, M., Eschelman, E. R., & McKay, M. (2008). *The relaxation and stress reduction workbook* (6th ed.). Oakland, CA: New Harbinger.

DelPozo, J., Gevirtz, R. N., Scher, B., & Guarneri, E. (2004). Biofeedback treatment increases heart rate variability in patients with known coronary artery disease. *American Heart Journal, 147*(3), E11.

Dominquez Trejo, B., Mascorra, G. E., Troncosa, C. H., Salazar, M. G., Lopez, Y. O., & Rangel Marquez, R. A. (2001). Psychophysiological monitoring, natural disasters, and post-traumatic stress. *Biofeedback, 29*(2), 12–17.

Dulicai, D., & Hill, E. S. (2007). Expressive movement. In L. L'Abate (Ed.), *Low-cost approaches to promote physical and mental health* (pp. 177–200). New York: Springer Science.

Edwards, C. E., & Murdock, N. L. (1994). Characteristics of therapist self-disclosure in the counseling process. *Journal of Counseling and Development, 72*(4), 384–389.

Emmons, R. A., & McCullough, M. E. (2003). Counting blessings versus burdens: An experimental investigation of gratitude and subjective well-being in daily life. *Journal of Personality and Social Psychology, 84*(2), 377–389.

Giardino, N. D., Chan, L., & Borson, S. (2004). Combined heart rate variability and pulse oximetry biofeedback for chronic obstructive pulmonary disease: Preliminary findings. *Applied Psychophysiology and Biofeedback, 29*(2), 121–133.

Gordon, J. S. (2008). *Unstuck: Your guide to the seven-stage journey out of depression*. New York: NY: Penguin.

Grant, J., Korenfeld, I., Wally, C., & Truitt, A. (2010). Inhalation-to-exhalation ratio affects HRV training success [Abstract]. *Applied Psychophysiology and Biofeedback, 35*(1), 181.

Grossman, P., Nieman, L., Schmidt, S., & Walach, H. (2004). Mindfulness based stress reduction and health benefits: A meta analysis. *Journal of Psychosomatic Research, 57*, 35–53.

Hammond, D. C. (2006). Quantitative electroencephalography patterns associated with medical conditions. *Biofeedback, 34*(3), 87–94.

Hassett, A. L., Radvanski, D. C., Vaschillo, E. G., Vaschillo, B., Sigal, L. H., Buyske, S., et al. (2007). A pilot study of the efficacy of heart rate variability (HRV) biofeedback in patients with fibromyalgia. *Applied Psychophysiology and Biofeedback, 32*, 1–10. doi:10.1007/s10484-006-9028-0.

Jacobs-Stewart, T. (2003). *Paths are made by walking*. New York: Warner Books.

Jourard, S. (1968). *Disclosing man to himself*. Princeton: Van Nostrand.

Jourard, S. (1971). *Self-disclosure: An experimental analysis of the transparent self*. New York: Wiley-Interscience.

Kabat-Zinn, J. (1994). *Wherever you go, there you are: Mindfulness meditation in everyday life*. New York: Hyperion.

Karavidas, M. K., Lehrer, P. M., Vaschillo, E., Vaschillo, B., Marin, H., Buyske, S., et al. (2007). Preliminary results of an open label study of heart rate variability biofeedback for the treatment of major depression. *Applied Psychophysiology and Biofeedback, 32*, 19–30.

Kleiger, R. E., Miller, J. P., Bigger, J. T., Moss, A. J., & The Multicenter Post-Infarction Research Group. (1987). Decreased heart rate variability and its association with increased mortality after acute myocardial infarction. *The American Journal of Cardiology, 59*, 256–262.

Kramer, A. F., & Erickson, K. I. (2007). Capitalizing on cortical plasticity: Influence of physical activity on cognition and brain function. *Trends in Cognitive Science, 11*(8), 342–348.

Kristeller, J. L. (2007). Mindfulness meditation. In P. M. Lehrer, R. L. Woolfolk, & W. E. Sime (Eds.), *Principles and practice of stress management* (3rd ed., pp. 393–427). New York: Guilford.

Kroger, W. S., & Schneider, S. A. (1959). An electronic aid for hypnotic induction: A preliminary report. *The International Journal of Clinical and Experimental Hypnosis, 7*, 93–98.

Lehrer, P. M., Vaschillo, E., & Vaschillo, B. (2000). Resonant frequency biofeedback training to increase cardiac variability. Rationale and manual for training. *Applied Psychophysiology and Biofeedback, 25*(3), 177–191.

Lehrer, P., Vaschillo, E., Vaschillo, B., Lu, S., Scardella, A., Siddique, M., et al. (2004). Biofeedback Treatment for Asthma. *Chest, 126*, 352–361.

References

Linden, W. (1990). *Autogenic training: A clinical guide*. New York: Guilford.

Linden, W. (2007). The autogenic training method of J. H. Schultz. In P. M. Lehrer, R. L. Woolfolk, & W. E. Sime (Eds.), *Principles and practice of stress management* (3rd ed., pp. 151–174). New York: Guilford.

Luthe, W. (1963). Autogenic training: Method, research, and application in medicine. *American Journal of Psychotherapy, 17*, 174–195.

Mahon, N. E. (1982). The relationship of self-disclosure, interpersonal dependency, and life change to loneliness in young adults. *Nursing Research, 31*(6), 343–347.

McGrady, A. (2007). Relaxation and meditation. In L. L'Abate (Ed.), *Low-cost approaches to promote physical and mental health* (pp. 161–175). New York: Springer Science.

Moss, D. (1999). The humanistic psychology of self-disclosure, relationship, and community. In D. Moss (Ed.), *Humanistic and transpersonal psychology: A historical and biographical sourcebook* (pp. 6–84). Westport, CT: Greenwood.

Moss, D. (2005). Expressive writing. *Biofeedback, 33*(4), 159.

Moss, D., Lehrer, P. M., & Gevirtz, R. (2008). Special issue: The emergent science and practice of heart rate variability biofeedback. *Biofeedback, 36*(1), 1–4.

Nahshoni, E., Aravot, D., Aizenberg, D., Sigler, M., Zalsman, G., Strasberg, B., et al. (2004). Heart rate variability in patients with major depression. *Psychosomatics, 45*(2), 129–134.

Nelson, C. (2009). Appreciating gratitude: Can gratitude be used a psychological intervention to improve individual well-being? *Counseling Psychology Review, 24*(3 & 4), 38–50.

Norris, P. A. (2008). Thermal biofeedback: The essential ingredient in self-regulation. Abstracts of scientific papers presented at the 12th Anniversary Meeting of the Biofeedback Foundation of Europe in Salzburg, Austria. *Applied Psychophysiology and Self-Regulation, 33*, 239–240.

Norris, P. A., Fahrion, S. L., & Oikawa, L. O. (2007). Autogenic biofeedback therapy and stress management. In P. M. Lehrer, R. L. Woolfolk, & W. E. Sime (Eds.), *Principles and practice of stress management* (3rd ed., pp. 175–208). New York: Guilford.

Nyklicek, I., & Kuijpers, K. F. (2008). Effects of mindfulness-based stress reduction intervention on psychological well-being and quality of life: Is increased mindfulness indeed the mechanism? *Annals of Behavioral Medicine, 35*, 331–340.

Oliveira, A., Gevirtz, R., & Hubbard, D. (2006). A psycho-educational video used in the emergency department provides effective treatment for whiplash injuries. *Spine, 31*(15), 1652–1657.

Pennebaker, J. W. (1997a). *Opening up: The healing power of expressing emotion*. New York: Guilford.

Pennebaker, J. W. (1997b). Writing about emotional experiences as a therapeutic process. *Psychological Science, 8*(3), 162–166.

Pennebaker, J. W. (1999). Health effects of expressive emotions through writing. *Biofeedback, 27*(2): 6–9, 14.

Pennebaker, J. W. (2002). *Emotion, disclosure, and health*. Washington, DC: American Psychological Association.

Pennebaker, J. W. (2004). *Writing to heal: A guided journal for recovering from trauma and emotional upheaval*. Oakland, CA: New Harbinger.

Pieron, H. (1982). Melanges dedicated to Monsieur Pierre Janet. *Acta Psychiatrica Belgica, 1*, 7–112.

Rasmussen, P., Brassard, P., Adser, H., Pedersen, M. V., Leick, L., Hart, E., et al. (2009). Evidence for a release of brain-derived neurotrophic factor from the brain during exercise. *Experimental Physiology, 94*(10), 1062–1069.

Rice, D. (1999). Sydney Jourard: Disclosing to ourselves and others. In D. Moss (Ed.), *Humanistic and transpersonal psychology: A historical and biographical sourcebook* (pp. 314–322). Westport, CT: Greenwood.

Rice, B. (2007a). Clinical benefits of training patients to voluntarily increase peripheral blood flow: The warm feet intervention. *The Diabetes Educator, 33*(3), 442–454.

Rice B. (2007b). *The WarmFeet® Kit. CD and/or cassette tape recording with instructions. A relaxation technique designed to improve blood flow to the feet and a thermometer for assisted biofeedback.* http://www.warmfeetkit.com/About_us.html .

Sarafino, E. P. (2011). *Self-management: Using behavioral and cognitive principles to manage your life.* Hoboken, NJ: Wiley.

Schultz, J. (1932). *Das Autogene Training-Konzentrative Selbstenspannung (The autogenic training: Concentrative self-relaxation).* Leipzig, Germany: Thieme.

Schultz, J., & Luthe, W. (1969). *Autogenic therapy: Vol. I. Autogenic methods.* New York: Grune & Stratton.

Sheese, B. E., Brown, E. L., & Graziano, W. G. (2004). Emotional expression in cyberspace: Searching for moderators of the Pennebaker disclosure effect via e-mail. *Health Psychology, 23*(5), 457–464.

Siever, D. (2003a). Audio-visual entrainment: History and physiological mechanisms. *Biofeedback, 31*(2), 21–27.

Siever, D. (2003b). Audio-visual entrainment: II. Dental disorders. *Biofeedback, 31*(3), 31–32.

Siever, D. (2004). The application of audio-visual entrainment for the treatment of seasonal affective disorder (part IV). *Biofeedback, 32*(4), 32–35.

Siever, D. (2007). Audio-visual entrainment: History, physiology, and clinical studies. In J. R. Evans (Ed.), *Handbook of neurofeedback: Dynamics and clinical applications* (pp. 155–183). Binghamton, NY: The Haworth Medical.

Smyth, J. M., Stone, A. A., Hurewitz, A. A., & Kaell, A. (1999). Effects of writing about stressful experiences on symptom reduction in patients with asthma or rheumatoid arthritis: A randomized trial. *The Journal of the American Medical Association, 281*(14), 1304–1309.

Stetter, F., & Kupper, S. (2002). Autogenic training: A meta-analysis of clinical outcome studies. *Applied Psychophysiology and Biofeedback, 27*, 45–98.

Widmaier, E. P., Raff, H., & Strang, K. T. (2006). *Vander, Sherman & Luciano's human physiology* (10th ed.). New York: McGraw Hill.

Zucker, T. L., Samuelson, K. W., Muench, F., Greenberg, M. A., & Gevirtz, R. N. (2009). The effects of respiratory sinus arrhythmia biofeedback on heart rate variability and post traumatic stress: A pilot study. *Applied Psychophysiology and Biofeedback, 34*(2), 135–143.

Chapter 17
Developing a Wellness Plan

Abstract The Pathways Model is applied to the case of a client who presents with a desire to improve his health and mental well-being. Imbalances in the clients' energy allocations and stated needs form the framework for implementation of the Pathways Model. Recommended approaches to this type of client, goal-setting strategies, and choice of interventions are discussed. Level One and Level Two interventions are implemented with good success.

Keywords Well being • Self explanatory model • Nutrition • Exercise • Happiness

Types of Wellness Programs

Wellness programs are very variable in structure, types of providers, techniques, and length. Some programs comprise standard interventions, such as weight loss strategies, exercise, and smoking cessation. Others are directed towards clients who are physically and emotionally well at the time but who seek improved well-being. The relatively recent focus on positive psychology leads still other clients to search for programs that concentrate on philosophical issues such as finding the meaning of life and increasing the experience known as "happiness" (McCullough, Emmons, & Tsang, 2002). Counseling wellness may focus on decreasing the effects of stress, and prevention of illness, based on understanding of brain functioning in health and disease. The neuroscience of perceived health and well-being remains in early stages, but initial studies suggest that there is overlap between basic sensory pleasures and higher level more abstract facets of happiness (Berridge & Kringelbach, 2011). An in-depth discussion of wellness programs is beyond the scope of this chapter; however, the case will illustrate the application of the Pathways Model. There are differences between interventions suited for the physically or emotionally ill client and those stating a *desire* (in contrast to a *need*) for improved well-being. Most clients seeking wellness understand that they will be advised to make changes; sometimes, they have already begun that process before contacting a provider. This is in stark contrast to some psychiatric clients who wish for pills, not skills. In the Pathways Model, there are commonalities between offering services to ill and well clients. In all clients, a careful evaluation is conducted, recommendations are made within a collaborative framework; short, long, and process goals are developed; and monitoring occurs throughout treatment (Bodenheimer, Davis, & Helman, 2007).

The Case of Philip

Philip was a 45-year-old man who came to the clinic seeking a wellness program. He worked as a software engineer at a local company whose major contracts were for the United States government. He found his job challenging and interesting most of the time. As projects proceeded towards completion and deadlines loomed, his work hours increased, reaching 60 h per week. Three mid level programmers were direct reports to Philip. Although these employees were qualified, Philip tended to over-instruct them and frequently double-checked their work, rarely finding a small error.

Philip stated that he wanted to get a fresh start on his health. One year ago, his marriage of 25 years had ended in divorce. There was mutual agreement between Philip and his wife (Margie) about the deterioration of their relationship; the common interests that they had shared were no longer topics of conversation. Although the divorce was mutually agreeable, Philip was lonely. He missed in-depth conversations about books and old movies that had drawn him and his wife together so many years ago. Philip could never discuss his work, which frustrated Margie, even though she understood the reasons for it. Their one daughter was born when they were both 17 years old, and she was now happily married. Their daughter stayed in touch with both parents and included them in summer cookouts and winter card nights, but these contacts never exceeded monthly visits. Margie and Philip were friendly during these events, exhibiting minimal tension.

Philip admitted that he felt much older than his 45 years. He questioned his ability to attain the next promotion at work, nor was he totally sure that he wanted to stay another 20 years until retirement. He endorsed feelings of sadness and a lack of fulfillment at times. He wanted to find new activities but didn't know where to start. He had considered a number of options—getting a personal trainer, looking for another job, and starting to go to church. But nothing really excited him. Was he too old for a new relationship? In sum, Philip felt sluggish physically and mentally. He was searching for ways for move off "dead center."

Assessment. The team recommended that Philip obtain a complete physical from his family doctor and approval for an exercise program. Philip did not participate in any aerobic activity, although he lifted weights several times a week. At the next appointment, the report from his doctor was reviewed. Philip was overweight by 10 lb. His blood pressure and cholesterol levels were normal, but blood glucose levels were prediabetic. He was approved to begin an aerobic exercise program. Philip was also evaluated using standard psychological inventories for mood and anxiety, and all his scores were in the normal range. There was no personal history of psychiatric or substance abuse problems. He did have risk factors for high blood pressure and diabetes and worried that his heredity would catch up with him soon. Caffeinated coffee was used in moderation (two cups per day), and alcohol was taken once or twice a week.

The first encounter with a client seeking a "wellness program" must be conducted with particular insight and skill on the part of the practitioner. Sometimes, the appointment is a vehicle for entry into psychotherapy, because the real problem is depression or anxiety that is interfering with functioning, and the request for wellness is a disguised cry for help. Some clinics offer only (what we have termed) the Level Three interventions and may be surprised by requests for wellness plans. If the evaluation does not reveal a psychological disorder, the provider should keep in mind that the client has decided to purchase this service, made the appointment and is seeking help. Sometimes, these clients are turned away by providers who state that "there is nothing wrong with you; what are you doing here?" or "we have so many really ill individuals" (unspoken—we have no time for you). In contrast, the Pathways Model suggests that the same seriousness used with depressed and anxious clients be applied to the stated goals of the client seeking to be more well than just physically well. In Philip's case, no physical problems or emotional diagnoses were found, so the therapist and Philip collaboratively agreed on goals and devised the wellness plan.

Goal setting. The goal-setting session with Philip identified his major objective as feeling happier and making good decisions for his future. The basic construct used in the goal-setting session was the Wheel of Wellness (Myers & Sweeney, 2005). Philip recognized that he was out of balance in all areas of his life. His work/career took up much of his time and energy but also provided satisfaction and challenge. In contrast, there were deficits in the social, spiritual, and activity domains. Philip had never heard of Maslow's self-actualization model (Ryan & Deci, 2000), but as the team explained the hierarchy of needs, Philip remarked with surprise: "I am living my life as if I am on the lowest level, focusing on survival. I think I can be more than that." In some aspects, Philip was an optimist; he believed that improvement in well-being was possible, he had choices to make, and those decisions affected outcome. In other situations, he characteristically took a negative view. Karren, Smith, Hafen, and Jenkins (2010) provide a discussion on the impact of explanatory style (mental habits by which people explain the events in their lives) on health and well-being. It was instructive for Philip to understand that thinking habits are learned and honed by experience, but are not necessarily permanent.

Level One interventions. First, Philip was taught the Level One mindful breathing technique with self-generated positive statements. Philip came up with "steady and calm." His homework was to begin to read the book by Kabat-Zinn (1994). The breathing techniques were easily learned and practiced several times per day. Discussing the readings in the book with the therapist brought recognition that indeed Philip always found himself "where he was." Even when he tried to escape, his struggles came back to him.

The therapist suggested that even an amicable divorce brings on a grieving period, since there was a loss of a relationship that once was nurturing and fulfilling. Philip was recommended to attend a divorce support group, which at first, he totally rejected. These groups were for people who "couldn't cope" or were "forced into a split." He didn't want to sit around with "a bunch of guys crying over their wives." Two weeks later, he decided to attend one introductory session and that was all he promised the team. To Philip's surprise, the group that he found through a local church turned out to be comprised of highly intelligent adults. When Philip said that he was a software engineer who couldn't talk about his work, there was understanding from another member, who happened to be a drug addiction counselor. The group shared activities, including two individuals that loved and attended old movies. When one of the members broke down, crying over her wrecked marriage and terrible divorce, Philip was not disgusted, but rather he understood her sadness and acknowledged that he too grieved aspects of his relationship with Marge.

A nutritional analysis of Philip's intake of carbohydrates, protein, and fat was conducted by the registered dietitian (Benson & Stuart, 1992). His protein and fat calories were within the recommended range, but the daily intake of carbohydrates was about 25% higher than what was appropriate based on his height and goal weight. A plan was developed for him, and he agreed, among other items, to increase his intake of omega 3 fatty acids (Ammerman, Lindquist, Lohr, & Hersy, 2002; Stoll, 2001). He was instructed to attend to the smell, appearance, and taste of the food that he cooked for himself to enhance his experience of (the Level One intervention) feeding. Since he cooked for himself several evenings a week, it was not too difficult to adjust his portions. Within 6 weeks, he noticed a small weight loss and felt more energetic. He looked forward to his healthy meals and enjoyed them more. During this period, Philip questioned the focus on basics such as breathing and feeding, since he was interested in "self-actualization." In response, the Pathways Model was described as sharing some concepts with Maslow, specifically that one begins at the beginning, certifying that biological rhythms are normalized before progressing to more complicated techniques.

Level Two interventions. Next, the Level Two intervention, aerobic exercise, was recommended to Philip. He replied that he would buy exercise equipment for his basement so he could use it any time that he wanted. The team considered this, but then talked to Philip about joining a local facility at least in the early stages of his program so that he would be around people and attend classes if they were appropriate for him. He did find a local facility and committed to an introductory program. Unfortunately, the trainers pushed him too hard; there was soreness in his shoulders after most of the sessions. He refused to go back; instead he requested an evaluation by an exercise physiologist which was made available by the cardiac unit. The result was a recommendation for walking and biking and continuing to lift weights. Philip soon became bored with the walking program, but enjoyed the biking very much and felt happier after an outing (Teychenne, Ball, & Salmon, 2010). At the 2-month appointment, he reported that he had found a group of guys who biked regularly and he decided to train with them for longer rides in the summer months.

Philip's negative thoughts about his future in the workplace were confronted, and Level Two cognitive restructuring (not the Level Three intervention: cognitive behavioral therapy) was begun (Young, 2005). Philip thought the counselor's analysis of his negative thoughts was too confrontational. He replied that everyone had concerns about their jobs and he was no different. His work was important, and he was successful. This was a difficult session which challenged the therapist to remember that highly intelligent individuals like Philip are going to need logical explanations for recommendations. Using Philip's own words, "I don't think I can achieve the next promotion" and "I can't keep doing the same thing for another 20 years," the negativity of these statements was explored and eventually countered by Philip himself. A trend towards a more optimistic explanatory style regarding his work was fostered. In the next month, he met with his direct supervisor and human resources to determine what the options were for the future. Both told Philip what he needed to do to achieve the next level and that it was very possible for him to meet those criteria within the next 2 years.

Philip came for appointments twice a month for 6 months. He lost 10 lb during that time and continued to exercise by biking indoors or outside, weather permitting. Weight lifting became a secondary, instead of a primary activity. His attitude about the future was more positive. He stated that the proportion of his time devoted to work was still "off balance," but the activity and social components had increased significantly. A curiosity about the spiritual life developed, and he had attended two church services led by a dynamic pastor. "The guy made me think" was interpreted as a high compliment. There were no dating relationships at that time, and Philip had not felt interested in anyone. With a smile, he said that he was still "grieving some of the time" and wasn't ready.

Philip continued to work as a software engineer; he had tried delegating some more tasks to the other people in his department. After some anxious weeks, he realized that they were capable of taking on more responsibility and performing well. He was pleased to be in more of a mentor role while working towards his own next promotion. Emphasis on personal growth not only increased the sense of well-being but built "emotional reserves" to be used in difficult times (Emmons & Crumpler, 2000). Philip's occasional 60-h weeks served as a good example of situations where in the past he felt continually stressed and fatigued. However, when Philip believed that he could prepare emotionally for these weeks, he felt less drained and more confident of his capacity to handle them. The final session was devoted to maintaining the new behaviors, reinforcing feelings of self-efficacy, and discussing personal growth as a lifelong process (Sarafino, 2011).

Case Summary

The wellness program designed for Philip was successful. The goals and objectives that had been developed at the beginning were met. He no longer attended the support group meetings, but continued his friendships with three of the people that he met there. Philip was more active in the physical health, social, and spiritual domains; he was much happier and felt more energetic. As this case illustrates, the Pathways Model can be applied to clients such as Philip who are not physically or emotionally ill and instead seek improved well-being. The providers are advised to be aware of applicable readings and community resources, such as support groups and exercise facilities. If the practice resides in a hospital setting, information about nutrition, complementary medicine, and exercise physiology services should also be on hand. The intervention team should be familiar with several wellness models, as each client will have different needs and goals.

References

Ammerman, A. S., Lindquist, C. H., Lohr, K. N., & Hersy, J. (2002). The efficacy of behavioral interventions to modify dietary fat and fruit and vegetable intake: A review of the evidence. *Preventive Medicine, 35*, 25–41.

Benson, H., & Stuart, E. M. (1992). *The wellness book* (pp. 129–153). New York: Simon & Schuster.

Berridge, K. C., & Kringelbach, M. L. (2011). Building a neuroscience of pleasure and well-being. *Psychology of Well Being., 1*(3), 1–26.

Bodenheimer, T., Davis, C., & Helman, H. (2007). Helping patients adopt healthier behaviors. *Clinical Diabetes., 25*(2), 66–70.

Emmons, R. A., & Crumpler, C. A. (2000). Gratitude as a human strength: Appraising the evidence. *Journal of Social and Clinical Psychology, 19*, 56–69.

Kabat-Zinn, J. (1994). *Wherever you go, there you are*. New York: Hyperion.

Karren, K. J., Smith, N. L., Hafen, B. Q., & Jenkins, K. J. (2010). *Mind/body health. The effects of attitudes, emotions and relationships* (4th ed.). San Francisco: Pearson.

McCullough, M. E., Emmons, R. A., & Tsang, J. (2002). The grateful disposition: A conceptual and empirical topography. *Journal of Personality and Social Psychology, 82*, 112–127.

Myers, J. E., & Sweeney, T. J. (2005). The wheel of wellness. In J. E. Myers & T. J. Sweeney (Eds.), *Counseling for wellness: Theory, research and practice* (pp. 15–38). Alexandria, VA: American Counseling Association.

Ryan, R., & Deci, E. (2000). Self-determination theory and the facilitation of intrinsic motivation, social development, and well-being. *American Psychologist, 55*(1), 68–78.

Sarafino, E. P. (2011). *Self management. Using behavioral and cognitive principles to manage your life*. New York: Wiley.

Stoll, A. L. (2001). *The omega-3 connection*. New York: Simon and Schuster.

Teychenne, M., Ball, K., & Salmon, J. (2010). Sedentary behavior and depression among adults: A review. *International Journal of Behavioral Medicine, 17*(4), 246–254.

Young, J. S. (2005). A wellness perspective on the management of stress. In J. E. Myers & T. J. Sweeney (Eds.), *Counseling for wellness: Theory, research and practice* (pp. 207–215). Alexandria, VA: American Counseling Association.

Chapter 18
Seeking Professional Help

Abstract In the Pathways Model, Level Three treatment planning calls for the use of health professionals for specific interventions. Finding a reliable, skilled professional to deliver a specialized intervention is a challenge. Physicians and pastors can often provide a referral. Physicians and behavioral health professionals can also coach patients to become active well-informed consumers of health-care services. Patients can learn to use online search pages to find specialists for therapies such as clinical hypnosis, biofeedback, acceptance and commitment therapy, life and health coaching, cognitive behavioral therapy, and mindfulness training. Communication skills also can assist patients to verify provider skills and training, and to take an active role in treatment planning.

Keywords Pathways Model • Referral • Informed health care consumer • Communication skills

Finding a Provider for Pathways Interventions

In the Pathways Model, the Level Three platform requires a skilled health professional to design and implement specialized interventions, ranging from biofeedback to hypnosis, to meditation, and to psychotherapy. Finding a reliable, well-trained professional, capable of delivering a specialized intervention, is often challenging. This is particularly true in the behavioral health and integrative health fields, where there is no standardization of graduate education to assure the consumer that all persons in a given profession will possess comparable skills. In seeking a psychotherapist, for example, one health insurance program reimburses only licensed psychologists, while the next provides an authorized "panel" of only social workers and licensed professional counselors. Even among psychologists, one psychotherapist will identify specific treatment goals, with a specified time frame, with the patient actively engaged in the process. The next psychologist may remain passive in the interview, provide minimal direction, and only nod empathetically when the patient expresses emotions. It is challenging for the patient and the patient's family to know which professional to choose and when to trust the professional. It is also a challenge for many physicians and mental health professionals to know where they can refer an individual with a chronic illness or complex medical problem to receive effective behavioral health and mind-body interventions.

In developing the Pathways Model, the authors advocate for a patient-centered collaborative model, in which patients take an active role and acquire knowledge and skills useful in pursuing health and wellness. The health professional need not know the Pathways Model, but the professional must be open to patient empowerment and active self-management of health. Otherwise, the professional can undermine patients' strategies for pursuing self-care, self-regulation, and self-efficacy. "Trust the doctor and let her make the decisions" is no longer a viable approach to health.

Sources for referrals. The primary care physician will often be a good source for a recommendation for a generalist psychologist or counselor. Physicians are generally practical individuals who are impressed by positive treatment outcomes and their patients' feedback about the interpersonal skills of the referred provider. Similarly, many clergy can recommend a counselor or psychologist; if patients are seeking a mental health provider whose orientation is that of a particular religious denomination, clergy is a good source of recommendations.

Identifying professionals qualified in specialized intervention. The first guideline in seeking a provider is to recognize when one is looking for a unique or highly specialized intervention. There are hundreds of thousands of psychotherapists in the USA and more worldwide. But if one is seeking to refer a patient to an Acceptance and Commitment Therapist, a Dialectical Behavioral Therapist, or a "Pelvic Floor Biofeedback" provider, these are specialties not covered in most graduate training. The first piece of evidence one might seek is whether the provider has a certification in the specialty. In an urban area with high population, it is easier to find professionals with certification in most specialized therapies. But in more remote areas, one may have to be content with a noncertified professional.

There are thousands of health professionals and behavioral professionals who have learned to provide various interventions without obtaining certification. But a professional who is dedicated to provide a type of intervention with skill, should be able to show evidence of training in the specialty, even if it is an occasional workshop at a professional society meeting.

Using an online directory. Many professional organizations maintain a list of providers organized by location and specialty areas. Such directories are helpful, because the providers listed often share some basic professional credential.

Examples are as follows:

1. Many state psychological, social work, or counseling associations maintain a list of members providing services by location.
2. The Biofeedback Certification International Alliance (BCIA) is the most respected certifying organization for biofeedback and neurofeedback practitioners. The BCIA website at www.bcia.org provides a "Find a Practitioner" online

search service, listing only certified practitioners, by location, and by certification area (general biofeedback, neurofeedback, or pelvic floor biofeedback).
3. The American Society for Clinical Hypnosis provides a "Member Referral Search," listing members by certification level, specialty, and location. The search page can be found at http://www.asch.net/Public/MemberReferralSearch/tabid/182/Default.aspx.
4. The International Coaching Federation (ICF) provides a "Find a Coach" online search service, which lists only individuals certified by the ICF as coaches. This service provides a search by specialty area such as personal coaching, career coaching, and small business coaching. The service can be found at http://www.coachfederation.org/find-a-coach/find-a-coach-now/coach-referral-service-search/.
5. The Association for Contextual Behavioral Science has a website, listing those of its members who provide Acceptance and Commitment Therapy. The website is at http://contextualpsychology.org/civicrm/profile?gid=17&reset=1&force=1.
6. The Association for Behavioral and Cognitive Therapy also has a website, with a "Find a Therapist" search service, searching by type of behavioral and cognitive therapy, age group served, zip code, and disorder. The service can be found at http://www.abct.org/Members/?m=FindTherapist&fa=FT_Form&nolm=1.
7. Psychology Today has a general online search service for "Find a Therapist," as well as specific pages for specialized therapies, such as "Mindfulness-based Cognitive Therapy." The general therapy search is at http://therapists.psychologytoday.com/rms/; this search service also allows the consumer to put in specialized forms of therapy or disorders for which one is seeking therapy. The Mindfulness-Based Cognitive Therapy search is at http://therapists.psychologytoday.com/rms/prof_search.php?s6=16.

The Well-Informed, Critical Health-Care Consumer

Personal referrals by physicians and pastors and the use of online search services are helpful in helping the individual find a professional in his or her geographic area providing specific services. Yet there are no guarantees associated with either a personal referral or the professional referral services. A physician- or pastor-generated referral may bring a qualified generalist who is unfamiliar with the patient's specific condition or problem. In many cases, membership in an association, or payment of a fee, is enough to qualify the professional for inclusion in an online search service. The listing of specialties often rests on the professional's own self-report. Those services that list a certification level are somewhat more helpful. Certification, for example, in biofeedback or hypnosis, does indicate that the professional has at least a minimal number of hours of training and in some cases that the person has passed an exam. This is a good starting point in seeking a professional, although the patient also needs to become an active and critical consumer of professional services.

Becoming an active, critical, and well-informed health-care consumer. The authors encourage all health professionals to help their patients to develop the orientation of an active, critical, and well-informed health-care consumer. Becoming actively involved in designing and selecting one's treatment empowers the patient and improves adherence to self-care. Obtaining professional services of high quality requires active engagement and communication skills on the patient's part. Primary care physicians, medical specialists, and behavioral health professions can directly assist the patient in seeking additional services, but even more important is coaching the patient in how to actively search and select new professionals. This is especially true in a community with limited resources. If the patient begins with only the family physician's recommendation or a yellow pages ad to start with, there are steps the patient can follow to gain some initial assurance about a new professional.

First, patients can conduct an Internet search for the provider's name. The provider probably has a website listing education, training, and any publications. If a provider is more active professionally, there may be many Google™ hits showing presentations the professional has given at association meetings or awards received. We encourage patients to read critically what the Internet shows. If the patient is a 50-year-old woman with fibromyalgia, and the web material only shows this provider treating adolescents with learning disabilities, there is an obvious mismatch between the patient's needs and this provider's specialty.

Second, we encourage patients to ask the receptionist at the provider's office: "Does Dr. Smith treat many patients with diabetes?" Or "does Dr. Smith have training in mindfulness?"

Third, we encourage patients to "interview" each new provider. Today, it is not unusual for a patient to ask a new provider for 5 minutes on the telephone prior to scheduling a first session. If this is not possible, the same questions can be posed during the first visit. The patient can ask about the provider's experience with his or her presenting problem. If the patient is requesting a specialized service, such as heart rate variability biofeedback or health coaching, he or she can ask the provider whether he/she provides this service, what training he/she has attended, and for how long he/she has provided this type of service. The patient can ask the provider which books or experts he or she has found most informative about the technique and any professional journals he or she reads. If the provider attended one workshop 10 years ago and cannot name a book or author, he/she is not maintaining expertise in the field, as is usually required for licensed professionals.

Fourth, we encourage patients to trust their emotional response. If a patient feels uncomfortable with the atmosphere of the office, the etiquette of the provider, or the emotional undertone of conversation, he or she should consider changing providers. We are not encouraging patients to be closed-minded, by any means. Some patients will be uncomfortable with any exploration of emotion with another person; in this case, the patient may request that the pace of therapy slow down and may coach him or herself to persist in spite of discomfort. Some individuals, with conservative religious backgrounds, might be uneasy seeing a Buddhist temple painting or a book on hypnosis in the consulting room. So patients need to find a balance, learning to be open to new learning experiences and to accept diversity, while still paying attention to any cues that this provider, as a person, is not good for this patient. For example, if a patient feels judged or put down, the patient should pay attention to this feeling and try to identify what the provider is doing to elicit this feeling.

Fifth, we encourage patients to ask the provider about the rationale for any treatment recommendations: Why is he or she recommending acupuncture or hypnosis, has this form of treatment been shown by good research to be helpful for patients with similar problems, or is the provider offering the only form of treatment he or she has bothered to learn, as if one size really would fit all? The patient can ask the provider to explain any recommended form of treatment and to suggest something the patient might read or access online about the treatment. Patients will engage more actively in their treatment if they clearly understand where it is going. If the provider becomes cool or abrupt when questions are asked, this is probably not the right therapist to engage in a collaborative Pathways Model treatment relationship.

Sixth, we encourage patients to feel free to change providers. The patient is paying for a professional consultation and has a right to seek a different professional. Patients can stop treatment at any time, or seek a second opinion and then return to a provider. Pathways Model treatment needs to be patient centered and patient driven, and patients are in charge of making that happen.

Finally, taking an empowered role in one's health care has many advantages, but there are occasionally costs as well. As medical corporations have consolidated much of medical and behavioral care in larger corporate entities, there are certain hazards for patients. This author has experienced several examples, where a patient's effort to ask questions about the recommended treatment has resulted in the physician discharging the patient. In two recent cases, the patient was then denied service by all affiliated practitioners within the larger corporation. One had been explicitly labeled in the clinic database as an uncooperative patient, who did not comply with recommended treatment. In geographic areas where one medical corporation enlists all or most providers, this is a serious concern. For this reason, we encourage patients to learn to be gently assertive and courteous, when raising questions. We also advise patients, who sense tensions or resentment building in the practitioner about the patient's approach or questions, to seek another provider themselves, before the provider takes action. Fortunately, today, more and more health professionals seem to respond positively to a patient who asks questions and actively participates in planning the treatment process.

About the Authors

Angele McGrady Ph.D., received her B.S. from Chestnut Hill College in Philadelphia, her Masters in Physiology from Michigan State University, and her Ph.D. in Biology from the University of Toledo. Later she completed a Masters in Guidance and Counseling. She is a licensed Professional Clinical Counselor and is certified by the Biofeedback Certification Institute of America. Currently Dr. McGrady is a professor and Director of Medical Education in the Department of Psychiatry at the University of Toledo. Dr. McGrady has extensive experience in all levels of teaching at the University of Toledo. In 1997, she was honored with the Dean's Award for Teaching Excellence. Dr. McGrady is a Past President of the Association for Applied Psychophysiology and Biofeedback and on the editorial board of the international journal *Applied Psychophysiology and Biofeedback*. Dr. McGrady lectures locally and nationally on topics related to Stress, Behavioral Medicine and Chronic Illness, Biofeedback and Wellness for Health Care Professionals. Her curriculum vitae lists 70 publications and 21 book chapters. She has coedited one book, *Handbook of Mind-Body Medicine for Primary Care*. In March 2000, Dr. McGrady received the Distinguished Scientist Award from the Association for Applied Psychophysiology and Biofeedback.

Donald Moss Ph.D., received his B.S. in International Relations from Georgetown University, his M.S. and Ph.D. in Clinical Psychology from Duquesne University. He is licensed in Clinical Psychology in the State of Michigan, certified as a Biofeedback Practitioner with the Biofeedback Certification Institute of America. He is a Training Consultant in Clinical Hypnosis, American Society of Clinical Hypnosis. Dr. Moss is Chair of the College of Mind-Body Medicine, at Saybrook University in San Francisco. He is past-president of Division 30 (hypnosis) of the American Psychological Association, past-president of the Association for Applied Psychophysiology and Biofeedback, current treasurer and certification chair for the Society of Clinical and Experimental Hypnosis, a SCEH delegate to the International Society for Hypnosis, a Board member of the Biofeedback Certification International Alliance, and an advisory board member for the International Network for Integrative Mental Health. He is co-editor of the *Handbook of Mind-Body Medicine for Primary*

Care (Sage Publications, 2003) and chief editor of *Humanistic and Transpersonal Psychology* (Greenwood Press, 1998), and of *Biofeedback: A Clinical Journal*, and consulting editor for *Journal of Neurotherapy*, *Psychophysiology Today*, and *Journal of Phenomenological Psychology*. Dr. Moss has published over 50 articles and chapters on consciousness, psychophysiology, spirituality in health, and integrative medicine. He operates two clinics in Michigan, providing hypnosis and other mind-body services for anxiety, PTSD, functional medical problems, and chronic pain.

Index

A
Acceptance and commitment therapy
 (ACT), 87, 151
Addiction, 96, 99–101, 203
Addictions model, 98
Adverse childhood events (ACEs), 32
Alcoholics Anonymous (AA), 104
Ambulatory blood pressure monitoring
 (AMBP), 162
American College of Rheumatology
 (ACR), 187
γ-Aminobutyric acid (GABA), 100
Amitryptaline, 190
Antispasmodics, 203
Anxiety
 adjustment disorder, 133
 amygdala, 139
 autogenic phrases and emotional
  journaling, 140–141
 CBT and SEMG biofeedback, 141–142
 emotion, 134
 functional impairment, 133
 hyper-excitability, 136
 hippocampus, 139
 intervention plan
  CBT, 137–138
  education, 136–137
  modified relaxation exercise, 137
 optimism, 139
 over-activation, 136
 pessimism, 139
 psychological and physiological
  characteristics, 135
 "relaxing sigh", 140
 stress management, 138
 stress responses systems, 136
 trauma, 134

Appetite, 23, 53, 121, 125, 133, 134, 184,
 195–198
Applied psychophysiological therapy
 biofeedback, 88
 guided imagery, 89
 hypnosis, 89
Assessment
 psychophysiological, 71
 professional, 66–67
 self, 64–66
 standardized tools, 68–69
Aquatherapy, 192
Audio-visual entrainment (AVE)
 caution, 235–236
 devices, 236
 history of, 235
 neurophysiological mechanisms, 236
 pathways interventions plan, 234
Autogenic training, 224–227
Autonomic nervous system (ANS) disorders
 etiology of, 163–164
 impending syncope, 164
 mindful breath exercise, 165
 progressive relaxation technique, 165
 psychodynamic psychotherapy, 166
 social interactions, 165
 symptoms, 164

B
BDNF. *See* Brain-derived neurotrophic
 factor (BDNF)
Beck Depression Inventory (BDI), 40, 52,
 120, 123, 124, 127, 159
Behavior, 35, 38–39, 56, 57, 67, 77–79,
 90, 117
Behavioral Risk Factor Surveillance System, 39

Benzodiazepines, 203
Biofeedback
 applied psychophysiological therapy, 88
 heart rate variability, 231–233
 neurofeedback, 104–106, 120, 224, 250
  (*see also* Electroencephalography (EEG))
 SEMG, 141–142
 thermal/temperature, 227–229
Bipolar disorder, 23, 212, 219
Blood pressure (BP), 11, 55, 65, 159–160, 213
Body mass index (BMI), 7, 33, 148
Brain-derived neurotrophic factor (BDNF), 21
Breathing, 125, 226
Brief dynamic psychotherapy, 87–88

C
Canadian Community Health Survey, 33
Catecholamines, 21, 49, 51, 54, 134, 135, 201
Catechol-o-methyltransferase (COMT), 21
Chronic disease, 48, 95, 99, 232
 genetic heritability, 99
 measurable pathophysiology, 99–100
 objective diagnostic criteria, 100–101
 personal responsibility, role of, 101
 relapsing and remitting course, 100
 treatment, 98
Circadian clock
 genetics, 25
 peripheral, 212
 suprachiasmatic nucleus, 55, 213
Cognitive behavioral therapy (CBT), 84, 87, 137, 162, 174, 188
Cognitive renewal, 82–83
Communication, 85–86
Complementary medicine, 248
Coping
 negative, 35
 positive, 38–39
Cortisol, 34, 49, 54, 55, 135, 147, 148, 213
C-reactive protein (CRP), 25, 52, 54
Crocus sativus, 118

D
Dance, 81, 117, 120, 127, 237
DBT. *See* Dialectical Behavioral Therapy (DBT)
Death
 causes, 5–6
Dehydroepiandrosterone (DHEA), 118

Depression
 breathing, 125
 clinical depression, 110–111
 emotional journaling, 125–126
 HRV biofeedback, 126
 hypnosis and hypnotherapy, 126–127
 initial visit and assessment, 122–124
 interventions
  exercise, 117
  integrative treatment, 121–122
  medication, 114–115
  mind-body therapies, 119–121
  nutrition, 117–119
  psychotherapy, 115–116
 mechanisms and models
  comorbidity, 112–113
  environmental factors, 112
  genetics, 111
  neurochemical and neuroscience models, 111–112
 medication, 124
 movement, 125
 self-soothing, 125
 sleep hygiene, 125
 support group, 126
 yoga, 125
DHEA. *See* Dehydroepiandrosterone (DHEA)
Diabetes and obesity
 assessment process, 149
 biofeedback and relaxation, 153
 breathing exercise, 150
 definitions and standard management, 145–146
 mindfulness meditation, 151
 progressive relaxation, 150
 psychophysiological etiology
  chronic stress, 146
  leptin, 147
  negative emotions, 146–147
  SES, 148
  sleep deprivation, 148
 stress, 149
 weight loss, 152
 yoga class, 150
Diabetes mellitus (DM), 100, 145
Diagnostic and Statistical Manual of Mental Disorders (DSM IV-TR), 50, 51, 64, 100
Dialectical Behavioral Therapy (DBT), 87
Diastolic BP (DBP), 158
Diet, 8, 12, 101, 118
Disability
 causes, 6–7
Disability-adjusted life years (DALY), 6
DM. *See* Diabetes mellitus (DM)

Index

E

Educational and community resources
 cognitive renewal, 82–83
 communication, 85–86
 mindfulness, 84
 movement, 80–81
 pause system, 83–84
 physical exercise, 82
 progressive relaxation, 82
Electroencephalography (EEG), 88, 100, 120, 188, 235, 236
Electromyography (EMG) biofeedback, 88
Emotional journaling
 instructions, 231
 self-disclosure and health, 229–230
Endocrine system, 48, 200
Exercise, 39, 65, 77, 80–82, 117, 140, 178, 206, 218, 225–227, 230

F

FAPS. *See* Functional abdominal pain syndrome (FAPS)
Fear-avoidance model, 176
Fibromyalgia syndrome
 achy soreness, 189
 aquatherapy, 192
 definition, 185–186
 EZ-Air Plus, 191
 HRV biofeedback, 192–193
 mechanisms and models, 187–189
 mild exercise, 191
 mindful breathing, 191
 muscle biofeedback, 193
 pathways treatment, 190–191
 prevalence, 186–187
 slow healing and soft tissue damage, 189
 symptoms, 190
 yoga, 176
Flexeril, 189
Functional abdominal pain syndrome (FAPS), 201
Functional medicine, 119

G

Gastrointestinal (GI) disorders
 anxiety and mood disorders, 202
 CBT, 207–208
 FAPS, 204–205
 functional dyspepsia, 204
 hypnosis, 207–208
 illness-related behaviors, 201
 irritable bowel syndrome
  antispasmodics, 203
  autogenic training, 204
  CBT, 203–204
  diagnosis, 202
  hypnotherapy, 203
  medical treatment, 202
  psychopharmacological treatment, 203
 joint psychotherapy, 207–208
 mindful breathing, 206
 overview of, 199–200
 progressive relaxation, 206–207
 stress sensitivity, 201
 visceral pain receptors, 201
General adaptation syndrome, 47
Genetic etiology
 alleles, 19
 environment, 22–23
 personality traits, 20–21
 phenotypes, 20
 physical illness, 24–25
 psychiatric illness, 23–24
 racial factors, 20
 risk, 21–22
Geography of Illness, 12–13
Guided imagery, 89

H

Hamilton Depression Scale, 120
Harvard School of Public Health, 6
HDL. *See* High-density lipoprotein (HDL)
Headache and back pain
 anxiety disorder, 178
 assessment, 173
 breathing based relaxation therapy, 178
 CBT, 174, 179
 chronic pain, 171–172
 cognitive factors, 177
 cognitive renewal, 174
 education, 178
 fear-avoidance model, 176
 hip and leg pain, 177
 Klonopin, 178
 medication reductions, 180
 migraine headache, 172
 mindful breathing practice, 174
 muscle tension, 174–175
 neuroticism, 176
 progressive relaxation, 174, 179
 research support, case interventions, 175–176
 self-soothing, 178–179
 tension-type headache, 173
Health problem model, 98–101

Health risk behavior, 35
Heart rate variability (HRV) biofeedback
  inexpensive tools, 232–233
  resonance frequency, 232
Heridity, 21, 23, 25, 70, 211, 245
High-density lipoprotein (HDL), 10
High risk model, 48
Holmes–Rahe Life Events scale, 31
Hyperexcitability, 51–52
Hypericum perforatum, 118
Hypertension
  cardiac rehabilitation, 161
  CBT techniques, 162
  HRV biofeedback, 162
  mindful breathing technique, 161
  myocardial infarction, 160
  prehypertension, 158
  psychosocial factors, 159–160
  regulation of, 158
  SBP and DBP, 158
  second heart attack, 160
  using alcohol, 161
Hypnosis
  hypnotherapy, 126–127
Hypocortisolism, 34
Hypothalamic–pituitary–adrenal axis (HPA), 53–55, 178

I
IBS. *See* Irritable bowel syndrome (IBS)
Imagery, 86–89, 228, 239
Immune system, 52–54
Individualized educational plan (IEP), 164
Inflammation, 34, 52–54, 187
Interleukin-6 (IL-6), 25, 52, 54
International Classification System (ICD), 50
Interventions
  applied psychophysiological therapy
    biofeedback, 88
    guided imagery, 89
    hypnosis, 89
  exercise, 117
  integrative treatment, 121–122
  Level One Interventions
    mindful breathing, 76–77
    movement, 80–81
    nutrition and feeding behavior, 77–78
    self-soothing, 79–80
    sleep and rest, 78–79
  Level Two interventions
    cognitive renewal, 82–83
    communication, 85–86
    mindfulness, 84
    movement, 80–81
    pause, 83–84
    physical exercise, 82
    progressive relaxation, 82
  Level Three interventions
    ACT, 87
    brief dynamic psychotherapy, 87–88
    CBT, 87
    DBT, 87
    medication, 114–115
    mind-body therapies, 119–121
    nutrition, 117–119
    readiness for change
      collaborative goal setting, 70–71
      education, 70
      ongoing assessment, 71
Interviewing, 69, 71, 149, 150
Irritable bowel syndrome (IBS)
  antispasmodics relax, 203
  autogenic training, 204
  CBT, 203–204
  diagnosis, 202
  hypnotherapy, 203
  medical treatment, 202
  psychopharmacological treatment, 203

K
Klonopin, 178

L
Lavandula, 118
Life events, 30–35, 48, 68, 112, 139, 201
Life stress, 3, 6, 38, 120, 147, 191, 228, 239
Lifestyle
  choices, 4, 6, 12, 47
Loneliness, 54, 66, 124, 217, 230
Long-term potentiation (LTP), 139
Loss, 31–32, 112

M
Major depressive disorder (MDD), 217
MAOIs. *See* Monoamine oxidase inhibitors (MAOIs)
Mean arterial pressure (MAP), 158
Medically unexplained symptoms (MUPS), 50–56
Memory, 51, 55–57, 139, 152
Mental illness, 9, 32
Migraine headache, 172
Mind–body interactions models
  personal mastery and optimism, 58
  psychological stress and illness, 49–50

Index 261

risk and resilience factors
    action representation mechanisms, 56
    lower social support, 57
    memory consolidation, 57
somatization
    circadian rhythms, 55–56
    DSM IV-TR, 50
    HPA axis, 53–55
    hyperexcitability, 51–52
    MUPS, 50
    regulatory systems, 52–53
Mindful breathing, 76–77, 103, 150, 206
Mindfulness, 84
Mindfulness meditation, 236–237
Monoamine oxidase inhibitors (MAOIs), 114
Mood disorders, 9, 24, 25, 110, 133
Motivational, 69, 71, 149, 150
Movement, 80–81
Multisite Cardiac Lifestyle Intervention
    Program, 118
Myocardial infarction (MI), 12, 113, 160

N
National Alliance on Mental Illness
    (NAMI), 110
National Comorbidity Survey (NCS), 32, 110
National Institute of Mental Health
    Epidemiological Catchment
    Area, 110
Negative affect, 35, 48
Negative coping, 35
Neurofeedback. *See* Biofeedback
Neurocardiogenic syncope. *See* Autonomic
    nervous system (ANS) disorders
Neurocircuitry models, 112
Neurons
    mirror, 56, 86
Neuroticism, 21
Nucleus cuneiformis (NCF), 51
Nutrition, 77–78, 117–119

O
Obesity. *See* Diabetes and obesity
Ornish program, 118

P
Pain, 21, 40–42, 138, 140, 171–181, 185–192,
    194, 195, 204, 205
Pathways model
    assessment goals, 63–64
    community-wide campaigns, 13

health and disease
    blood pressure, 11
    continuum, 9–11
    cross-cultural comparisons, 11
    low-sodium diet, 11
    salt, 11
illness
    acute medical conditions, 4
    death, causes of, 5–6
    disability, 6–7
    emotional illness, 8–9
    homeostasis and health, 4
    lifestyle factors, 8
    obesity, inactivity and smoking, 7–8
    women's roles, 5
intervention
    collaborative goal setting, 70–71
    education, 70
    ongoing assessment, 71
positive psychology, 14
professional assessment
    medical assessment, 67
    standardized tests, 66–67
self-assessment
    behavioral diary, 65
    data collection, 64
    Internet resources, 65
Western health risks
    Call center employees, 12
    clean water, 12
    Oriental diet, 12
    Prudent diet, 12
    UNICEF, 12
    workplace stress, 13
Pause, 83–84
Peniston Protocol, 100, 105
Physical exercise, 82
Plasminogen activator inhibitor type 1
    (PAI-1), 22
Positive psychology, 14
Posttraumatic stress disorder (PTSD), 34, 51,
    105, 123, 127, 134
Postural orthostatic tachycardia (POTS), 24
Premenstrual dysphoric disorder
    (PMDD), 134
Professional assessment
    medical assessment, 67
    standardized tests, 66–67
Professional help
    active, critical and well-informed
        health-care consumer
    costs, 253
    internet search, 252
    interview, 252

Professional help (*cont.*)
    receptionist, 252
        treatment recommendations, 253
        trust emotion, 252
    online directory, 250
    sources for referrals, 250–251
    specialized intervention, 250234
Progressive relaxation, 82
Psychoeducation, 238
Psychophysiological etiology
    allostatic load, 48
    general adaptation syndrome, 47
    mind–body interactions models
        personal mastery and optimism, 58
        psychological stress and illness, 49–50
        risk and resilience factors, 56–58
        somatization, 50–56
    psychiatric disorders, 48
    stress-related disorders, 48
Psychosocial etiology
    health risk behaviors, 35
    health supportive behaviors, 38–39
    initial visit and assessment
        depression, 40
        hypnotic pain treatment, 41
        readiness for change, 41
        relevant pathways, 41
    negative coping, 35
    positive coping, 38–39
    psychosomatic history, 30–31
    risky lifestyles, 35
    social activity, 42
    social supports, 36–37
    soothing, 42
    stressful life events and health, 31–32
    trauma
        adverse childhood events (ACEs), 32
        childhood maltreatment, 32
        chronic illness, 34
        mechanisms, 34
        migraine headache, 33
        path analytic statistical model, 33
        PTSD diagnoses, 33
    well lifestyles, 38–39
Psychosomatic diagnosis, 30
Psychosomatic history, 30–31
Psychotherapy
    ACT, 87
    brief dynamic psychotherapy, 87–88
    CBT, 87
    DBT, 87
PTSD. *See* Posttraumatic stress disorder (PTSD)

R
Relaxation, 65, 81, 137, 141
Resilience, 56–58, 153
Risky lifestyles, 35

S
Salvia officinalis, 118
Schizophrenia, 23
Selective serotonergic reuptake inhibitor (SSRI), 111
Self-Disclosure and Health, 229
Self-regulation therapies (SRT), 181
Self-soothing, 79–80
SEMG. *See* Surface electromyography (SEMG)
Separation, 31–32, 112
Simple Pathways techniques
    audio-visual entrainment, 234–236
    autogenic training, 224–227
    emotional journaling, 229–231
    expressive dance, 237
    heart rate variability biofeedback
        inexpensive tools, 232–233
        resonance frequency, 232
    mindfulness meditation, 236–237
    psychoeducation, 238
    thermal/temperature biofeedback, 227–229
Sleep disorders
    breathing and soothing exercises, 215
    CBT, 215, 218
    communication and movement, 217–218
    falling asleep, 211
    good habits, 215
    HRV biofeedback, 218
    hypothesis testing, 215
    insomnia, 212
    loneliness, 217
    major depressive disorder (MDD), 217
    medication, 218
    normal sleep, 211–212
    progressive relaxation and exercise, 218
    self-soothing and mindful breathing, 214
    sleep deprivation and effects, 211
Sleep hygiene, 79, 214, 215
Socialization, 159
Social Readjustment Scale, 48
Social support, 36–37
Socioeconomic status (SES), 148

Somatization, 50–56
SRT. *See* Self-regulation therapies (SRT)
SSRI. *See* Selective serotonergic reuptake inhibitor (SSRI)
Stages of Change, 41, 68, 124
Stress-buffering hypothesis, 36
Stress-related disorder, 14, 45
Substance abuse disorders
    AA sessions, 104
    acute *vs.* chronic disease model
        genetic heritability, 99
        measurable pathophysiology, 99–100
        objective diagnostic criteria, 100–101
        personal responsibility, role of, 101
        relapsing and remitting course, 100
        treatment, 98
    alcohol and cocaine abuse, 102
    biofeedback, 104
    caffeine use, 103
    cultivated mindfulness, 103
    EEG neurofeedback, 104
    irregular work, 102
    mindful breathing, 103
    paradigms, 97–98
    prevalence and costs, 96–97
    sleep problems, 102
Suicide, 67, 124, 178
Surface electromyography (SEMG), 151
Systolic BP (SBP), 158

T
Tension-type headache, 173
Thyroid-stimulating hormone (TSH), 9
Total peripheral resistance (TPR), 158
Trauma, 30–35

W
Ways of Coping Scale (WOCS), 38
Wellness
    counseling, 243
    plans, 243–248
    Wheel of Wellness, 245
Wellness plan
    aerobic exercise, 246
    assessment, 244–245
    emotional reserves, 247
    goal setting, 245
    mindful breathing technique, 245
    negative thoughts, 247
    nutritional analysis, 246
    types of, 243–244
Whitehall studies, 13
World Health Organization (WHO), 6, 8, 96, 110
World Mental Health Survey, 113

Y
Yoga, 103, 104, 125, 192

Made in the USA
Thornton, CO
05/05/24 11:56:04

18d48da9-287b-4214-a0ca-fb6f3059d74dR01